PROGRESS IN
CLINICAL NEUROSCIENCES

VOLUME 23

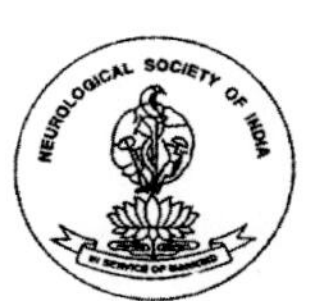

Neurological Society of India

PROGRESS
IN
CLINICAL
NEUROSCIENCES

VOLUME 23

Editors

VEDANTAM RAJSHEKHAR

KALYAN B BHATTACHARYYA

BYWORD BOOKS™

ISBN 978-81-8193-044-6

Cover design
NETRA SHYAM

Published by
BYWORD BOOKS PRIVATE LIMITED
Virat Bhavan, Mukherjee Nagar Commercial Complex, Delhi 110009
email: bywordbooks@gmail.com
website: www.bywordbooks.in

Printed at
Indraprastha Press (CBT), New Delhi 110002

Contents

EPILEPSY

Preface

We have continued the theme-based Continuing Medical Education (CME) programme of the Neurological Society of India. The common session features talks on issues in the basic neurosciences including clinical applications of stem cell therapy for neurological disorders. The neurology sessions are focused on neuroinfections and epilepsy; the neurosurgery sessions are in the areas of spinal and functional neurosurgery. As in the past two years, the neurosurgery sessions include the popular 'Controversies in Neurosurgery' debates.

This is the third year for both of us as Conveners of the CME programme and we would like to thank the Society for providing us this platform to realize our vision for this programme. The major changes that we implemented in the programme were the introduction of theme-based programmes and having this book published professionally. We hope that the members approve of these efforts. As we hand over the responsibility to our successors, we would like to thank all the speakers at this and the previous two years' CME programmes for their cooperation.

We would also like to record our appreciation of the efforts of the staff at Byword Books, New Delhi in bringing out this book on time. The publication of this book takes nearly 6 months from commissioning the authors, getting the chapters from them, getting the proofs corrected by the authors to final publication. We would appreciate your feedback on this book or any other aspect of the CME programme so that we can pass on your suggestions to our successors.

14 November 2008

VEDANTAM RAJSHEKHAR
Convener, CME
KALYAN B BHATTACHARYYA
Co-convener, CME

Contributors

P. DAVID ADELSON
Department of Neurosurgery, Children's Hospital of Pittsburgh, 3705, Fifth Avenue, Pittsburgh, Pennsylvania, USA, 15213; david.adelson@chp.edu

A. BATLA
Department of Neurology, G.B. Pant Hospital, New Delhi 110002

DHANANJAYA I. BHAT
Department of Neurosurgery, National Institute of Mental Health and Neurosciences (NIMHANS), Bangalore, Karnataka

DEBASIS BASU
Department of Neuromedicine, BSMCH, Bankura, West Bengal

RIVU BASU
Intern, Department of Medicine, Medical College, Kolkata, West Bengal; go4rivu@hotmail.com

MALLA BHASKARA RAO
Division of Neurosurgery, Department of Clinical Neurosciences, Riyadh Military Hospital, Post Box: 7897-B99, Riyadh 11159, Kingdom of Saudi Arabia; brmalla@yahoo.com

KALYAN B. BHATTACHARYYA
Department of Neurology, Burdwan Medical College and Hospital, Burdwan, West Bengal; kalyanbrb@gmail.com

ARI G. CHACKO
Section of Neurosurgery, Department of Neurological Sciences, Christian Medical College, Vellore 632004, Tamil Nadu; agchacko@cmcvellore.ac.in

ROY T. DANIEL
Section of Neurosurgery, Department of Neurological Sciences, Christian Medical College, Vellore 632004, Tamil Nadu

KAMALESH DAS
Department of Neurology, Burdwan Medical College and Hospital, Burdwan, West Bengal;
drkamaleshdas@rediffmail.com

PARESH K. DOSHI
Stereotactic and Functional Neurosurgical Program, Jaslok Hospital and Research Centre,
Mumbai 400026, Maharashtra; pareshkd@vsnl.com

RAMAKRISHNA EASWARAN
Consultant Neurosurgeon, Maruti Hospital, 95, Pattabhiraman St., Tennur, Tiruchirappalli 620017,
Tamil Nadu; drrke12@yahoo.co.in

ATUL GOEL
Department of Neurosurgery, King Edward Memorial Hospital and Seth G.S. Medical College, Parel,
Mumbai 400012, Maharashtra; atulgoel62@hotmail.com

BHAGAVATULA INDIRA DEVI
Department of Neurosurgery, National Institute of Mental Health and Neurosciences (NIMHANS),
Bangalore, Karnataka; bindira@nimhans.kar.nic.in

SHAILESH JAIN
Department of Neurosurgery, Neurosciences Centre, All India Institute of Medical Sciences, Ansari Nagar,
New Delhi 110029

MATHEW JOSEPH
Section of Neurosurgery, Department of Neurological Sciences, Christian Medical College, Vellore 632004,
Tamil Nadu

VIVEK B. JOSEPH
Section of Neurosurgery, Department of Neurological Sciences, Christian Medical College, Vellore 632004,
Tamil Nadu

J. KALITA
Department of Neurology, Sanjay Gandhi PGIMS, Raebareily Road, Lucknow 226014, Uttar Pradesh

SUBHASH KAUL
Department of Neurology, Nizam's Institute of Medical Sciences, Panjagutta, Hyderabad 500082,
Andhra Pradesh; subashkaul@hotmail.com

P. MEHNDIRATTA
Intern, Aligarh Muslim University, Aligarh, Uttar Pradesh

M.M. MEHNDIRATTA
Department of Neurology, G.B. Pant Hospital, New Delhi110002; mmehndi@hotmail.com

U.K. MISRA
Department of Neurology, Sanjay Gandhi PGIMS, Raebareily Road, Lucknow 226014, Uttar Pradesh;
ukmisra@sgpgi.ac.in; drukmisra@rediffmail.com

MANISH MODI
Department of Neurology, PGIMER, Chandigarh; modim72@yahoo.com

RANJITH K. MOORTHY
Department of Neurological Sciences, Christian Medical College, Vellore 632004, Tamil Nadu;
ranjith@cmcvellore.ac.in

ARABINDA MUKHERJEE
Department of Neurology, Vivekananda Institute of Medical Sciences, Kolkata, West Bengal;
mukherjee31@yahoo.com

M.V. PADMA SRIVASTAVA
Department of Neurology, All India Institute of Medical Sciences, Ansari Nagar, New Delhi 110029;
vasanthapadma123@gmail.com

S. PRABHAKAR
Department of Neurology, PGIMER, Chandigarh; sudeshprabhakar@gmail.com

C. PRADHAN
Department of Neurology, National Institute of Mental Health and Neurosciences (NIMHANS),
Bangalore, Karnataka

VEDANTAM RAJSHEKHAR
Department of Neurological Sciences, Christian Medical College, Vellore 632004, Tamil Nadu;
rajshekhar@cmcvellore.ac.in

BRIG P.K. SAHOO
Department of Neurosurgery, Neurosciences Centre, Command Hospital (SC), Pune 411040,
Maharashtra; prafullksahoo@hotmail.com

P. SARAT CHANDRA
Department of Neurosurgery, Neurosciences Centre, All India Institute of Medical Sciences, Ansari Nagar,
New Delhi 110029; saratpchandra@gmail.com

P. SATISHCHANDRA
Department of Neurology, National Institute of Mental Health and Neurosciences (NIMHANS),
Bangalore, Karnataka

T.N. SATHYAPRABHA
Department of Neurophysiology, National Institute of Mental Health and Neurosciences (NIMHANS),
Deemed University, Bangalore, Karnataka; drpsatishchandra@yahoo.com

VOLKER SEIFERT
Department of Neurosurgery, Goethe-University, Frankfurt/Main, Germany

A.V. SRINIVAS
Department of Neurology, Madras Institute of Neurology, Chennai, Tamil Nadu

S. SUNDARRAJAN
Consultant Orthopaedic Surgeon, Maruti Hospital, 95, Pattabhiraman St, Tennur
Tiruchirappalli 620017, Tamil Nadu; sundarortho@rediffmail.com

MANJARI TRIPATHI
Department of Neurology, Neurosciences Centre, All India Institute of Medical Sciences, Ansari Nagar,
New Delhi 110029

CHRISTIAN ULRICH
Department of Neurosurgery, Goethe-University, Frankfurt/Main, Germany; ulrich@med.uni-frankfurt.de

1

Paediatric TBI Guidelines: Optimizing the outcome in the post-injury phase

P. DAVID ADELSON

Abstract

Traumatic brain injury in children is the foremost cause of morbidity and mortality in this population. Evidence-based guidelines for the management of acute paediatric traumatic brain injury have been developed as a guide to patient care using a multidisciplinary team approach by clinicians and researchers. While these guidelines highlight the lack of data from well-designed, controlled studies resulting in few treatment standards, they provide a starting point for the development of protocols for optimizing outcome by creating an environment for recovery of the brain in the secondary phase. Recognizing the limitations of understanding of the patho-physiological response and often limited avail-ability of resources in this field, it is necessary to define realistic goals for the future and delineate areas for focused study.

Introduction

At the present time, data from well-designed, controlled studies on acute management of traumatic brain injury (TBI) in the paediatric population is sparse and lacking. In 2003, the *Guidelines for the acute medical management of severe traumatic brain injury in infants, children and adolescents* were published as a multi-disciplinary team effort by a group of clinicians and researchers, to highlight the known scientific literature in this field.[1] This provided evidence-based strategies for the management of children following TBI by analysing the current knowledge base. Systematic review of the methodology used for treating paediatric TBI showed significant dependence on information derived from the adult population or low levels of classes of data in children[1] that lack strength to definitively support existing management. The guidelines aimed to bridge this gap and will be an ongoing project with revisions and additions in the future.

The present guidelines use standard evidence-based methodology that evaluates the literature in support of a specific clinical question. Each individual study that is evaluated is categorized by the strength of the science and methodology. Studies included in class I evidence are those that were performed as well-designed, randomized, controlled clinical trials. Class II evidence is the next level and consists of less rigorous clinical trials or other reliable, retrospective series including observational, cohort, or case–control studies. Finally, there is class III evidence that includes small or unreliable retrospective observational studies and case reports. The available evidence on each individual topic is then used to define whether an intervention meets the criteria for a 'standard', a 'guideline', or an 'option', and has been more recently supplanted by levels I through III recommendations, respectively. A level I recommendation is an accepted principle of patient management derived from class I or strong class II data. A level II recommendation reflects moderate clinical certainty and is derived from class II or ample class III data. Level III recommendations have an unclear clinical certainty and are based on class III data. The goal of classifying data and providing levels of recommendations help clinicians identify well-proven interventions. Currently, the paediatric TBI guidelines have only three standards or level I recommendations. These include avoiding propofol as a continuous infusion, avoiding hyperventilation and the lack of benefit of using anti-epileptic drugs to prevent late (>7 days) seizures. The rest mostly consists of level II or III recommendations. The paucity of management standards provided the motivation to insert further 'expert' recommendations for research within each chapter under the subtopic *Key areas for future investigation*.

Primary management goal: Prevention of second insults

Like any other form of traumatic injury, the best treatment of severe paediatric TBI lies in prevention. In addition, specific goals of management following severe TBI include forestalling second insults and minimizing secondary injury. Second insults are potentially avoidable outcomes of injury and management, and may include hypotension or conversely, severe hypertension, hyper- or hypocarbia and hypoxia that can occur following the primary injury (the injury that occurs at the time of impact). These second insults, on top of the primary injury, can worsen the outcome by potentiating the secondary injury response and can be avoided by strict adherence to a meticulous treatment protocol. Secondary injuries, on the other hand, are secondary mechanisms resulting from the cascade of physiological and pathophysiological events following the primary injury and any additional second insults. Some of these secondary injury responses include compromise of cerebral autoregulation, breakdown of the blood–brain barrier, inflammation cascade, oxidative stress pathways, excitotoxicity and apoptosis or delayed cell death. The resultant tissue damage to the already injured brain causes both local and diffuse intracellular and extracellular oedema, and further ischaemic brain injury. With our current knowledge base, secondary injuries are difficult to prevent and thus their study provides the greatest potential for advancements in the treatment of TBI in the future. Ideally, a standardized protocol is started at the earliest possible time of intervention, i.e. at the scene and is continued throughout the acute, subacute and chronic phases to optimize outcome by providing an optimal milieu for brain recovery. While the ideal or optimal treatment paradigm remains undetermined, the present-day approach to severe TBI management utilizes a multidisciplinary dedicated team with an optimal environment for cerebral recovery, minimizing second insults and preventing secondary injury responses.

Overview of guidelines, key findings and results

The paediatric TBI guidelines[1] aimed to be a comprehensive document reviewing the literature on all aspects of paediatric head injury management. A breadth of the issues discussed ranged from public policy to acute pre-hospital care to medical and surgical management of these patients. In a review of the recommendations, organization of paediatric trauma systems is encouraged since these can facilitate delivery and lead to better care. Transferring children with TBI to a paediatric trauma centre leads to decreased morbidity and mortality. If this is not possible, they should be transported to an adult trauma centre capable of treating paediatric patients.

All aspects of care of the critically injured children should be optimized from the initial phases starting from pre-hospital management. Attention to detail in the delivery of care throughout transportation and admission to the hospital setting is imperative. At the scene, the primary goal is initial resuscitation including maintaining a stable airway and circulation to prevent second insults. As hypoxia leads to a worse neurological outcome, it should be prevented at all times during pre-hospital and in-hospital care. Depending on the expertise, supplemental oxygen, bag–valve–mask ventilation and endotracheal intubation can be used to improve oxygenation. Intubation is the only means of securing the airway, which reduces the likelihood of aspiration and provides a route to deliver medications. Although detrimental if applied poorly, intubation should be utilized in children with a Glasgow Coma Score (GCS) <9. As right mainstem and oesophageal intubation are common in paediatric patients, specialized training and the use of end-tidal CO_2 monitors should be employed. Thus, the optimal method for providing adequate oxygenation and ventilation depends on the expertise.[2]

Sedation, analgesia and neuromuscular blockade can be used to facilitate management. Although no specific drugs are recommended, the Food and Drug Administration recommends against using continuous infusions of propofol in the paediatric population due to evidence of unexplained metabolic acidosis and increased mortality with its use. Appropriate sedation and analgesia with selective agents can prevent fluctuations in intracranial pressure (ICP) and blood pressure. Similarly, events such as coughing, bucking and straining can be avoided by the use of paralytic agents. Hypotension also adds to ischaemic brain injury and adverse neurological outcomes, and should be prevented. Resuscitation fluids should be administered early as children can rapidly develop hypotensive shock.

ICP-directed therapy

As sustained ICP >20 mmHg has been shown to be associated with worse outcomes,[3,4] a potential advantage of ICP-guided therapy to maintain the ICP below this level may exist in the paediatric population. An intraventricular pressure transducer is the most accurate and reliable method for monitoring the ICP. Although useful, parenchymal monitors are prone to measurement drift and lack the benefit of cerebrospinal fluid (CSF) drainage. Currently, the goal of therapy in children with severe TBI is to keep the ICP <20 mmHg and cerebral perfusion pressure (CPP) in the 40–65 mmHg range. A recent paper by Adelson *et al.*[4] showed that, regardless of treatment, an ICP <20 mmHg and CPP >50 mmHg were associated with good outcomes. The critical value of ICP for different ages at injury remains unclear.

First-tier therapy

Initial measures to avoid and/or treat elevated ICP include elevating the head of the bed to a 30° angle, preventing obstruction to venous outflow, avoiding hyperthermia, and minimizing stimulation. First-tier therapy for persistent ICP elevation includes sedation, paralytics, mild-to-moderate hypocapnia (30–35 mmHg), and hyperosmolar therapy (Fig. 1). Another strategy that is an option or level III recommendation includes CSF drainage via an external ventricular drain. (Use of a lumbar drain for CSF drainage, provided there is no radiological evidence of intracranial mass lesion or focal herniation, open basal cisterns and a functioning ventricular drain, is a second-tier option.)

Although early literature supported the use of prophylactic hyperventilation to counter 'hyper-aemia' following severe TBI, current evidence shows a low incidence of hyperaemia and thus vasoconstriction from hyperventilation may be more harmful than beneficial. The use of mild-to-moderate hypocapnia ($PaCO_2$ 30–35 mmHg)

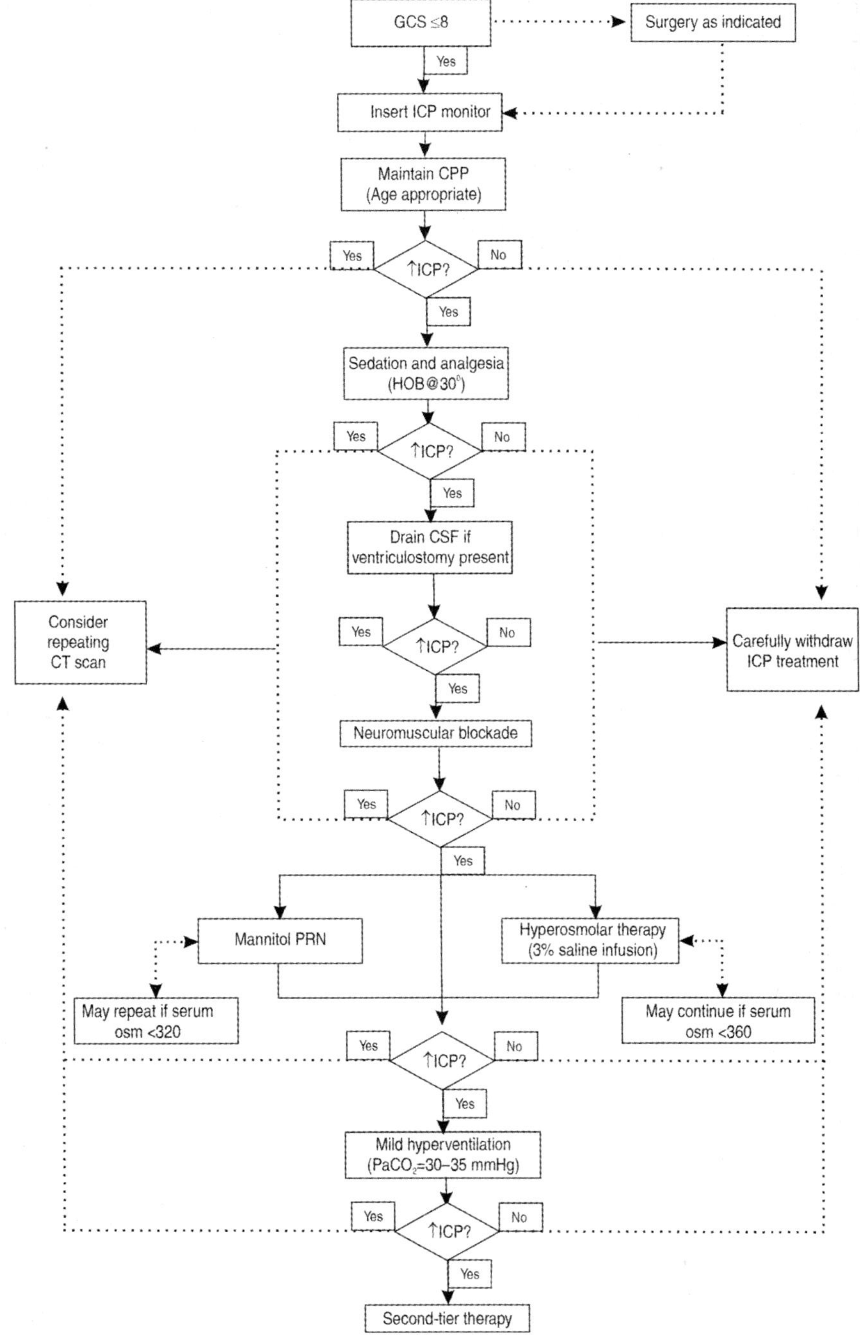

Fig. 1. First-tier. Glasgow Coma Scale (GCS); intracranial pressure (ICP); cerebral perfusion pressure (CPP); head of bed (HOB); cerebrospinal fluid (CSF); computed tomography (CT); PRN, as needed. *(Reprinted with permission from Lippincott Williams & Wilkins)*

is an option to lower the ICP but should be minimized. As aggressive hyperventilation ($PaCO_2$ <30 mmHg) has the potential of reducing cerebral blood flow to ischaemic levels, it is reserved as a second-tier option for the management of refractory intracranial hypertension. It should only be utilized as a temporary measure and is to be used with brain tissue oxygen monitoring to avoid ischaemia. Various modalities for brain oxygenation or delivery including brain tissue oxygen probes, cerebral blood flow imaging, or jugular venous oxygen monitoring can be used.

Another effective first-line option for controlling the ICP is hyperosmolar therapy. Euvolaemic hyperosmolarity is favoured based on the current principles of management. There are no data to prove if either hypertonic saline or mannitol is superior to the other. Mannitol has been used for more than half a century and has a two-fold effect. It lowers cerebral blood volume and ICP by reducing blood viscosity, while augmenting cerebral blood flow because of higher blood flow velocity. It also osmotically dehydrates the brain with a resultant decrease in intracranial volume and pressure. In addition, mannitol may potentiate metabolic autoregulation. Mannitol can be titrated to a serum osmolarity of 320 mOsm/L, with a concern that higher osmolarity may be associated with renal failure. Although there is more evidence to support its use, hypertonic saline has only recently been taken up at many centres. Its mode of action is similar to mannitol, and it also has the potential advantages of restoring resting membrane potential at a cellular level, stimulating the release of atrial natriuretic peptide, inhibiting the inflammatory cascade and augmenting cardiac output. There is also evidence that it can augment ICP reduction in patients refractory to infusion of mannitol. Hypertonic saline may be used with a serum osmolarity of up to 360 mOsm/L. The difference in end-points for serum osmolarity was only based on the available literature for each modality and not by direct knowledge of the likelihood of renal failure.

Except for the proven instances of hypocortisolaemia, the literature did not support the use of steroids in the management of paediatric severe TBI. Use of steroids does not improve outcomes, suppresses endogenous corticosteroid production and increases the risk of infection. Thus, steroids are not recommended in the acute injury period.

Second-tier therapy

After the first tier of therapeutic interventions have been exhausted, the second tier of treatment comes into play for managing persistently elevated ICP. These include the use of high-dose barbiturates, decompressive surgical procedures, lumbar drain CSF diversion, hypothermia and aggressive hyperventilation (Fig. 2). These are high-risk interventions and require a careful assessment of the risk–benefit ratio before any of these is administered.

The commonly used barbiturate is pentobarbital at a loading dose of 10 mg/kg over a 30-minute period, followed by a maintenance dose of 1 mg/kg/hour that can be titrated for burst suppression on continuous electroencephalographic (EEG) monitoring. A decrease in blood pressure is common in children receiving high-dose barbiturates and pharmacological intervention is usually required to maintain the CPP >40 mmHg.

Surgical procedures including decompressive craniectomy, duraplasty and lobectomy are options to lower ICP refractory to medical management. This can be especially useful in patients with expanding mass intracranial lesions or diffuse cerebral oedema at initial evaluation, GCS >3 subsequent to injury, or worsening within 48 hours of admission. A lumbar drain for CSF drainage can also be used, as mentioned above.

Hypothermia is another second-tier option. Hyperthermia leads to poor outcomes by potentiating the acute pathophysiological response to injury. Hypothermia can reduce secondary

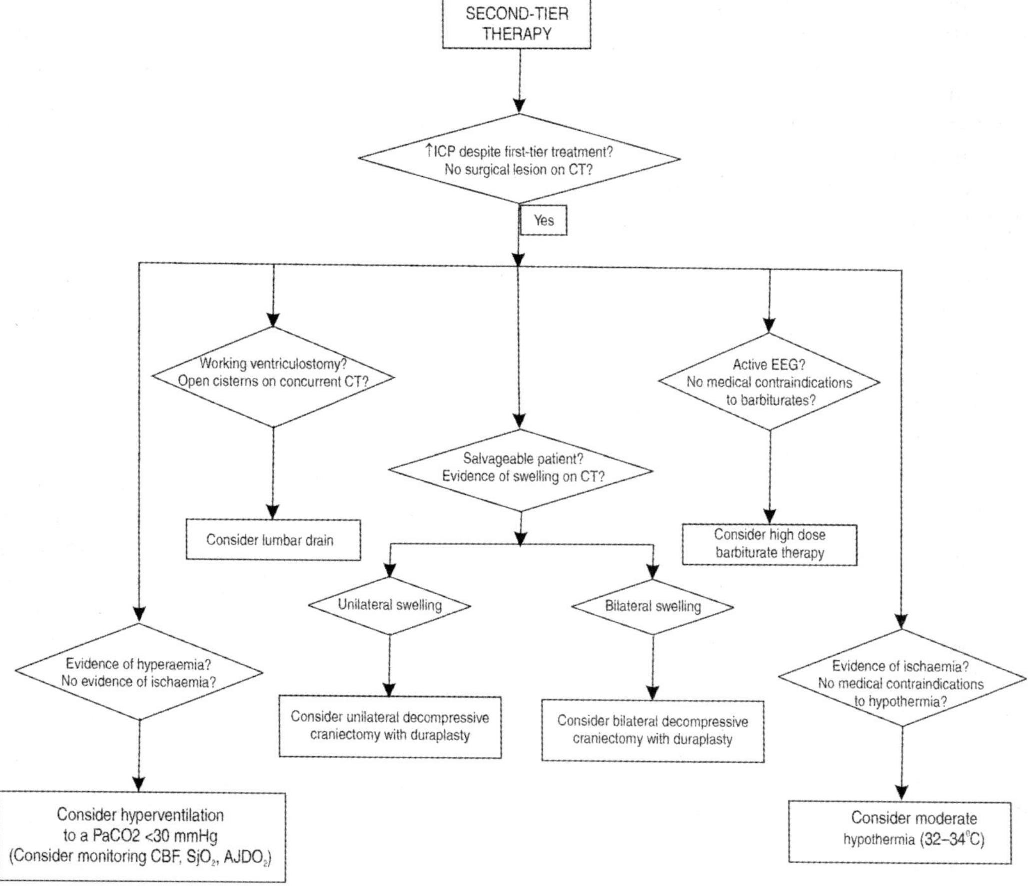

Fig. 2. Second-tier. intracranial pressure (ICP); computed tomography (CT); electroencephalography (EEG); cerebral blood flow (CBF); jugular venous oxygen saturation (SjO$_2$); arterial–jugular venous difference in oxygen (AJDO$_2$) content. (*Reprinted with permission from Lippincott Williams & Wilkins*)

injury responses as well as seizures. Currently, there is no definitive evidence for the use of hypothermia in children. Based on adult data,[3] reduction of core body temperature below 35°C is considered an option. A phase II trial[4] showed potentially lower mortality and improved outcome, but as the study had too few patients and limitations in study design, the results do not allow anything more than a level III recommendation at this time. In a recent phase III trial of hypothermia following severe TBI in children, Hutchison *et al.*[5] reported that hypothermia initiated within 8 hours of injury, continued for 24 hours and followed by rapid rewarming does not improve neurological outcome and may increase mortality after TBI in children. They concluded that 'this particular hypothermia protocol was not warranted for the treatment of severe head injury in children' and 'further research is necessary to determine whether earlier implementation or more prolonged therapy would improve the outcome in children with severe traumatic brain injury'. A US-based phase III trial for the study of 48 hours of hypothermia initiated within 6 hours of injury, with a slow rewarming period in paediatric TBI, are ongoing at the present time (PD Adelson; personal communication).

The incidence of post-traumatic seizures in infants and children is high. Anti-epileptic medications decrease the incidence of seizures that occur within 7 days of the initial event. However, they offer no protection against chronic post-traumatic seizures or epilepsy of late onset. The drugs with the most data to support their use are phenytoin and carbamazepine.

Nutrition also plays an important part in the care of children with severe TBI, as a high rate of metabolism is noted in these patients. With no one method of administering calories proven to be better than others, nutritional supplementation, in one form or another, should begin within 72 hours of the initial injury, with the goal of providing 130%–160% of resting metabolism expenditure.

Key areas of future investigation

Several key areas of research and investigation have also been outlined in the guidelines. The goal is to individualize care for patients at risk, prevent primary injury and avoid second insults (and secondary injury), and to develop environments conducive for recovery of the injured brain. Some of these key areas include measures for primary prevention of TBI (such as raising public awareness), development of protocols for early and accurate assessment of paediatric TBI, development of treatment algorithms guided by individualized monitoring of pathophysiological and biochemical processes, better anatomical and functional imaging, and development of comprehensive physical, cognitive and behavioural assessment scales for evaluating children with severe TBI.

Conclusions

The paediatric TBI guidelines seek to provide a detailed, evidence-based system for management of children with severe TBI. By focusing on the key areas provided in the guidelines, breakthrough discoveries in the understanding and treatment of paediatric TBI can be expected, along with development of new therapeutic interventions. These may also guide the way for newer, scientifically sound principles of management, with the possibility of individualization of care in the paediatric population, as realistic goals for study are defined while maintaining direction.

References

1. Adelson PD, Bratton SL, Carney NA, *et al.* Guidelines for the acute medical management of severe traumatic brain injury in infants, children and adolescents. *Crit Care Med* 2003;**31** (Suppl 6):S407–S491.
2. Wang H, Cassidy L, Peitzman A, *et al.* Out-of-hospital endotracheal intubation is associated with adverse outcome after traumatic brain injury. *Ann Emerg Med* 2004;**44**:439–50.
3. Brain Trauma Foundation; American Association of Neurological Surgeons; Congress of Neurological Surgeons; Joint Section on Neurotrauma and Critical Care, AANS/CNS. Guidelines for the management of severe traumatic brain injury. *J Neurotrauma* 2007;**24** (Suppl 1):S1–S106.
4. Adelson PD, Ragheb J, Muizelaar JP, *et al.* Phase II clinical trial of moderate hypothermia after severe traumatic brain injury in children. *Neurosurgery* 2005;**56**:740–54.
5. Hutchison JS, Ward RE, Lacroix J, *et al.* For the Hypothermia Paediatric Head Injury Trial Investigators and the Canadian Critical Care Trials Group: Hypothermia therapy after traumatic brain injury in children. *N Engl J Med* 2008;**358**:2447–56.

2

Experimental stem cell therapy in acquired neurological illnesses: Current status

RANJITH K. MOORTHY, VEDANTAM RAJSHEKHAR

Current management paradigms have resulted in the reduction of mortality due to several neurological illnesses, such as stroke or head injury, with the result that there has been an increase in the number of patients who may survive with significant disability. Since the primary pathology in many acquired and degenerative neurological illnesses involves the loss of neurons or their connections, cell replacement therapy seems to be the ideal choice for restoring function in such cases. In an organ system such as the skin or gastrointestinal tract, there is constant renewal and replenishment of lost cells. On the other hand, although recent studies and reviews have reported the presence of endogenous regeneration of cells within the mature adult central nervous system, the mechanisms involved seem to be inadequate in achieving the final goal of improving neurological deficits and thereby restoring function.[1–6] Hence, it would seem that the administration of exogenous cells, derived from embryonic as well as adult sources, could result in repopulation of the lost neurons and establishment of appropriate connections that could restore neurological function.[7–13] This review discusses various stem cell transplant strategies that are evolving for the treatment of acquired neurological disorders, with particular emphasis on traumatic brain injury (TBI), spinal cord injury (SCI), stroke and brain tumours.

What are stem cells?

A stem cell, by definition, should have two properties: self-renewal and differentiation. It should also be capable of asymmetric division: a stem cell divides to give rise to another stem cell as well as a progenitor cell. A stem cell such as the blastomeric cell, which can give rise to an entire organism, is totipotent. Pluripotent stem cells, such as embryonic stem cells, are able to produce all tissues.[8] Multipotent stem cells, such as haematopoietic and mesenchymal stem cells (MSCs), are able to produce many cell types.[7,11] Progenitor cells such as neural stem cells (NSCs) are able to produce a restricted number of cell types, with a limited capacity for self-renewal.[4,7]

Embryonic stem cells

Embryonic stem cells are pluripotent and are

derived from the inner cell mass in the blastocyst stage.[8] These cells are able to differentiate into tissues of all three germ layers, but cannot produce another embryo because of their inability to give rise to the placenta and supporting tissues.[9] They have been shown to be able to replicate indefinitely. Several investigators have isolated multiple types of neurons, neural stem cell populations, astrocytes and oligodendrocyte precursors from embryonic stem cells.[8]

The critical issues involved in the use of embryonic stem cells for transplant are: (i) ethical concerns regarding the procurement of these cells, (ii) the risk of tumour formation due to the presence of even a small population of persistently undifferentiated cells despite rigorous purification, (iii) contamination of the cells with animal molecules from the medium or feeder layers that are used during the culture of these cells, and (iv) immunological rejection, as these cells express major histocompatibility complex (MHC) molecules according to the information carried by their own genome.[8]

Stem Cell Inc. (Palo Alto, California, USA) is conducting a trial in which human embryonic stem cells are being transplanted in patients with neuronal ceroid lipofuchsinosis (www.stemcellsinc.com, www.clinicaltrials.gov).

Adult stem cells

If one uses adult stem cells, one can surmount several of the problems arising from the use of embryonic stem cells. The problem of immune rejection can be overcome by obtaining autologous cells from the patient. Due to their restricted lineage, these cells are far less likely to induce tumours.[4–7,10–13] Further, haematopoietic stem cells have been used to treat haematological disorders for the past few decades, proving the safety of the use of adult stem cells in clinical practice. Two main classes of adult stem cells hold promise as putative sources of transplant for neurological disorders: MSCs and NSCs, also called neural progenitor cells.[4–6,11,13]

Mesenchymal stem cells or bone marrow stromal cells are the non-haematopoietic bone marrow fraction that provides structural and functional support to haematopoietic stem cells.[11] By using a variety of mitogens as well as chemicals, such as retinoic acid, fibroblast growth factor, platelet-derived growth factor, epidermal growth factor and β-mercaptoethanol, neuronal differentiation has been induced *in vitro* in MSC cultures.[7,10,11]

Reynolds *et al.*[14] reported in 1992 the presence of NSCs in adult and embryonic mice. Further studies have shown that NSCs lie in the subventricular zone (SVZ) around the lateral ventricle in humans.[15] These cells have been isolated from neurosurgical specimens obtained from adult brains. It must be emphasized here that these adult NSCs are different from those found in the embryonic brain. Successful uptake of the neural progenitor cells derived from the foetal brain following transplant, as well as their morphological maturation into neurons, astrocytes and oligodendrocytes, has been reported.[16] The graft-derived neurons have also been found to form synapses. It has been reported that progenitor cells derived from the brain survive longer than those derived from the spinal cord.[17] The other advantage of using these cells is the lack of an immune response in the recipient. Further, there is no risk of tumour formation or localization of cells to unwanted sites.[16]

Other adult stem cells that could serve as a source of neuronal-like cells and astrocytes include umbilical cord blood, adipocytes, and dermis, muscle and amniotic epithelial cells.[7,9] The experimental evidence pertaining to the use of these cells or their properties is beyond the scope of this review.

Mechanisms of inducing functional improvement

Several mechanisms have been postulated for the restoration of function or improvement in neurological deficits following stem cell transplant in neurological illnesses. The most attractive phenomenon thought to be responsible is that of transdifferentiation of the stem cell into a neuronal phenotype, as evidenced by immunostaining for neural markers.[7,13,16,18–20] However, as research progressed, it was observed that very few of the stem cells showed evidence of double staining for the stem cell marker as well as neuronal markers.[7,19,21] Moreover, it was observed by several authors that a greater number of cells expressed markers for astrocytes.[22–25] On the basis of current evidence, it appears that trans-differentiation plays a minor role, if any, in inducing improvement in function following adult stem cell transplant.

Several reports have suggested that MSCs could induce angiogenesis, improving the vascularity and facilitating the recovery of the existing neurons.[5] It has also been thought that fusion of the stem cell with the existing cell could result in the restoration of function by improving the microenvironment.[13] Reduction of apoptosis has also been postulated. The transplant of MSCs and NSCs has been reported to result in the activation of endogenous neuronal precursors, as well as the proliferation of other progenitor cells.[5,20] It has also been reported to lead to an increase in the production of growth factors.[5] The production of growth factors, along with modulation of inflammation by the transplanted cells, could enhance the survival of the surviving neurons, thus restoring function. The improve-ment in function that has been observed following stem cell transplant seems to be an incompletely understood phenomenon and is likely to be multifactorial, with trophic and humoral components playing a greater role than transdifferentiation of the transplanted cell into a functional neuron.[2,4–6,11,13]

Mode of delivery

Preclinical studies have reported various modes of delivery of cells into the central nervous system. In a review of the methods of delivery, it has been suggested that the mode of delivery could be determined by the cell type used for transplant as well as the mechanism of action.[5] Intravenous administration is the easiest and safest route, considering that stem cells have the property of migrating to the site of injury. This migration is probably secondary to the action of cytokines released into the site of injury. However, there is considerable loss of cells as they pass through the pulmonary circulation. Intra-arterial injections have been tried to bypass the pulmonary circulation.[13] Intracerebral or intraventricular injections into the brain and intramedullary injections or lumbar puncture to deliver cells to the spinal cord are other strategies that have been reported.[5,12,26] PET scans and MRI are being investigated as methods of monitoring the progress of cells transplanted in a non-invasive manner, and this would be important in clinical trials.

Stem cell transplant in spinal cord injury (SCI)

Numerous molecular and biochemical cascades are triggered off following the initial mechanical insult that results in SCI. These cascades result in lipid peroxidation, production of reactive oxygen species, glutaminergic excitotoxicity and calcium-mediated damage to the cell membrane structure and physiology, resulting in cell death.[3,12] These non-mechanical effects extend to a few segments above and below the level of the injury. A glial scar forms as a part of the repair mechanism to contain the injury. The glial scar, as well as the release of myelin-associated glycoprotein, oligo-dendrocyte myelin protein and Nogo-A, are a few oligodendrocyte-derived inhibitors of axonal regrowth across the site of injury. Following cell death, the endogenous stem/progenitor cells within the adult spinal cord proliferate. This proliferative activity is too limited to support significant self-repair.[12] Thus, various cellular transplantation strategies have been adopted in models of SCI.

Using NSCs derived from embryonic stem cells, Kimura *et al.*[22] showed improved behavioural function in a mouse model of SCI. Pallini *et al.*[27] reported that following the transplant of embryo-derived NSCs into the injured spinal cord of mice after dorsal funiculotomy, the transplanted cells tended to differentiate into immature astrocytes. They observed an improvement in function in these mice and suggested that the immature astrocytes (which are typically seen during the early phase of injury) could permit the regeneration of axons. The use of the C17.2 clone of NSCs led to functional improvement, but the animals experienced allodynia.[28]

Several authors have reported enhanced locomotor function, as well as an improvement in sensory function and electrophysiological para-meters, following intravenous MSC transplant in rodent models with SCI.[23–25,29] In the wake of the observation that transplanted MSCs differentiated predominantly into the oligodendrocyte lineage, it has been postulated that MSC transplant improves function perhaps by promoting remyelination of the spared white matter tracts.[23] In one study, MSC transplant was combined with the infusion of fibroblast growth factor (βFGF) and it was suggested that the improvement in function could be due to the growth factor rather than the presence of transplanted cells.[24] In a recent study, intralesionally transplanted MSCs survived more than 6 weeks, but induced no significant functional recovery in nude rats with SCI.[30] It was also reported recently that in rats with SCI, those which were given exercise training along with parenchymal MSC infusion showed greater improvement in function than those which remained sedentary.[31]

Glial differentiation of transplanted adult NSCs has been reported in animal models of SCI, but no significant improvement in the locomotor rating scales has been observed.[17,32–34] In order to improve survival, adult neural progenitor cells from the brain and spinal cord were seeded into extramedullary chitosan channels. The cells derived from the brain had better survival, and showed predominant glial differentiation, but there was no improvement in functional outcomes.[17] It has been observed that transplanted neural progenitor cells survive long-term with predominant glial differentiation and are able to remyelinate the axons in the presence of post-transplantation delivery of growth factors in subacute transplantation following SCI, while survival is poor in chronic SCI.[12]

Few studies have been reported following SCI in humans. The ones that have been carried out are non-randomized and are essentially phase I trials. Lima *et al.*[35] reported that olfactory mucosa auto-transplantation into the injured human spinal cord many months after SCI is feasible, relatively safe and potentially beneficial. Chernykh *et al.*[36] reported similar findings, following intralesional and parenchymal transplant of autologous bone marrow stem cells in chronic SCI. Sykova *et al.*[37] reported that implantation of autologous bone marrow cells appears to be safe, with improvements being observed in patients who received acute versus late transplant. However, as their study lacked controls, it is not possible to derive definitive conclusions and the improvement in function could be a result of the natural history of the illness.

A review of preclinical studies suggests that the use of autologous or allogeneic MSCs rather than adult neural progenitor cells seems to improve function following SCI. It seems that stem cell transplant is more likely to have beneficial results when the implantation is performed in the subacute phase rather than the chronic phase. The use of growth factors or polymer scaffolds could promote survival of the transplanted cells, which may or may not translate into functional improvement. There is a risk of developing allodynia following stem cell therapy. Randomized clinical trials in humans are essential before the use of stem cell transplant can be considered as the 'standard of care' in human SCI.

Stem cell transplant in traumatic brain injury (TBI)

Several authors have reported that following TBI, there is generation of neurons and proliferation of neuronal precursors in the subventricular zone, dentate gyrus of the hippocampus, as well as the cortex. Studies in rodents have demonstrated that in the subgranular zone of the dentate gyrus in the adult, there is continuous generation of neurons, which migrate into the granule cell layer and can functionally integrate into the hippocampal circuitry.[1] This endogenous cell proliferation can be augmented by the addition of growth factors, as well as agents such as S100B and erythropoietin.[1] Although there is literature supporting the induction of endogenous cell proliferation in the hippocampus and the SVZ, this is obviously insufficient for regaining function as most patients with moderate and severe head injury have residual cognitive or other neurological deficits. The use of growth factors has been reported to induce the proliferation of endogenous cells and enhance the survival of the graft, besides promoting neuronal differentiation.

Significant improvement in neurological function was observed in rodents following transplant of foetal cortical tissue into a cortical lesion.[38] Rodent NSCs have been shown to survive for more than a year. They migrate to the areas of injury and enhance motor and cognitive recovery.[39] Differentiation and functional integration of embryo-derived NSCs has been reported following TBI in rodents.[13] The problems that need to be tackled before this cell type can be considered for human use include reduced survival of grafted NSCs in severe forms of TBI (compared with mild TBI), and the likely need for immunosuppression as well as apoptosis of the grafted neural progenitor cells.[13,21,40]

In a series of publications starting in 2001, Chopp and co-workers have reported successful outcomes following the transplant of bone marrow-derived mononuclear cells and MSCs in rodents with cortical impact injury.[13,18–20,41] In their experiments, the transplanted cells were shown to migrate to the site of injury, irrespective of the mode of delivery, and a proportion of the cells expressed neuronal markers. The experiments demonstrated the efficacy of transplant at 24 hours and 7 days after the cortical impact injury, and the transplanted cells were surviving 3 months after the transplant. According to Chopp and co-workers,[18–20] the spontaneous recovery that appears to occur in neurological function seems to be enhanced by the use of cell transplant. It has been suggested that the transplantation of MSCs could induce cellular proliferation within the recipient brain.[20] Recently, Chopp and co-workers have reported that the neurological improvement conferred by the transplantation of MSCs can be enhanced by using a collagen scaffold to aid the delivery of the cells.[41]

No clinical studies of stem cell transplant for human TBI have been reported. On the basis of preclinical studies, it seems that MSCs derived from bone marrow are an attractive candidate and these may be tested in phase I trials in the future. A phase I clinical trial approved by the US Food and Drug Administration (FDA) in Texas is currently recruiting paediatric patients with severe head injury for the transplantation of autologous mononuclear cell fraction derived from the bone marrow within 36 hours of the injury.

Stem cell therapy in ischaemic stroke

Current experimental cellular replacement strategies for promoting neurological recovery following experimental stroke focus on two issues: augmentation or increase of the survival and differentiation of endogenous stem cells, the proliferation of which is stimulated following ischaemia, and replacement of cells from exogenous sources.[2,4–7] The use of embryo-derived NSCs as well as MSCs to improve neurological function following experimental middle cerebral artery occlusion has been reported.[7,42,43] These cells have been found to survive over a long period of time, and to express glial as well as neuronal markers. What remains to be seen is how many functional neurons can be produced in the setting of ischaemia, particularly as a large area of the cortex is lost following middle cerebral artery occlusion. On the basis of the number of surviving cells and degree of differentiation noted, it appears that these cells are likely to influence improvement by humoral mechanisms, facilitating survival of the neurons spared from injury and reducing inflammation.

Trials of intrastriatal transplant of post-mitotic mature neuron cells derived from an immortalized cell line in patients who had stable motor deficits for 6 months to 6 years showed that cell transplant was safe, but there was no significant improvement in functional outcomes.[5] Another phase I trial of the transplantation of porcine embryo-derived neural cells for chronic stroke in humans was terminated by the US FDA, with no significant functional improvement being reported in patients who received the cells at 2 years' follow-up.[5,6] On the basis of the experience with these trials, it seems that transplantation is feasible but poses the risks of seizures, subdural haematoma and venous occlusion.[6] Two trials studying the intra-arterial autologous CD34+ (haematopoietic stem cells) cell transfusion in cases of middle cerebral artery stroke are currently enrolling patients (www. clinicaltrials.gov).

On the basis of a review of the literature, stem cell transplant in the setting of experimental stroke is safe. The cells survive in the long-term and there is partial restoration of function. The transplanted cells seem to act like 'biological mini-pumps', with a small number of the exogenous cells differentiating into neurons.

Stem cells in the management of brain tumour

The treatment of malignant gliomas and metastases in the brain is impeded by the inability to achieve ablation of every last tumour cell with current surgical or chemotherapeutic strategies. The inability of several chemotherapeutic agents to cross the blood–brain barrier effectively and the systemic toxicity of these agents necessitate a search for better treatment strategies. It has been demonstrated that MSCs and NSCs possess a remarkable tumour tropism that is mediated through a variety of cytokines, growth factors and receptors.[44–46] The migration of the infused cells into the tumour helps to overcome the blood–brain barrier while ensuring the presence of cells only at the target site, thus avoiding unnecessary side-effects. These cells have also been shown to migrate along the infiltrating tumour cells and satellite tumour nodules, which have been the bane of successful treatment of malignancies.[45]

In preclinical studies, both MSCs and NSCs have been genetically manipulated to: (i) secrete excess prodrug-activating enzymes, such as cytosine deaminase;[44] (ii) deliver immunomodulatory interleukins, such as IL-4, IL-12 and IL-23, or immunomodulatory molecules, such as interferon-β;[44,46,47] (iii) deliver oncolytic adenoviruses;[48] and (iv) deliver apoptosis-promoting proteins, such as tumour necrosis factor-related apoptosis-inducing ligand (TRAIL).[45] Studies on the use of genetically manipulated MSCs in brain tumour models in rodents have reported a 70%–90% reduction in the size of the tumour, associated with extended survival of the animals. Future strategies are likely to focus on the use of engineered MSCs as this can help one avoid the use of immunosuppression, which may be required if allogeneic foetal derived-NSCs are employed as vehicles for the delivery of any of the agents mentioned above. A cause of concern in relation to the use of NSCs in brain tumour therapy is their potential tumorigenicity.

Appraisal of literature

Most of the published studies report that stem cell transplant is associated with positive results for various disorders. Adult stem cells are being used clinically for several cardiac conditions. For neurological illnesses, most of the research is still preclinical, with proof of principle still being demonstrated on the safety and efficacy of the use of these cells. Table 1 summarizes some important points one should consider while evaluating any study publishing the results of stem cell transplant. It is important to analyse these results critically, as spontaneous recovery is a part of the natural history of several acquired neurological illnesses. In several studies, growth factors have been used to enhance graft survival and the beneficial effects could be a result of these agents alone, rather than that of the transplanted cells.

Ethical challenges

Current experimental evidence suggests that the use of stem cells may be beneficial in certain neurological disorders. It is tempting to see if stem cell transplant would be beneficial in cases in which all current lines of treatment have failed. However, there are several ethical concerns regarding their use in human trials. Unlike a drug which has the same chemical composition batch after batch, the later passages of stem cells are unlikely to be genetically identical to the earlier passages in culture. This could result in altered phenotypic expression, which might have deleterious consequences. Further, it is not clear if the use of stem cells could result in cognitive or affective disorders in the long term, as such disorders cannot be adequately evaluated in animal models. Finally, studies of appropriate animal models are lacking for several disorders for which stem cells could prove beneficial.

With regard to the patients to be included in trials, there is no justification for using healthy volunteers as controls in early trials. While trials in the sickest patients may be scientifically and ethically justifiable, these may be the patients who benefit the least from any therapy and this could result in a false impression that the trial intervention provides no benefit. Due to the hype surrounding the use of stem cells and the lack of knowledge regarding long-term consequences,

Table 1. Issues to be addressed while reporting or evaluating literature on stem cell therapy

- *Animal-related issues*
  —Species, number and age
  —Injury mechanism and severity

- *Issues related to cell transplant*
  —Type of cell used: embryonic/adult
  —Source of cell used: commercially available cell lines or cell lines generated for study
  —Cell labelling for follow-up:
    Bromodeoxyuridine
    Green fluorescent protein
    Markers for chemilumiscence
    Beta galactosidase (LacZ)
    Supermagnetic iron oxide particles
  —Mode of delivery:
    Intravenous
    Intra-arterial
    Intracerebral/intramedullary
    CSF-based approaches
  —Associated use of growth factor
  —Associated immunosuppression
  —Timing of cell transplant in relation to injury

- *Issues regarding mechanism of action*
  —Histopathology evidence:
    Presence of cells at site of injury
    Co-labelling of neuronal/glial markers using immunostaining
    Change in lesion volumes compared to controls
  —Biochemical assays for quantification of trophic factors

- *Neurological function assessment*
  —Objective tool used
  —Whether or not assessor is blinded to the intervention received
  —Spontaneous recovery observed in control vs. experimental group

providing accurate information about their use to a potential recipient before obtaining informed consent will itself be a challenge. Interdisciplinary groups composed of neuroscientists, cell biologists and lawyers have discussed these aspects in detail and certain broad guidelines have been suggested.[49] However, it is lamentable that there are no guidelines governing clinical trials of stem cells in India, where stem cell therapy is advertised by various institutions without adequate preclinical data.[50]

From bench to bedside?

On the basis of this review, it may be surmised that, in the backdrop of very few clinical trials, there is still some time to go before stem cell therapy for neurological disorders can reach the clinic. Although the survival of transplanted cells has been demonstrated in various animal models of neurological diseases, the functional improvement reported is modest. The details of approved clinical trials using stem cell transplant in neurological disorders besides those discussed here are available at www.clinicaltrials.gov. The use of stem cell therapy in the clinic should be withheld till the results of these approved clinical trials are reported and evaluated.

According to various strategies evolving in preclinical trials, it appears that a combination of growth factors and stem cells or the use of cells that are genetically modified to secrete certain trophic factors will be the ideal paradigm for the treatment of acquired neurological illnesses. On the basis of the current knowledge, MSCs derived from bone marrow seem to hold the greatest promise for clinical use.

Conclusion

Stem cell transplant seems to be relatively safe and holds the promise of restoring neurological function, albeit partly, through multifactorial mechanisms that are not completely understood. Very few clinical trials have been approved for stem cell-based therapy for stroke and TBI. The use of stem cells by neurologists and neurosurgeons must be withheld till such time as the results of approved clinical trials in humans are reported.

References

1. Richardson RM, Sun D, Bullock MR. Neurogenesis after traumatic brain injury. *Neurosurg Clin North Am* 2007;**18**:169–81.
2. Kalluri HSG, Dempsey RJ. Growth factors, stem cells and stroke. *Neurosurg Focus* 2008;**24**:E13.
3. Bambakidis NC, Butler J, Horn EM, *et al.* Stem cell biology and its therapeutic applications in the setting of spinal cord injury. *Neurosurg Focus* 2008;**24**:E20.
4. Kornblum HI. Introduction to neural stem cells. *Stroke* 2007;**38**:810–16.
5. Bliss T, Guzman R, Daadi M, *et al.* Cell transplantation therapy for stroke. *Stroke* 2007;**38**:817–26.
6. Savitz SI, Dinsmore JH, Wechsler LR, *et al.* Cell therapy for stroke. *NeuroRx* 2004;**1**:406–14.
7. Corti S, Locatelli F, Strazzer S, *et al.* Neuronal generation from somatic stem cells: Current knowledge and perspectives on the treatment of acquired and degenerative central nervous system disorders. *Curr Gene Ther* 2003;**3**:247–72.
8. Choong C, Rao MS. Human embryonic stem cells. *Neurosurg Clin North Am* 2007;**18**:1–14.
9. Cogle CR, Guthrie SM, Sanders RC, *et al.* An overview of stem cell research and regulatory issues. *Mayo Clin Proc* 2003;**78**:993–1003.
10. Woodbury D, Schwarz EJ, Prockop DJ, *et al.* Adult rat and human bone marrow stromal cells differentiate into neurons. *J Neurosci Res* 2000;**61**:364–70.
11. Hardy SA, Maltman DJ, Przyborski SA. Mesenchymal stem cells as mediators of neural differentiation. *Curr Stem Cell Res Ther* 2008;**3**:43–52.
12. Eftekarpour E, Karimi-Abdolrezaee S, Fehlings MG. Current status of experimental cell replacement approaches to spinal cord injury. *Neurosurg Focus* 2008;**24**:E19.
13. Harting MT, Baumgartner JE, Worth LL, *et al.* Cell therapies for traumatic brain injury. *Neurosurg Focus* 2008;**24**:E17.
14. Reynolds BA, Weiss S. Generation of neurons and astrocytes from isolated cells of the adult mammalian central nervous system. *Science* 1992;**255**:1707–10.
15. Quinones-Hinojosa A, Sanai N, Gonzalez-Perez O, *et al.* The human brain subventricular zone: Stem cells in this niche and its organization. *Neurosurg Clin North Am* 2007;**18**:15–20.
16. Lepore AC, Neuhuber B, Connors TM, *et al.* Long-term fate of neural precursor cells following trans-

plantation into developing and adult CNS. *Neuroscience* 2006;**142**:287–304.

17. Nomura H, Zahir T, Kim H, *et al.* Extramedullary chitosan channels promote survival of transplanted neural stem and progenitor cells and create a tissue bridge after complete spinal cord transaction. *Tissue Eng Part A* 2008 (Epub ahead of print).

18. Lu D, Mahmood A, Wang L, *et al.* Adult bone marrow stromal cells administered intravenously to rats after traumatic brain injury migrate into brain and improve neurological outcome. *Neuroreport* 2001;559–63.

19. Mahmood A, Lu D, Qu C, *et al.* Long-term recovery after bone marrow stromal cell treatment of traumatic brain injury in rats. *J Neurosurg* 2006;**104**:272–7.

20. Mahmood A, Lu D, Chopp M. Marrow stromal cell transplantation after traumatic brain injury promotes cellular proliferation within the brain. *Neurosurgery* 2004;**55**:1185–93.

21. Wennersten A, Meier X, Holmin S, *et al.* Proliferation, migration and differentiation of human neural stem/progenitor cells after transplantation into a rat model of traumatic brain injury. *J Neurosurg* 2004;**100**:88–96.

22. Kimura H, Yoshikawa M, Matsuda R, *et al.* Transplantation of embryonic stem cell-derived neural stem cells for spinal cord injury in adult mice. *Neurol Res* 2005;**27**:812–19.

23. Cizkova D, Rosocha J, Vanicky I, *et al.* Transplants of human mesenchymal stem cells improve functional recovery after spinal cord injury in the rat. *Cell Mol Neurobiol* 2006;**26**:1167–80.

24. Kim KN, Oh SH, Lee KH, *et al.* Effect of human mesenchymal stem cell transplantation combined with growth factor infusion in the repair of injured spinal cord. *Acta Neurochir Suppl* 2006;**99**:133–6.

25. Lee KH, Suh-Kim H, Choi JS, *et al.* Human mesenchymal stem cell transplantation promotes functional recovery following acute spinal cord injury in rats. *Acta Neurobiol Exp (Wars)* 2007;**67**:13–22.

26. Bakshi A, Barshinger AL, Swanger SA, *et al.* Lumbar puncture delivery of bone marrow stromal cells in spinal cord contusion: A novel method for minimally invasive cell transplantation. *J Neurotrauma* 2006;**23**:55–65.

27. Pallini R, Vitiani LR, Bez A, *et al.* Homologous transplantation of neural stem cells to the injured spinal cord of mice. *Neurosurgery* 2005;**57**:1014–25.

28. Macias MY, Syring MB, Pizzi MA, *et al.* Pain with no gain: Allodynia following neural stem cell transplantation in spinal cord injury. *Exp Neurol* 2006;**201**:335–48.

29. Urdzikova L, Jendelova P, Glogarova K, *et al.* Transplantation of bone marrow stem cells as well as mobilisation by granulocyte-colony stimulating factor promotes recovery after spinal cord injury in rats. *J Neurotrauma* 2006;**23**:1379–91.

30. Sheth RN, Manzano G, Li X, *et al.* Transplantation of human bone marrow-derived stromal cells into the contused spinal cord of nude rats. *J Neurosurg Spine* 2008;**8**:153–62.

31. Carvalho KA, Cunha RC, Vialle EN, *et al.* Functional outcome of bone marrow stem cells ('CD45(+)/CD34(-)) after cell therapy in acute spinal cord injury: In exercise training and sedentary rats. *Transplant Proc* 2008;**40**:847–9.

32. Pfiefer K, Vroemen M, Caioni M, *et al.* Autologous adult rodent neural progenitor cell transplantation represents a feasible strategy to promote structural repair in the chronically injured spinal cord. *Regen Med* 2006;**1**:255–66.

33. Parr AM, Kulbatski I, Tator CH. Transplantation of adult rat spinal cord stem/progenitor cells for spinal cord injury. *J Neurotrauma* 2007;**24**:835–45.

34. Webber DJ, Bradbury EJ, McMohan SB, *et al.* Transplanted neural progenitor cells survive and differentiate but achieve limited functional recovery in the lesioned adult rat spinal cord. *Regen Med* 2007;**2**:929–45.

35. Lima C, Pratas-Vital J, Escada P, *et al.* Olfactory mucosa autografts in human spinal cord injury: A pilot clinical study. *J Spinal Cord Med* 2006;**29**:191–203.

36. Chernykh ER, Stupak VV, Muradov GM, *et al.* Application of autologous bone marrow stem cells in the therapy of spinal cord injury patients. *Bull Exp Biol Med* 2007;**143**:543–7.

37. Sykova E, Homola A, Mazanec R, *et al.* Autologous bone marrow transplantation in patients with subacute and chronic spinal cord injury. *Cell Transplant* 2006;**15**:675–87.

38. Sinson G, Voddi M, McIntosh TK. Combined fetal neural transplantation and nerve growth factor infusion effects on neurological outcome following fluid–percussion brain injury in the rat. *J Neurosurg* 1996;**84**:655–62.

39. Shear DA, Tate MC, Archer DR, *et al.* Neural progenitor cell transplants promote long-term functional recovery after traumatic brain injury. *Brain Res* 2004;**1026**:11–22.

40. Bakshi A, Keck CA, Koshkin VS, *et al*. Caspase-mediated cell death predominates following engraftment of neural progenitor cells into traumatically injured rat brain. *Brain Res* 2005;**1065**:8–19.

41. Lu D, Mahmood A, Qu C, *et al*. Collagen scaffolds populated with human marrow stromal cells reduce lesion volume and improve functional outcome after traumatic brain injury. *Neurosurgery* 2007;**61**:596–603.

42. Horita Y, Honmou O, Harada K, *et al*. Intravenous administration of glial cell line-derived neurotrophic factor gene-modified human mesenchymal stem cells protects against injury in a cerebral ischemia model in the adult rat. *J Neurosci Res* 2006;15:**84**:1495–1504.

43. Buhnemann C, Scholz A, Bernreuther C, *et al*. Neuronal differentiation of transplanted embryonic stem cell-derived precursors in stroke lesions of adult rats. *Brain* 2006;**129**:3238–48.

44. Aboody KS, Najbauer J, Danks MK. Stem and progenitor cell-mediated tumor selective gene therapy. *Gene Ther* 2008;**15**:739–52.

45. Mapara KY, Stevenson CB, Thompson RC, *et al*. Stem cells as vehicles for the treatment of brain cancer. *Neurosurg Clin North Am* 2007;**18**:71–80.

46. Nakamizo A, Marini F, Amano T, *et al*. Human bone marrow derived mesenchymal stem cells in the treatment of gliomas. *Cancer Res* 2005;**65**:3307–18.

47. Beneditti S, Pirola B, Pollo B, *et al*. Gene therapy of experimental brain tumors using neural progenitor cells. *Nat Med* 2000;**6**:447–50.

48. Sonabend AM, Ulasov IV, Tyler MA, *et al*. Mesenchymal stem cells effectively deliver an oncolytic adenovirus to intracranial glioma. *Stem Cells* 2008;**26**:831–41.

49. Mathews DJH, Sugarman J, Bok H, *et al*. Cell-based interventions for neurologic conditions: Ethical challenges for early human trials. *Neurology* 2008;**71**:288–93.

50. Pandya SK. Stem cell transplantation in India: Tall claims, questionable ethics. *Indian J Med Ethics* 2008;**5**:15–17.

3

Primary prevention of stroke

SUBHASH KAUL

Stroke is a major public health problem in India.[1] A recent community survey in the eastern Indian city of Kolkata showed the prevalence rate of stroke to be 545 per 100,000 population.[2] The average annual incidence rate of stroke in the same study was 145 per 100,000 persons per year.[2] These rates, age-standardized to world standard population, are similar to or higher than those in many western nations.[3] These rates are also much higher than those reported previously from other parts of India.[4,5] The stroke burden in India has been rising in the past few decades in contrast to developed countries, where the prevalence of stroke has decreased or plateaued.[6,7]

Why primary prevention?

Despite modern methods of treatment, stroke remains a major cause of mortality and morbidity. The best option is to prevent the first attack itself. This is particularly true in India, where the average age of stroke patients is at least one decade lower than patients in western countries, affecting people in the prime of their careers.[8,9] Primary prevention strategies are designed to prevent the first attack of stroke. This chapter provides an evidence-based update on the pathophysiology and management of selected risk factors for the primary prevention of stroke. For each risk factor, data on strength of association and recommendations for stroke prevention are described.

Conspiracy of risk factors

Many factors can contribute to a person's stroke risk, and some persons have more than one risk factor. Although most risk factors have an independent effect, interactions between individual factors can compound the risk. As per a statement from the American Stroke Association, independent stroke predictors include age, systolic blood pressure, hypertension, diabetes mellitus, current smoking, established cardiovascular disease, congestive heart failure, atrial fibrillation and left ventricular (LV) hypertrophy on ECG.[10] In 1989, the Indian Council of Medical Research (ICMR) found hypertension, diabetes mellitus, tobacco use and low concentration of normal haemoglobin as the most important risk factors for ischaemic strokes in India.[11] The World Health Organization (WHO) Task Force Report on Stroke (1989) found that hypertension, smoking, elevated blood lipid levels and diabetes were important modifiable risk factors for ischaemic stroke in India.[12]

Other reasons contributing to a rise in stroke burden in India include increasing longevity and changes in lifestyle accompanying urbanization. Indians may also be genetically prone to stroke due to a high prevalence of the metabolic syndrome, which comprises central obesity, high levels of triglycerides, and low levels of high-density lipoprotein (HDL) cholesterol with or without glucose intolerance.[13] It is useful to conceptualize the risk factors as non-modifiable and modifiable. The identification of non-modifiable risk factors helps to identify those who are at highest risk of stroke and who may benefit from rigorous prevention or treatment of modifiable risk factors.

Non-modifiable risk factors

Age

The cumulative effects of ageing on the cardiovascular system and the progressive nature of stroke risk factors over a prolonged period of time substantially increase stroke risk. The risk of stroke doubles for each successive decade after the age of 55 years.[14,15] In India, the average life expectancy rose from 41.2 years in 1951–1961 to 61.4 years in 1991–1996, which is one of the reasons for the rise in incidence of stroke.[13]

Sex

Stroke is more prevalent in men than in women.[14] Men generally also have higher age-specific stroke incidence rates than women.[16] Exceptions are those in the age group of 35–44 years and >85 years of age. In these age groups, women have a slightly greater age-specific incidence of stroke than men. Factors such as oral contraceptive use and pregnancy contribute to the increased risk of stroke in young women.[17–19]

Genetic factors

Both paternal and maternal history of stroke have been associated with an increased stroke risk.[20,21] This increased risk is mediated through a variety of mechanisms including genetic heritability of stroke risk factors, inheritance of susceptibility to the effects of such risk factors, familial sharing of cultural/environmental and lifestyle factors, and the interaction between genetic and environmental factors.[22] Twin studies provide strong data suggestive of a familial inheritance of stroke risk. Concordance rates for stroke are markedly higher in monozygotic than in dizygotic twins, with a nearly five-fold increase in stroke prevalence among monozygotic compared with dizygotic twins.[23]

Genetic influences on stroke risk can be considered on the basis of individual risk factors, genetics of common stroke types, and uncommon or rare familial stroke types. Many of the established and emerging risk factors such as hypertension, diabetes and hyperlipidaemia have genetic and environmental/behavioural components.[24–26] In some cases, elevation of blood homocysteine is due to one or more mutations in the methylene tetrahydrofolate reductase gene.[27–29] Many coagulopathies are inherited as autosomal dominant traits.[30] These disorders, including protein C and S deficiencies, factor V Leiden mutations, and various other factor deficiencies can lead to an increased risk of venous thrombosis.[31–36] Some apparently acquired coagulopathies, such as the presence of a lupus anticoagulant or anticardiolipin antibody, can be familial in 10% of cases.[37,38] Inherited disorders of various clotting factors (i.e. factors V, VII, X, XI and XII) are autosomal recessive traits and can lead to cerebral haemorrhage in childhood or the neonatal period. Arterial dissections, moyamoya syndrome and fibromuscular dysplasia have a genetic or familial component in 10%–20% of cases.[39,40]

The DeCode genetics group (Iceland) has reported genetic linkage of phosphodiesterase 4D (chromosome 5g12) and 5-lipoxygenase activating protein (chromosome 13q12–13) to common forms of ischaemic stroke.[41,42] In both cases, there appears to be an association between several specific genetic haplotypes and stroke, although no pathogenic mutations have been identified.

Several rare genetic disorders have been associated with stroke. Cerebral autosomal dominant arteriopathy with subcortical infarcts and leukoencephalopathy (CADASIL) is characterized by subcortical infarcts, dementia and migraine headaches.[43] CADASIL can be caused by any of a series of mutations in the *Notch3* gene.[43,44] Acetazolamide may reduce migraine headaches in patients with CADASIL.[45] Marfan syndrome (due to mutations in the fibrillin gene) and neurofibromatosis types I and II are associated with an increased risk of ischaemic stroke. Gene transfer therapy has been attempted to correct the genetic defect.[46] Fabry disease is a rare inherited disorder that can lead to ischaemic stroke.

Recommendations

Referral for genetic counselling may be considered for patients with rare genetic causes of stroke (Class IIb; level of evidence C).

Modifiable risk factors

An important risk factor for a first stroke is the presence of atherosclerotic vascular disease in another vascular bed. Those with a history of cardiovascular disease have a significantly increased risk of a first stroke as compared with those without such a history, after adjustment for other risk factors.[47] Treatments used in the management of these other conditions may also reduce the risk of stroke. The risk factors for first stroke and the risk factors for cardiovascular disease overlap.

Recommendations

Persons with evidence of non-cerebrovascular atherosclerotic vascular disease are at increased risk for a first stroke. Treatments used in the management of these other conditions can reduce the risk of stroke.

Hypertension

Hypertension is a major risk factor for both cerebral infarction and intracerebral haemorrhage.[48] The relationship between blood pressure and cardiovascular risk is continuous, consistent and independent of other risk factors.[49] The higher the blood pressure, the greater the stroke risk.[50] Blood pressure, particularly systolic blood pressure, increases with increasing age. There is strong evidence that the control of high blood pressure contributes to the prevention of stroke as well as to the prevention or reduction of other target-organ damage, including congestive heart failure and renal failure.[51] A meta-analysis of 18 long-term randomized trials found that both beta-blocker therapy and treatment with diuretics were effective in preventing stroke.[52] Overall, antihypertensive therapy is associated with a 35%–44% reduction in the incidence of stroke.[53] Recent national guidelines recommend lowering blood pressure to <140/90 mmHg (with lower targets in some subgroups, such as individuals with diabetes).[51]

Several categories of antihypertensive agents, including thiazide diuretics, angiotensin-converting enzyme inhibitors (ACEIs), angiotensin-receptor blockers (ARBs), beta-adrenergic receptor blockers, and calcium-channel blockers, reduce cardiovascular risk including the risk of stroke in patients with hypertension.[54,55] Blood pressure control can be achieved in most patients, but the majority require combination therapy with two or more antihypertensive agents.[56,57] Direct comparisons among the various types of antihypertensives are limited. It remains unsettled whether specific classes of antihypertensive agents offer special protection against stroke in addition to their blood pressure-lowering effects in other settings. Controlling isolated systolic hypertension (systolic blood pressure >160 mmHg and diastolic blood pressure <90 mmHg) in the elderly is also important. The Systolic Hypertension in Europe Trial randomized 4595 patients with isolated systolic hypertension to active treatment with a calcium-channel blocker or placebo and showed a 42% risk reduction in the actively treated group.[58] The Systolic Hypertension in the Elderly Program (SHEP) Trial found a 36% reduction in the incidence of stroke following treatment with a thiazide diuretic with or without a beta-blocker.[59] In short, the benefit of hypertension treatment for primary prevention of stroke is established beyond doubt. The choice of a specific regimen must be individualized, but reduction in blood pressure is generally more important than the specific agent used to achieve this goal.

Recommendations

Regular screening for hypertension and appropriate management (Class I; level of evidence A), including dietary changes, lifestyle modification and pharmacological therapy as summarized in JNC 7, are recommended.

Cigarette smoking

All the major multivariate studies have identified cigarette smoking as a potent risk factor for ischaemic stroke, associated with an approximate doubling of ischaemic stroke risk. In addition, smoking has been clearly associated with a two- to four-fold increased risk for haemorrhagic stroke.[60,61] Based on the available evidence, in 1989, the US Surgeon-General concluded that a definite relationship exists between smoking and both ischaemic and haemorrhagic stroke, particularly at young ages.[62]

Several studies suggest that environmental tobacco smoke (passive cigarette smoke) is also a risk factor for stroke.[63,64] Smoking is likely to contribute to increased stroke risk through both acute effects on the risk of thrombus generation in narrowed arteries and chronic effects related to an increased burden of atherosclerosis. In addition to placing individuals at increased risk for both thrombotic and embolic stroke, cigarette smoking approximately triples the risk of cryptogenic stroke among individuals with low atherosclerotic burdens and no evidence of cardiac sources of emboli.[65]

Recommendations

Abstention from cigarette smoking and smoking cessation for current smokers is recommended. Avoidance of environmental tobacco smoke for stroke prevention should also be considered. The use of counselling, nicotine replacement and oral-smoking cessation medications has been found to be effective for smokers.

Diabetes

Case–control studies of stroke patients and prospective epidemiological studies have confirmed an independent effect of diabetes on ischaemic stroke, with an increased relative risk in persons with diabetes ranging from 1.8-fold to nearly six-fold.[66] The Heart Outcomes Prevention Evaluation (HOPE) Study compared the addition of an ACEI to the current medical regimen of high-risk patients. The substudy of 3577 diabetic patients (of a total population of 9541 participants in the HOPE Study) showed a reduction in the primary combined outcome of myocardial infarction (MI), stroke and cardiovascular death by 25%, and stroke by 33% as compared with controls.[67] Whether these benefits were a specific effect of the ACEI or an effect of blood pressure lowering has been the subject of debate. The Medical Research Council/

British Heart Foundation Heart Protection Study (HPS) found that the addition of a statin to existing treatments in 5963 diabetic individuals resulted in a 22% reduction in the rate of major vascular events, and a 24% reduction in strokes.[68] The Collaborative Atorvastatin Diabetes Study (CARDS) reported that in subjects with type 2 diabetes who had at least one additional risk factor and a low-density lipoprotein (LDL) cholesterol level <160 mg/dl, but without a prior history of cardiovascular disease, treatment with a statin resulted in a 48% reduction in stroke.[69]

Recommendations

It is recommended that hypertension be tightly controlled in patients with either type 1 or type 2 diabetes (the JNC 7 recommendation of <130/80 mmHg in diabetic patients is endorsed) as part of a comprehensive risk-reduction programme (Class I; level of evidence A). Treatment of adults with diabetes, especially those with additional risk factors, with a statin to lower the risk of a first stroke is recommended (Class I; level of evidence A). The recommendation to consider treatment of patients of diabetes with an ACEI or ARB is endorsed.

Atrial fibrillation

Patients with paroxysmal or persistent atrial fibrillation and valvular heart disease such as mitral stenosis are at the highest risk for future embolic events and should be anticoagulated (Class I). Atrial fibrillation alone is associated with a three- to four-fold increased risk of stroke.[70] Among those without a prior transient ischaemic attack (TIA) or stroke, 2%–4% per year have an ischaemic stroke.[71,72] Randomized clinical trials have firmly established the value of antithrombotic therapies for reducing the risk of stroke in patients with atrial fibrillation. The risk is reduced by 60% with adjusted-dose warfarin and by 20% with aspirin.[73] The absolute risk of stroke varies twenty-fold among patients with atrial fibrillation, according to age and associated vascular diseases. The threshold of absolute stroke risk warranting anticoagulation is importantly influenced by the estimated bleeding risk if anticoagulated, patient preferences and access to high-quality anticoagulant monitoring. The reader is referred to some important publications for risk stratification.[74,75] Most patients with atrial fibrillation who are <75 years of age without prior stroke or TIA have a relatively low risk of stroke if given aspirin, and they do not benefit sufficiently from anticoagulation to warrant its use for primary stroke prevention.[76,77] It is generally agreed that patients with atrial fibrillation whose estimated stroke risk exceeds 4% per year should be anticoagulated in the absence of contraindications.[78] It has been observed that anticoagulation is particularly underused in elderly patients with atrial fibrillation.[79] Although the attributable risk of stroke associated with atrial fibrillation increases with age,[80] elderly patients (>75 years of age) with atrial fibrillation have about twice the risk of serious bleeding complications during anticoagulation as compared with the younger population.[81] Nevertheless, anticoagulation is still warranted if their risk of ischaemic stroke without warfarin is greater than their risk of bleeding. In addition to age, poorly controlled hypertension and concomitant aspirin or non-steroidal anti-inflammatory drug use confer higher bleeding risk during anticoagulation.

Recommendations

Anticoagulation of patients with atrial fibrillation who have valvular heart disease (particularly those with mechanical heart valves) is recommended (Class I; level of evidence A). Antithrombotic therapy (warfarin or aspirin) is recommended to prevent stroke in patients with non-valvular atrial fibrillation according to assessment of their absolute stroke risk, estimated bleeding risk, patient preferences and access to high-quality anticoagulation monitoring (Class I; level of evidence A). Warfarin (INR 2.0–3.0) is recommended for high-risk (>4% annual risk of stroke) patients with atrial fibrillation who have no clinically significant contraindications to oral anticoagulants (Class I; level of evidence A).

Other cardiac conditions

Other types of cardiac diseases that can contribute to the risk of thromboembolic stroke include dilated cardiomyopathy, valvular heart disease and intracardiac congenital defects. The incidence of stroke is inversely proportional to the cardiac ejection fraction. Patients with myocardial infarction who have an ejection fraction <29% have a relative risk of stroke of 1.86 as compared with patients who have an ejection fraction of >35%.[82]

Recommendations

In addition to atrial fibrillation, a variety of cardiac conditions have been associated with an increased risk of stroke. Various practice guidelines recommend strategies to reduce the risk of stroke in patients with a variety of cardiac conditions. These include the management of patients with valvular heart disease,[83] unstable angina,[84] chronic stable angina[85] and acute myocardial infarction.[86] Strategies to prevent postoperative neurological injury and stroke in patients undergoing surgical revascularization for atherosclerotic heart disease are discussed in detail in the recently published *Coronary bypass graft surgery guidelines.*[87] It is reasonable to prescribe warfarin to patients who have post-ST segment elevation MI with LV dysfunction and extensive regional wall-motion abnormalities (Class IIa; level of evidence A), and warfarin may be considered in patients with severe LV dysfunction, with or without congestive heart failure (Class IIb; level of evidence C).[88]

Dyslipidaemia

Three prospective studies in men have shown increases in ischaemic stroke rates at higher levels of total cholesterol, particularly for levels above 240–270 mg/dl.[89–91] The US Women's Pooling Project found a 25% increased risk of fatal ischaemic stroke for each 1 mmol/L increase in total cholesterol in women 30–54 years of age.[92] Therefore, there does appear to be a close relationship between dyslipidaemia and risk of ischaemic stroke in both men and women.

HMG-CoA reductase inhibitors (statins) have received regulatory approval for the prevention of ischaemic stroke in patients with coronary artery disease (CAD); the approval was based on consistent benefits in large randomized trials using these agents.[93,94]

Recommendations

The National Cholesterol Education Programme III Guidelines for the management of patients who have not had a cerebrovascular event and have elevated total cholesterol or non-HDL cholesterol in the presence of hypertriglyceridaemia are endorsed.[95,96] It is recommended that patients with known CAD and high-risk hypertensive patients, even with normal LDL cholesterol levels, be treated with lifestyle measures and a statin (Class I; level of evidence A). Suggested treatments for patients with known CAD and low HDL cholesterol include weight loss, increased physical activity, cessation of smoking, and possibly niacin or gemfibrozil (Class IIa; level of evidence B).

Asymptomatic carotid artery stenosis

It is recommended that patients with asymptomatic carotid artery stenosis be screened for other treatable causes of stroke and that intensive therapy of all identified stroke risk factors be pursued (Class I; level of evidence C). The use of aspirin is recommended unless contraindicated. Prophylactic carotid endarterectomy is recommended in highly selected patients with high-grade symptomatic carotid stenosis performed by surgeons with <3% morbidity/mortality rates (Class I; level of evidence A). Patient selection should be guided by an assessment of co-morbid conditions and life expectancy as well as other individual factors, balanced by an understanding of the overall impact of the procedure if all-cause mortality is considered as one of the end-points, and includes a thorough discussion of the risks and benefits of the procedure with an understanding of the patient's preferences. Carotid angioplasty–stenting might be a reasonable alternative to endarterectomy in asymptomatic patients at high risk for the surgical procedure (Class IIb; level of evidence B); however, given the reported periprocedural and overall one-year event rates, it remains uncertain whether this group of patients should have either procedure.

Diet and nutrition

In observational studies, diet has been shown to have an effect on stroke risk. A generally consistent body of evidence from prospective studies has documented that increased fruit and vegetable consumption is associated with a reduced risk of stroke in a dose–response fashion. In ecological[97] and some prospective studies,[98,99] a higher level of sodium intake is associated with an increased risk of stroke. A higher level of potassium intake is also associated with a reduced risk of stroke in prospective studies.[100,101] The potential effects of sodium and potassium on stroke risk appear to be at least partially mediated through blood pressure. However, there is a reasonable biological basis, and some empirical evidence from animal studies, which suggests that the effects of sodium and potassium on stroke are also mediated through mechanisms that are independent of blood pressure.[102]

Recommendations

A reduced intake of sodium and increased intake of potassium is recommended to lower blood pressure (Class I; level of evidence A), which may thereby reduce the risk of stroke. The recommended sodium intake is <2.3 g/day and that for potassium is >4.7 g/day. Diets rich in fruits and vegetables, including the Dietary Approaches to Stop Hypertension (DASH) diet, which emphasizes fruits, vegetables and low-fat dairy products and a reduction in saturated and total fat, also lowers blood pressure and is recommended (Class I; level of evidence A).

Physical inactivity

The beneficial effects of physical activity for stroke prevention have been documented.[103] The protective effect of physical activity may be partly mediated through its role in reducing blood pressure[103] and controlling other risk factors for cardiovascular disease,[104,105] diabetes[103] and increased body weight. Other biological mechanisms have also been associated with physical activity, including reductions in plasma fibrinogen and platelet activity, and elevations in plasma tissue plasminogen activator (TPA) activity and HDL concentration.[106–108] A sedentary lifestyle is associated with an increased risk of stroke. Guidelines endorsed by the Centers for Disease Control and Prevention (CDC) and the National Institutes of Health (NIH) recommend moderate exercise (at least 30 minutes) on most, and preferably all, days of the week.[109,110]

Recommendations

Increased physical activity is recommended because it is associated with a reduction in the risk of stroke (Class I; level of evidence B). Exercise guidelines recommended by the NIH of regular exercise (>30 minutes of activity of moderate intensity daily) as part of a healthy lifestyle are reasonable (Class IIa; level of evidence B).

Obesity and body fat distribution

The traditional classification of weight status is defined by body mass index (BMI: weight in kilograms divided by the square of the height in metres). Persons with a BMI of 25–29.9 kg/m^2 are classified as being overweight, and those with a BMI of >30 kg/m^2 are classified as being obese.[111] Abdominal obesity is commonly measured by either the waist-to-hip ratio or waist circumference. Clinically, abdominal obesity is defined by a waist circumference of >102 cm (40 inches) in men and 88 cm (35 inches) in women.[111]

Recommendations

There is enough evidence from large-scale prospective studies that increased weight is associated with an increased risk of stroke. Weight reduction is recommended because it lowers blood pressure (Class I; level of evidence A) and may thereby reduce the risk of stroke.

Metabolic syndrome

The National Cholesterol Education Programme Adult Treatment Panel III (ATP III) defined the metabolic syndrome as the presence of >3 of the following: (i) abdominal obesity as determined by waist circumference >102 cm or >40 inches for men and >88 cm or >35 inches for women; (ii) triglycerides >150 mg/dl; (iii) HDL cholesterol <40 mg/dl for men and <50 mg/dl for women; (iv) blood pressure >130/>85 mmHg; and (v) fasting glucose >110 mg/dl.[112] WHO modified the definition for epidemiological studies with the addition of hyperinsulinaemia.[113] Obesity and a sedentary lifestyle coupled with diet and other factors interact to produce the metabolic syndrome.

Recommendations

Management of individual components of the metabolic syndrome, including lifestyle measures and pharmacotherapy as recommended by the National Cholesterol Education Programme ATP III[112] and JNC 7,[51] are endorsed. Lifestyle management should include exercise, appropriate weight loss and proper diet. Pharmacotherapy may include medications to lower the blood pressure and lipid levels, achieve glycaemic control and treat microalbuminuria or proteinuria. Antiplatelet therapy (e.g. aspirin) is prescribed according to the individual circumstances and risk.

Alcohol abuse

Strong evidence indicates that alcoholism and heavy drinking are risk factors for all stroke subtypes. The majority of studies have suggested a J-shaped relationship between alcohol consumption and ischaemic stroke risk with a protective effect in light and moderate drinkers and an elevated risk with heavy alcohol consumption.[114,115] Light-to-moderate alcohol consumption can increase HDL cholesterol, reduce platelet aggregation and lower plasma fibrinogen concentration.[116] Heavy alcohol consumption can lead to hypertension, hyper-coagulability, reduced cerebral blood flow and a greater likelihood of atrial fibrillation.[117]

Recommendations

For those who consume alcohol, a recommendation of <2 drinks per day for men and <1 drink per day for non-pregnant women best reflects the state of science for alcohol and stroke risk. However, non-drinkers should not be encouraged to begin drinking, as it is well established that alcohol can induce dependence and that alcoholism is a major public health problem.

Oral contraceptive use

Some groups of women appear to be at higher risk for stroke associated with the use of oral contraceptives. Women who are >35 years of age, smoke cigarettes, have hypertension, diabetes, migraine, or have had prior thrombo-embolic events may be at increased risk for stroke if they use oral contraceptives.[118] The absolute increase in stroke risk with low-dose oral contraceptives is small.[119]

Recommendations

The incremental risk of stroke associated with the use of low-dose oral contraceptives in women without additional risk factors appears low (Class III; level of evidence B).[120] It is suggested that oral contraceptives be discouraged in women with additional risk factors (cigarette smoking or prior thromboembolic events) (Class III; level of evidence C).[121] For those who elect to assume the increased risk, aggressive therapy of stroke risk factors may be useful (Class IIb; level of evidence C).[121]

Sleep-disordered breathing

Epidemiological studies suggest that habitual snoring is a risk factor for ischaemic stroke and is independent of confounding factors such as hypertension, ischaemic heart disease, obesity and age.[122,123] Consistent with these observations, a case–control study of 181 patients found that excessive daytime sleepiness likely due to obstructive sleep apnoea was associated with stroke.[124] Snoring may be a marker for sleep-disordered breathing (SDB), which can secondarily increase stroke risk by leading to or worsening hypertension and heart disease, and possibly by causing a reduction in cerebral blood flow, altered cerebral autoregulation, impaired endothelial function, accelerated atherogenesis, hypercoagulability, inflammation and paradoxical embolism in patients with a patent foraman ovale (PFO).[125–127]

Treatment of SDB must be individualized and can include continuous positive airway pressure (CPAP) ventilation, bi-level positive airway pressure and automatic control of airway pressure delivery with CPAP devices. A variety of surgical interventions and prosthetic oral devices are available.

Recommendations

Questioning bed partners and patients, particularly those with abdominal obesity and hypertension, about symptoms of SDB and referral to a sleep specialist for further evaluation as appropriate may be reasonable, especially in the setting of drug-resistant hypertension (Class IIb; level of evidence C).

Migraine

Migraine headache has been most consistently associated with stroke in young women.[128] Specific data showing that migraine prophylaxis decreases stroke risk are lacking. No proven primary prevention strategies exist for patients with migraine and/or PFO.

Recommendations

There are insufficient data to recommend a specific treatment approach that would reduce the risk of first stroke in women with migraine, including migraine with aura.

Hyperhomocysteinaemia

Epidemiological and prospective studies show a positive relationship between blood homocysteine levels and stroke risk. Prospective trials designed to determine whether pharmacological lowering of total homocysteine reduces the risk of first stroke are needed.

Recommendations

Recommendations to meet the current guidelines for daily intake of folate (400 g/day), B_6 (1.7 mg/day), and B_{12} (2.4 mg/day) by consumption of vegetables, fruits, legumes, meats, fish, and fortified grains and cereals may be useful for reducing the risk of stroke (Class IIb; level of evidence C). There are insufficient data to recommend a specific treatment approach that would reduce the risk of first stroke in patients with elevated homocysteine levels. In the interim, use of folic acid and B vitamins in patients with known elevated homocysteine levels may be useful, given their safety and low cost (Class IIb; level of evidence C).

References

1. Poungvarin N. Stroke in the developing countries. *Lancet* 1998;**352**:(SIII) 19–22.
2. Das SK, Banerjee TK, Biswas A, *et al.* A prospective community-based study of stroke in Kolkata, India. *Stroke* 2007;**38**:906–10.
3. Feigin VL, Lawes CM, Bennet DA, *et al.* Stroke epidemiology: A review of population-based studies of incidence, prevalence, and case fatality in the late 20th century. *Lancet Neurol* 2003;**2**:43–53.
4. Abraham J, Rao PSS, Imbraj SG, *et al.* An epidemiological study of hemiplegia due to stroke in South India. *Stroke* 1970;**1**:477–81.
5. Anand K, Chowdhury D, Singh KB, *et al.* Estimation of mortality and morbidity due to strokes in India. *Neuroepidemiology* 2001;**20**:208–11.
6. Garraway WM, Whisnant JP, Drury I. The continuing decline in the incidence of stroke. *Mayo Clin Proc* 1983;**58**:520–3.
7. Bonita R, Beaglehole R. The enigma of the decline in stroke deaths in the United States—the search for an explanation. *Stroke* 1996;**27**:370–2.
8. Kaul S, Sunitha P, Suvarna A, *et al.* Subtypes of ischaemic stroke in Hyderabad (South India): Data from a hospital-based stroke registry. *Neurol India* 2002;**50**:S8–S14.
9. Dalal PM. Burden of stroke: Indian perspective. *International Journal of Stroke* 2006;**1**:164–6.
10. Goldstein LB, Adams R, Alberts JM, *et al.* Primary prevention of ischemic stroke: A guideline from the American Heart Association/American Stroke Association Stroke Council: Co-sponsored by the Atherosclerotic Peripheral Vascular Disease Interdisciplinary Working Group; Cardiovascular Nursing Council: Clinical Cardiology Council; Nutrition, Physical Activity, and Metabolism Council; and the Quality of Care and Outcomes Research Interdisciplinary Working Group. *Circulation* 2006;**113**:e873–e923.
11. Dalal PM, Dalal KP, Rao SP, *et al.* Strokes in west–central India: A prospective case–control study of 'risk factors' (a problem of developing countries). In: Bartko B (ed). *Neurology in Europe*. London: John Libbey and Co.; 1989:16–20.
12. WHO Task Force on Stroke and other Cerebrovascular disorders: Recommendations on stroke prevention, diagnosis and therapy. *Stroke* 1989;**20**: 1407–31.
13. Reddy KS, Yousuf S. Emerging epidemic of cardiovascular disease in developing countries. *Circulation* 1998;**97**:596–601.
14. Brown RD, Whisnant JP, Sicks JD, *et al.* Stroke incidence, prevalence and survival: Secular trends in Rochester, Minnesota through 1989. *Stroke* 1996;**27**: 373–80.
15. Wolf PA, D'Agostino RB, O'Neal MA, *et al.* Secular trends in stroke incidence and mortality: The Framingham Study. *Stroke* 1992;**23**:1551–5.
16. Sacco RL, Boden-Albala B, Gan R, *et al.* Stroke incidence among white, black and Hispanic residents of an urban community: The Northern Manhattan Stroke Study. *Am J Epidemiol* 1998;**147**:259–68.
17. Kittner SJ, Stern BJ, Feeser BR, *et al.* Pregnancy and the risk of stroke. *N Engl J Med* 1996;**332**:768–74.
18. Qureshi AI, Giles WH, Croft JB, *et al.* Number of pregnancies and risk for stroke and stroke subtypes. *Arch Neurol* 1997;**54**:203–6.
19. Mosca L, Manson JE, Sutherland SE, *et al.* Cardiovascular disease in women: A statement for healthcare professionals from the American Heart Association. *Circulation* 1997;**96**:2468–82.
20. Welin L, Svardsudd K, Larsson B, *et al.* Analysis of

risk factors for stroke in a cohort of men born in 1913. *N Engl J Med* 1987;**317**:521–6.

21. Kiely DK, Wolf PA, Cupples LA, *et al.* Familial aggregation of stroke: The Framingham Study. *Stroke* 1993;**24**:1366–71.

22. Liao D, Myers R, Hunt S, *et al.* Familial history of stroke and stroke risk: The Family Heart Study. *Stroke* 1997;**28**:1908–12.

23. Brass LM, Isaacsohn JL, Merikangas KR, *et al.* A study of twins and stroke. *Stroke* 1992;**23**:221–3.

24. Rubattu S, Stanzione R, Gigante B, *et al.* Genetic susceptibility to cerebrovascular accidents. *J Cardiovasc Pharmacol* 2001;**38** (Suppl 2):S71–S75.

25. Nicolaou M, DeStefano AL, Gavras I, *et al.* Genetic predisposition to stroke in relatives of hypertensive patients. *Stroke* 2003;**31**:487–92.

26. Tuner ST, Boerwinke E. Genetics of blood pressure, hypertensive complications, and antihypertensive drug responses. *Pharmacogenomics* 2003;**4**:53–65.

27. Hasan A, Hunt BJ, O'Sullivan M, *et al.* Homocysteine is a risk factor for cerebral small vessel disease, acting via endothelial dysfunction. *Brain* 2004;**127** (pt 1):212–19.

28. Scott CH, Sutton MS. Homocysteine: Evidence for a causal relationship with cardiovascular disease. *Cardiol Rev* 1997;**7**:101–7.

29. Fodinger M, Horl WH, Sunder-Plassmann G. Molecular biology of 5,10-methylenetetrahydrofolate reductase. *J Nephrol* 2000;**13**:20–33.

30. Ortel TL. Genetics of coagulation disorders. In: Alberts MJ (ed). Genetics of cerebrovascular disease. Armonk, NY: Futura Publishing; 1999:129–56.

31. De Lucia D, Renis V, Belli A, *et al.* Familial coagulation-inhibiting and fibrinolytic protein deficiencies in juvenile transient ischemic attacks. *J Neurosurg Sci* 1996;**40**:25–35.

32. Bertina RM, Koeleman BP, Koster T, *et al.* Mutation in blood coagulation factor V associated with resistance to activated protein C. *Nature* 1994;**369**:64–7.

33. Ridker PM, Hennekens CH, Lindpaintner K, *et al.* Mutation in the gene coding for coagulation factor V and the risk of myocardial infarction, stroke, and venous thrombosis in apparently healthy men. *N Engl J Med* 1995;**332**:912–17.

34. Hillier CE, Collins PW, Bowen DJ, *et al.* Inherited prothrombotic risk factors and cerebral venous thrombosis. *QJM* 1998;**91**:677–80.

35. Kuwahara S, Abe T, Uga S, *et al.* Superior sagittal sinus and cerebral cortical venous thrombosis caused by congenital protein C deficiency: Case report. *Neurol Med Chir* 2000;**40**:645–9.

36. Deschiens MA, Conard J, Horellou MH, *et al.* Coagulation studies, factor V Leiden, and anticardiolipin antibodies in 40 cases of cerebral venous thrombosis. *Stroke* 1996;**27**:1724–30.

37. Weber M, Hayem G, DeBandt M, *et al.* The family history of patients with primary or secondary antiphospholipid syndrome (APS). *Lupus* 2000;**9**:258–63.

38. Goldberg SN, Conti-Kelly AM, Greco TP. A family study of anticardiolipin antibodies and associated clinical conditions. *Am J Med* 1995;**99**:473–9.

39. Begelman SM, Olin JW. Fibromuscular dysplasias. *Curr Opin Rheumatol* 2000;**12**:41–7.

40. Shetty-Alva N, Alva S. Familial moyamoya disease in Caucasians. *Pediatr Neurol* 2000;**23**:445–7.

41. Gretarsdottir S, Thorleifsson G, Reynisdottir ST, *et al.* The gene encoding phosphodiesterase 4D confers risk of ischemic stroke [published correction appears in *Na Genet* 2005;**37**:555]. *Nat Genet* 2003:**35**:131–8.

42. Helgadottir A, Manolescu A, Thorleifsson G, *et al.* The gene encoding 5-lipoxygenase activating protein confers risk of myocardial infarction and stroke. *Nat Genet* 2004;**36**:233–9.

43. Tournier-Lasserve E, Joutel A, Chabriat H. Clinical phenotypes and genetic data in 15 unrelated families. *Neurology* 1995;**45**(Suppl 4):A273.

44. Kalimo H, Vitanen M, Amerla K, *et al.* CADASIL: Hereditary disease of arteries causing brain infarcts and dementia. *Neuropathol Appl Neurobiol* 1999;**25**:257–65.

45. Forteza AM, Brozman B, Rabinstein AA, *et al.* Acetazolamide for the treatment of migraine with aura in CADASIL. *Neurol* 2001;**57**:2144–5.

46. Durlach J. A possible advance in arterial gene therapy for aortic complications in the Marfan syndrome by local transfer of an antisense Mg-dependent hammerhead ribozyme. *Magnes Res* 2001;**14**:64–7.

47. D'Agnostino RB, Wolf PA, Belanger AJ, *et al.* Stroke risk profile: Adjustment for antihypertensive medication. The Framingham Study. *Stroke* 1994;**25**:40–3.

48. Fields LE, Burt VL, Cutler JA, *et al.* The burden of adult hypertension in the United States 1999 to 2000: A rising tide. *Hypertension* 2004;**44**:398–404.

49. Wolf PA. Cerebrovascular risk. In: Izzo JLJ, Black HR (eds). *Hypertension primer: The essentials of high*

blood pressure. Baltimore, MD: Lippincott, Williams and Wilkins; 1999:239.

50. Lewington S, Clarke R, Qizilbash N, *et al.* Age-specific relevance of usual blood pressure to vascular mortality: A meta-analysis of individual data for one million adults in 61 prospective studies [published correction appears in *Lancet* 2003;**361**:1060]. *Lancet* 2002;**360**:1903–13.

51. Chobania AV, Bakris GL, Black HR, *et al.* National Heart Lung, and Blood Institute Joint National Committee on Prevention, Detection, Evaluation, and Treatment of High Blood Pressure: National High Blood Pressure Education Program Coordinating Committee. The Seventh Report of the Joint National Committee on Prevention, Detection, Evaluation, and Treatment of High blood Pressure: The JNC 7 report [published correction appears in *JAMA* 2003;**290**:197]. *JAMA* 2003;**289**:2560–72.

52. Psaty BM, Smith NL, Siscovick DS, *et al.* Health outcomes associated with antihypertensive therapies used as first-line agents. A systematic review and meta-analysis. *JAMA* 1997;**277**:739–45.

53. Neal B, McMahon S, Chapman N. Blood Pressure Lowering Treatment Trialists' Collaboration. Effects of ACE inhibitors, calcium antagonists, and other blood-pressure-lowering drugs: Results of prospectively designed overviews of Randomized Trialists' Collaboration. *Lancet* 2000;**356**:1955–64.

54. ALLHAT Officers and Coordinators for the ALLHAT Collaborative Research Group. Major outcomes in high-risk hypertensive patients randomized to angiotensin-converting enzyme inhibitor or calcium channel blocker *vs* diuretic: The Antihypertensive and Lipid-Lowering Treatment to Prevent Heart Attack Trial (ALLHAT) [published corrections appear in JAMA 2003;**289**:178 and *JAMA* 2004;**18**:2196] *JAMA* 2003;**288**:2981–97.

55. Turnbull F. Blood Pressure Lowering Treatment Trialists' Collaboration. Effects of different blood-pressure-lowering regimens on major cardiovascular events: Results of prospectively-designed overviews of randomized trials. *Lancet* 2003;**362**:1527–35.

56. Black HR, Elliott WJ, Neaton JD, *et al.* Baseline characteristics and early blood pressure control in the CONVINCE Trial. *Hypertension* 2001;**37**:12–18.

57. Cushman WC, Ford CE, Cutler JA, *et al.* Success and predictors of blood pressure control in diverse North American settings: The antihypertensive and lipid-lowering treatment to prevent heart attack trial (ALLHAT). *J Clin Hypertension* 2002;**4**:393–404.

58. Staessen JA, Fagard R, Thijs L, *et al.* Randomized double-blind comparison of placebo and active treatment for older patients with isolated systolic hypertension: The Systolic Hypertension in Europe (Syst-Eur) Trial Investigators. *Lancet* 1997;**350**:757–64.

59. SHEP Cooperative Research Group. Prevention of stroke by antihypertensive drug treatment in older persons with isolated systolic hypertension: Final results of the Systolic Hypertension in the Elderly Program (SHEP). *JAMA* 1991;**265**:3255–64.

60. Kurth T, Kase CS, Berger K, *et al.* Smoking and risk of hemorrhagic stroke in women. *Stroke* 2003;**34**:2792–5.

61. Broderick JP, Viscoli CM, Brott T, *et al.* Stroke Project Investigators. Major risk factors for aneurysmal subarachnoid hemorrhage in the young are modifiable. *Stroke* 2003;**34**:1375–81.

62. The Centers for Disease Control. The Surgeon General's 1989 Report on reducing the health consequences of smoking: 25 years of progress. *MMWR Morb Mortal Wkly Rep* 1989;**38** (Suppl 2):1–32.

63. Bonita R, Duncan J, Truelsen T, *et al.* Passive smoking as well as active smoking increase the risk of acute stroke. *Tob Control* 1999;**8**:156–60.

64. You RX, Thrift AG, Mc Neil JJ, *et al.* Ischemic stroke risk and passive exposure to spouses' cigarette smoking. Melbourne Stroke Risk Factor Study (MERS) Group. *Am J Public Health* 1999;**89**:572–5.

65. Karttunen V, Alfthan G, Hiltunen L, *et al.* Risk factors for cryptogenic ischemic stroke. *Eur J Neurol* 2002;**9**:625–32.

66. US Preventive Services Task Force. *Guide to clinical preventive services.* 2nd ed. Baltimore, MD: Williams and Wilkins; 1996.

67. Effect of ramipril on cardiovascular and microvascular outcomes in people with diabetes mellitus: Results of the HOPE study and MICRO-HOPE substudy. Heart Outcomes Prevention Evaluation Study Investigators [published correction appears in *JAMA* 1997;**277**:1356]. *JAMA* 1996;**276**:1886–92.

68. Collins R, Armitage J, Parish S, *et al.* Heart Protection Collaborative Group. MRC/BHF Heart Protection Study of cholesterol lowering with simvastatin in 5963 people with diabetes: A randomized placebo-controlled trial. *Lancet* 2003;**61**:2005–16.

69. Colhoun HM, Betteridge DJ, Durrington PN, *et al.*

CARDS investigators. Primary prevention of cardio-vascular disease with atorvastatin in type2 diabetes in the Collaborative Atorvastatin Diabetes Study (CARDS): Multicentre randomized placebo-controlled trial. *Lancet* 2004;**364**:685–96.

70. Wolf PA, Abbott RD, Kannel WB. Atrial fibrillation as an independent risk factor for stroke: The Framingham Study. *Stroke* 1991;**22**:983–8.

71. Go AS, Hylek EM, Chang Y, *et al*. Anticoagulation therapy for stroke prevention in atrial fibrillation: How well do randomized trials translate into clinical practice? *JAMA* 2003;**290**:2685–92.

72. van Walraven C, Hart RG, Singer DE, *et al*. Oral anticoagulants vs aspirin in nonvalvular atrial fibrillation: An individual patient meta-analysis. *JAMA* 2002;**288**:2441–8.

73. Hart RG, Benavente O, McBride R, *et al*. Antithrombotic therapy to prevent stroke in patients with atrial fibrillation: A meta-analysis. *Ann Intern Med* 1999;**131**:492–501.

74. Gage BF, van Walraven C, Pearce L, *et al*. Validation of clinical classification schemes for predicting stroke: Results from the National Registry of Atrial Fibrillation. *JAMA* 2001;**285**:2864–70.

75. Hart RG, Halperin JL, Pearce LA, *et al*. Stroke prevention in Atrial Fibrillation Investigators. Lessons from the Stroke Prevention in Atrial Fibrillation Trials. *Ann Intern Med* 2003;**138**:831–8.

76. van Walraven C, Hart RG, Wells GA, *et al*. A clinical prediction rule to identify patients with atrial fibrillation and a low risk for stroke while taking aspirin. *Arch Intern Med* 2003;**163**:936–43.

77. Patients with nonvalvular atrial fibrillation at low risk of stroke during treatment with aspirin: Stroke Prevention in Atrial Fibrillation III Study. The SPAF III Writing Committee for the Stroke Prevention in Atrial Fibrillation Investigators. *JAMA* 1998;**279**:1273–7.

78. Fuster V, Ryde LE, Asinger RW, *et al*. American Collge of Cardiology/American Heart Association/European Society of Cardiology Board ACC/AHA/ESSC guidelines for the management of patients with atrial fibrillation: Executive American College of Cardiology/American Heart Association Task Force on Practice Guidelines and the European Society of Cardiology Committee for Practice Guidelines and Policy Conferences (Committee to Develop Guidelines for the Management of Patients With Atrial Fibrillation): Developed in collaboration with the North American Society of Pacing and Electrophysiology. *J Am Coll Cardiol* 2001;**38**:1231–66.

79. Hart RG. Warfarin in atrial fibrillation: Underused in the elderly, often inappropriately used in the young. *Heart* 1999;**82**:539–40.

80. Bonow RO, Carabello B, de Leon AC Jr, *et al*. ACC/AHA guidelines for the management of patients with valvular heart disease: A report of the American College of Cardiology/American Heart Association Task Force on Practice Guidelines (Committee on Management of Patient with Valvular Heart Disease). *J Am Coll Cardiol* 1998;**32**: 1486–588.

81. Bleeding during antithrombotic therapy in patients with atrial fibrillation. The Stroke Prevention in Atrial Fibrillation Investigators. *Arch Intern Med* 1996;**156**:409–16.

82. Loh E, Sutton MS, Wun CC, *et al*. Ventricular dysfunction and the risk of stroke after myocardial infarction. *N Engl J Med* 1996;**335**:251–7.

83. Cannegieter SC, Rosendaal FR, Briet E. Thrombo-embolic and bleeding complications in patients with mechanical heart valve prostheses. *Circulation* 1994;**89**:635–41.

84. Braunwald E, Antaman EM, Beasley JW, *et al*. American College of Cardiology/American Heart Association Task Force on Practice Guidelines (Committee on the Management of Patients With Unstable Angina). ACC/AHA 2002 guideline update for the management of patients with unstable angina and non-ST-segment elevation myocardial infarction: A report of the American College of Cardiology/American Heart Association Task Force on Practice Guidelines (Committee on the Management of Patients with Unstable Angina). *Circulation* 2002;**106**:1893–1900.

85. Gibbons RJ, Abrams J, Chatterjee K, *et al*. American College of Cardiology; American Heart Association Task Force on Practice Guidelines. Committee on the Management of Patients with Chronic Stable Angina. ACC/AHA guidelines for the management of patients with chronic stable angina: A report of the American College of Cardiology/American Heart Association Task Force on Practice Guidelines (Committee to Update the 1999 Guidelines for the Management of patients with Chronic Stable Angina). *Circulation* 2003;**107**:149–58.

86. Antman EM, Abe DT, Armstrong PW, *et al*. ACC/AHA 2004 guideline update for the manage-ment of patients with ST-elevation myocardial infarction: A report of the American College of

Cardiology/American Heart Association Task Force on Practice Guidelines (Committee to Revise the 1999 Guidelines for the Management of patients with acute myocardial infarction). *J Am Coll Cardiol* 2004;**44**:E1–E211.

87. Eagle KA, Guyton RA, Davidoff R, *et al*. ACC/AHA 2004 guideline update for coronary artery bypass graft surgery: A report of the American College of Cardiology/American Heart Association Task Force on Practice Artery Bypass Graft Surgery. *Circulation* 2004;**110**:e340–e347.

88. Antman EM, Anbe DT, Armstrong PW, *et al*. American College of Cardiology; American Heart Association Task Force Practice Guidelines; Canadian Cardiovascular Society. ACC/AHA guidelines for the management of patients with ST-elevation myocardial infarction: A report of the American College of Cardiology/American Heart Association Task Force on Practice Guidelines (Committee to Revise the 1999 guidelines for the Management of Patients with Acute Myocardial Infarction) [published correction appears in *Circulation* 2005; **111**:2013–4]. *Circulation* 2004;**110**: e82–e292.

89. Iso H, Jacobs DR Jr, Wentworth D, *et al*. Serum cholesterol levels and six-year mortality from stroke in 350,977 men screened for the multiple risk factor intervention trial. *N Engl J Med* 1989;**320**:904–10.

90. Kagan A, Popper JS, Rhoads GG. Factors related to stroke incidence in Hawaii Japanese men. The Honolulu Heart Study. *Stroke* 1980;**11**:14–21.

91. Leepala JM, Virtama J, Fofelholm R, *et al*. Different risk factors for different stroke subtypes: Association of blood pressure, cholesterol, and antioxidants. *Stroke* 1999;**30**:2535–40.

92. Horenstein RB, Smith DE, Mosca L. Cholesterol predicts stroke mortality in the Women's Pooling Project. *Stroke* 2002;**33**:1863–8.

93. Crouse JR III, Byington RP, Bond MG, *et al*. Pravastatin, Lipids, and Atherosclerosis in the Carotid Arteries (PLAC-II). *Am J Cardiol* 1995;**75**: 455–9.

94. Sacks FM, Pfeffer MA, Moye LA, *et al*. The effect of pravastatin on coronary events after myocardial infarction in patients with average cholesterol levels. Cholesterol and Recurrent Event Trial investigators. *N Engl J Med* 1996;**335**:1001–9.

95. National Institutes of Health. Adult Treatment Panel III: Detection, Evaluation, and Treatment of High Blood Cholesterol in Adults. Bethesda, MD: National Institutes of Health; 2002.

96. Grundy SM, Cleeman JI, Merz CN, *et al*. Coordinating Committee of the National Cholesterol Education Program. Implications of recent clinical trials for the National Cholesterol Education Program Adult Treatment Panel III guidelines. *Arterioscler Thromb Vasc Biol* 2004;**24**:e149–e161.

97. Perry IJ, Beevers DG. Salt intake and stroke: A possible direct effect. *J Hum Hypertens* 1992;**6**:23–5.

98. He J, Ogden LG, Vupputuri S, *et al*. Dietary sodium intake and subsequent risk of cardiovascular disease in overweight adults. *JAMA* 1999;**282**:2027–34.

99. Nagata C, Takatsuka N, Shimuzu N, *et al*. Sodium intake and risk of death from stroke in Japanese men and women. *Stroke* 2004;**35**:1543–7.

100. Khaw KT, Barrett-Connor E. Dietary potassium and stroke-associated mortality. A 12-year prospective population study. *N Engl J Med* 1987;**316**:235–40.

101. Ascherio A, Rimm EB, Herna MA, *et al*. Intake of potassium magnesium, calcium and fiber and risk of stroke among US men. *Circulation* 1998;**98**:1198–204.

102. Tobian L, Lange JM, Ulm KM, *et al*. Potassium prevents death from strokes in hypertensive rats without lowering blood pressure. *J Hypertens* 1984; **2**(Suppl):S363–S366.

103. Manson JE, Colditz GA, Stampfer MJ, *et al*. A prospective study of maturity-onset diabetes mellitus and risk of coronary heart disease and stroke in women. *Arch Intern Med* 1991;**151**:1141–7.

104. Blair SN, Kampert JB, Kohl HW 3rd, *et al*. Influences of cardiorespiratory fitness and other precursors on cardiovascular disease and all-cause mortality in men and women. *JAMA* 1996;**276**:205–10.

105. Kokkinos PF, Holland JC, Pittaras AE, *et al*. Cardiorespiratory fitness and coronary heart disease risk factor association in women. *J Am Coll Cardiol* 1995;**26**:358–64.

106. LakkaTA, Salonen JT. Moderate to high intensity conditioning leisure time physical activity and high cardiorespiratory fitness are associated with reduced plasma fibrinogen in eastern Finnish Men. *J Clin Epidemiol* 1993;**46**:1119–27.

107. Williams PT. High-density lipoprotein cholesterol and other risk factors for coronary heart disease in female runners. *N Engl J Med* 1996;**334**:1298–303.

108. Wang HY, Bashore TR, Friedman E. Exercise reduces age-dependent decrease in platelet protein kinase C activity and translocation. *J Gerontol A Biol Sci Med Sci* 1995;**50A**:M12–M16.

109. NIH develops consensus statement on the role of physical activity for cardiovascular health. *Am Fam*

Physician 1996;**54:**763–64, 67.

110. Pate RR, Pratt M, Blair SN, *et al.* Physical activity and public health: A recommendation from the Centers for Disease Control and Prevention and the American College of Sports Medicine. *JAMA* 1995;**273:**402–7.

111. Novak K. NIH increase efforts to tackle obesity. *Nat Med* 1998:**4:**752–3.

112. Executive Summary of the Third Report of the National Cholesterol Education, and Treatment of High Blood Cholesterol in Adult (Adult Treatment Panel III). *JAMA* 2001;**285:**2486–7.

113. Lakka HM, Laaksonen DE, Lakka TA, *et al.* The metabolic syndrome and total and cardiovascular disease mortality in middle-age men. *JAMA* 2002;**288:**2709–16.

114. Hillbom M, Numminen H, Juvela S. Recent heavy drinking of alcohol and embolic stroke. *Stroke* 1999;**30:**2307–12.

115. Gill JS, Zezulka AV, Shipley MJ, *et al.* Stroke and alcohol consumption. *N Engl J Med* 1986;**315:**1041–6.

116. Gazino JM, Buring JE, Breslow JL, *et al.* Moderate alcohol intake, increased levels of high-density lipoprotein and its subfractions, and decreased risk of myocardial infarction. *N Engl J Med* 1993;**329:**1829–34.

117. Djousse L, Levy D, Benjamin EJ, *et al.* Long-term alcohol consumption and the risk of atrial fibrillation in the Framingham study. *Am J Cardiol* 2004;**93:**710–13.

118. Lidegaard O. Oral contraceptives, pregnancy and the risk of cerebral thromboembolism: The influence of diabetes, hypertension, migraine and previous thrombotic disease. *Br J Obstet Gynaecol* 1995;**102:**153–9.

119. Guillum LA, Mamidipudi SK, Johnston SC. Ischemic stroke risk with oral contraceptives: A meta-analysis. *JAMA* 2000;**284:**72–8.

120. Siritho S, Thrift AG, Mc Neil JJ, *et al.* Melbourne Risk Factor Study (MERFS) Group. Risk of ischemic stroke among users of the oral contraceptive pill: The Melbourne Risk Factor Study (MERFS) Group. *Stroke* 2003;**34:**1575–80.

121. Bousser MG, Conard J, Kittner S, *et al.* Recommendations on the risk of ischemic stroke associated with use of combined oral contraceptives and hormone replacement therapy in women with migraine. The International Headache Society Task Force on Combined Oral Contraceptives and Hormone Replacement Therapy. *Cephalalgia* 2000;**20:**155–6.

122. Partinen M, Palomaki H. Snoring and cerebral infarction. *Lancet* 1985;**2:**1325–6.

123. Palomaki H, Partinen M, Erkinjuntti T, *et al.* Snoring sleep apnea syndrome, and stroke. *Neurology* 1992;**42** (7 Suppl 6):75–81, discussion 82.

124. Davies DP, Rodgers H, Walshaw D, *et al.* Snoring daytime sleepiness and stroke: A case–control study of first-ever stroke. *J Sleep Res* 2003;**12:**313–18.

125. Culebras A. Cerebrovascular disease and sleep. *Curr Neurol Neurosci Rep* 2004;**4:**164–9.

126. Yaggi H, Mohsenin V. Sleep-disordered breathing and stroke. *Clin Chest Med* 2003;**24:**223–37.

127. Hermann DM, Bassetti CL. Sleep-disordered breathing and stroke. *Curr Opin Neurol* 2003;**16:**87–90.

128. Oral contraceptives and stroke in young women: Associated risk factors. *JAMA* 1975;**231:**718–22.

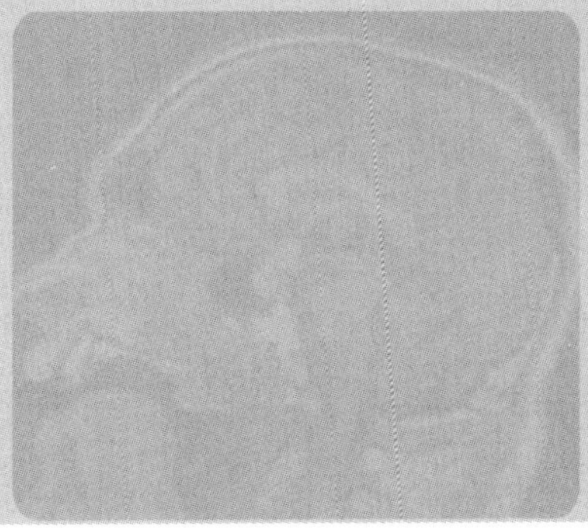

Neuroinfections

4

Neurocysticercosis: Trends in management
A continuing debate in the past decade

KAMALESH DAS, KALYAN B. BHATTACHARYYA

Introduction

Neurocysticercosis is an endemic disease and a major cause of acquired seizure disorder in developing countries, including India and the Latin American countries.[1] Massive immigration of people from endemic to non-endemic areas has recently produced an increase in the prevalence of neurocysticercosis in the North American and some European countries, where this disease was rare earlier.[2] Neurocysticercosis causes more than 50,000 deaths every year globally. Fifty million patients are affected globally and while many survive the disease, they are left with irreversible brain damage.[3] Some common clinical manifestations of neurocysticercosis are seizure disorder with a tendency towards recurrent attacks, encephalopathy (with headache, vomiting, convulsions and altered sensorium), meningitis and hydrocephalus. Worldwide, seizures have been observed in 70%–90% of patients with neurocysticercosis.[4] Neurocysticercosis is a major public health problem in developing countries as most of the affected people are in the productive age group.

The parasite

Taenia solium is a two-host zoonotic cestode. The adult stage is a 2–4 metre-long tapeworm that lives in the small intestine of humans. *Taenia solium* is not known to have any other final host in nature. The gravid proglottids at the terminal end of the worm contain eggs. The eggs and the larvae can cause cysticercosis.

The natural intermediate host is the pig, which harbours the larval cysts in its body. Humans beings become infected with the cyst either by consuming undercooked pork, or by the accidental ingestion of *T. solium* eggs through the faecal–oral route.

Aetiopathogenesis

Cysticercosis, including neurocysticercosis, occurs when human beings become the intermediate hosts in the life cycle of *T. solium* by ingesting its eggs with contaminated food or water (i.e. faecal–oral route of transmission), or by eating pork that is undercooked.

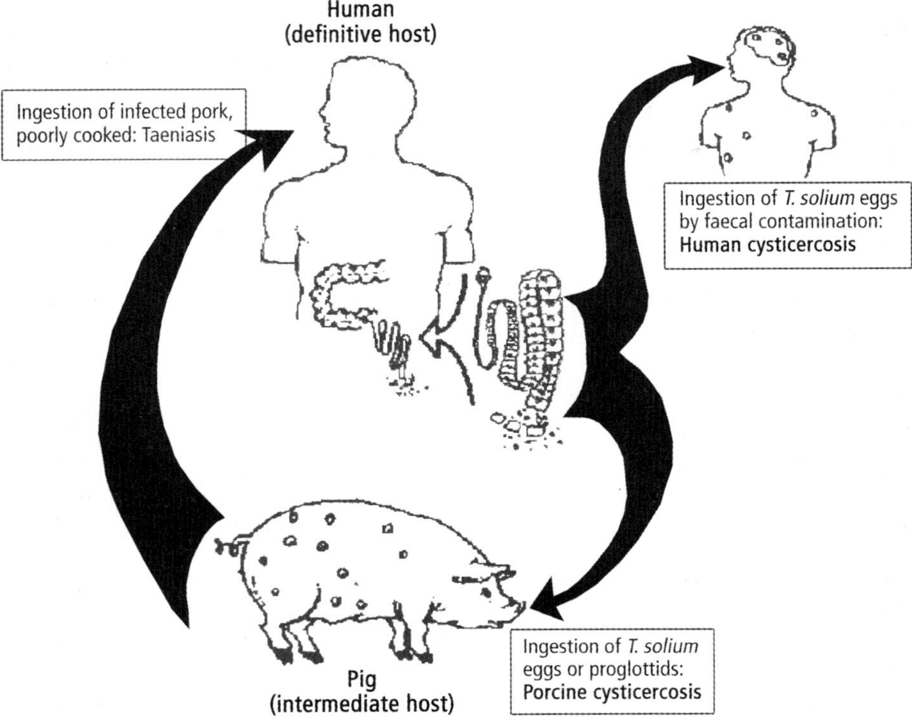

Fig. 1. Life cycle of *T. solium* (reproduced from *Clinical Microbiology Review* 2002;15(4)

On reaching the intestine, the eggs hatch into oncospheres, which can cross the intestinal wall to enter the blood circulation. They are then carried into the tissues, where the larvae (cysticerci) develop. Any organ in the host may be affected, but the main target organs are the skeletal muscles and the nervous system. In the nervous system, cysticerci may lodge in the brain parenchyma, subarachnoid space, ventricular system and spinal cord. Cysticerci are vesicle-like structures with two main parts—the vesicular wall and the scolex. The structure of the scolex is similar to that of the adult *T. solium*. It includes a rostellum armed with suckers and hooks.

The physical appearance of cysticerci varies according to their location in the nervous system. Brain parenchymal cysts, which lodge in the cerebral cortex or basal ganglia due to the abundance of blood supply in these areas, usually measure <20 mm. Subarachnoid cysticerci are usually located within the cortical sulci or in the cerebrospinal fluid (CSF) cisterns at the base of the brain. Cysticerci located at the cortical surface of the brain are small, but those within the CSF cisterns may attain a size of 50 mm or more. In the racemose form, the scolices cannot be identified as they are composed of several membranes that are attached to each other. Ventricular cysts may be small or large and may have no scolex. These cysts may be freely floating within the ventricular cavities or may be attached to the choroid plexus.

After entering the nervous system, the cysticerci elicit an inflammatory reaction in the surrounding areas. At this stage (vesicular stage), the parasites have a clear vesicular fluid and a normal scolex. The cysticerci may remain viable for years or may be attacked by complex immunological processes of the host and undergo degeneration, ending in death. The first stage of involution is the colloidal stage, in which the vesicular fluid becomes turbid and the scolex shows signs of degeneration. Colloidal cysticerci are surrounded by a thick collagen capsule, and the surrounding brain parenchyma shows astrocytic gliosis and diffuse oedema. Ultimately, the wall of the cyst thickens and the scolex is transformed into coarse, mineralized granules. This stage is called the granular stage. The next stage is the calcified stage, in which the remnants of the parasite appear as a mineralized nodule. During the granular and calcified stage, the oedema subsides, but the astrocytic changes surrounding the lesions become more intense than during the preceding stages.

Meningeal cysticerci may cause intense inflammation in the subarachnoid space, with the formation of dense exudates consisting of collagen fibres, lymphocytes, multinuclear giant cells and hyalinized parasitic membrane, leading to leptomeningeal thickening. The optic nerve and other cranial nerves may be encased in these exudates. The outlet channels of the ventricular system, i.e. the foramen of Luschka and the foramen of Magendie, may be occluded by the thickened leptomeninges. This subsequently leads to the development of hydrocephalus. The inflammatory reaction may affect small arteries of the brain, causing occlusion of the lumen of the vessels and cerebral infarctions.

Ventricular cysts may elicit an inflammatory reaction. If they are attached to the choroid plexus or the ventricular wall, the ependymal lining is disturbed and the ependymal cells are replaced by subependymal glial cells. The latter protrude towards the ventricular cavities and block the transit of CSF, particularly at the foramina of Monro or cerebral aqueduct, causing hydrocephalus.

Clinical manifestations

The clinical presentation of neurocysticercosis is highly variable due to individual differences in the number and location of lesions. Seizure disorder is the most common clinical manifestation, occurring in 70%–90% of patients.[4,5] Seizures are most often generalized tonic–clonic, simple partial or partial with secondary generalization. Some patients may present with complex partial seizures.

Focal neurological deficits related to the number and location of lesions have been observed in patients with neurocysticercosis. Focal deficits or signs usually follow a subacute or chronic course which resembles that taken by a brain tumour. Some patients may present with acute symptoms caused by cerebrovascular events following occlusion of the vascular lumen and the attendant immunological process. Intracranial hypertension has been observed in some cases of neurocysticercosis. This may be associated with seizures, dementia, focal signs, headache, vomiting and hydrocephalus due to basal arachnoiditis.

Intracranial hypertension may also occur in patients with giant cysts and in those with cysticercotic encephalitis. Cysticercotic encephalitis, which is mostly due to infection with a large number of cysticerci and the host's poor immune response, is the most important and gravest manifestation of neurocysticercosis. The leakage of toxic material from the cysticerci sets off an immune reaction which results in inflammation of the brain parenchyma. The usual symptoms of encephalopathy are headache, vomiting and altered sensorium, with seizures.

Patients with intrasellar cysticerci may present with opthalmological and endocrine disturbances, resembling those caused by a pituitary adenoma. Patients with spinal cord cysticercosis usually present with root pain or motor and sensory deficit, which vary according to the level of the lesion. Transverse myelopathy is a common clinical presentation of spinal cord cysticercosis. Patients with ocular cysticercosis usually present with decreased visual acuity, defects in the visual field and raised intraocular tension. A large number of cysticercal infections in the striated muscles may cause generalized weakness, associated with progressive muscle enlargement.

Diagnosis

As can be gleaned from the above discussion, neurocysticercosis has diverse clinical presentations. In fact, some infections are asymptomatic. The diagnosis of neurocysticercosis is, therefore, often difficult and challenging. In the case of hospitalized patients undergoing sophisticated diagnostic tests, diagnostic confusion may occur because of the lack of specificity of some neuroimaging abnormalities, as well as the number of false-positive and false-negative results yielded by the most commonly used immunological tests.[6] An international consensus conference in 1996 proposed diagnostic guidelines based on clinical, radiological, immunological and epidemiological criteria,[7] and revised guidelines were recommended by a consensus conference in 2001 to provide more reliable and convenient diagnostic criteria.[8] The new guidelines proposed two levels of diagnostic certainty—definite and probable, on the basis of four categories of diagnostic criteria (absolute, major, minor and epidemiological) (Table 1). Absolute criteria allow unequivocal diagnosis of neurocysticercosis. Major criteria strongly suggest the diagnosis, but cannot be used alone to confirm the disease. Minor criteria are frequent, but non-specific manifestations of the disease and epidemiological criteria refer to circumstantial evidence that favour the diagnosis (Table 2).

Neuroimaging diagnosis

Computed tomography (CT) and magnetic resonance imaging (MRI) provide objective evidence for the number and location of intracranial cysticerci, their viability and the severity of the host's inflammatory reaction against the parasite.[10]

It is claimed that CT has a sensitivity and specificity of over 95% for the diagnosis of neurocysticercosis, but its sensitivity is much lower for the ventricular or cisternal forms of the disease. The most accurate technique to assess

Table 1. Proposed diagnostic criteria for neurocysticercosis

Absolute criteria

- Histological demonstration of the parasite from a biopsy of a brain or spinal cord lesion
- Cystic lesions showing the scolex on CT or MRI
- Direct visualization of subretinal parasite by fundoscopic examination

Major criteria

- Lesions highly suggestive of neurocysticercosis on neuroimaging studies
- Positive serum immunoblot for detection of anticysticercal antibodies
- Resolution of intracranial cystic lesion after therapy with albendazole or praziquantel
- Spontaneous resolution of small single enhancing lesions

Minor criteria

- Lesions compatible with neurocysticercosis on neuroimaging studies
- Clinical manifestations suggestive of neurocysticercosis
- Positive CSF ELISA for detection of anticysticercal antibodies or cysticercal antigens
- Cysticercosis outside the central nervous system

Epidemiological criteria

- Evidence of a household contact with *T. solium* infection
- Individuals coming from or living in an area where cysticercosis is endemic
- History of frequent travel to disease-endemic areas

Table 2. Degrees of diagnostic certainty

Definite diagnosis

- Presence of one absolute criterion
- Presence of two major plus one minor and one epidemiological criteria

Probable diagnosis

- Presence of one major plus two minor criteria
- Presence of one major plus one minor and one epidemiological criteria
- Presence of three minor plus one epidemiological criteria

Adapted from Del Brutto *et al.*[9]

the degree of infection, and the location and evolutionary stage of the parasites, is MRI. It allows good visualization of the perilesional oedema and the degenerative changes of the parasite, as well as small cysts or those located in the ventricles, brain stem, cerebellum, base of the brain, eye and spinal cord. It allows visualization of a scolex as well. Parenchymal cysts are usually 5–20 mm in diameter and round in contour, while cyst fluid is isodense with CSF. On imaging studies performed during the active, viable stage of the cyst, its complete protective mechanism exists which may interfere with the development of the enhancing ring around it and one may perceive little or no cerebral oedema surrounding it. Symptomatic cysts invariably have a rim of enhancement that extends at least partly around them and there is oedema in the adjacent white matter. When the scolex of a non-inflamed or non-enhanced cyst is visible as a small dense knob, with a diameter of 2–3 mm in the middle, the image is diagnostic or pathognomonic. MRI is superior to CT scan if one wants to observe the general resolution and details of staging and, in particular, it is more sensitive for visualizing the scolex.

Cysticerci within the basilar cisterns can usually be identified by MRI. The findings may be subtle and not visible by CT scan. The most common CT finding in subarachnoid neurocysticercosis is hydrocephalus due to fibrous arachnoiditis. This may be visible (both by CT scan and MRI) as abnormal leptomeningeal enhancement at the base of the brain.

The cerebrovascular complications of neurocysticercosis are well visualized both by CT scan and MRI. On neuroimaging, the appearance of cysticerci-related cerebral infarction is the same as that of cerebral infarction due to other causes.

Serological tests

Most of the serological tests for the diagnosis of cysticercosis have poor sensitivity and specificity. Enzyme-linked immunosorbent assay (ELISA) is a common serological method used for the detection of either cysticercal antigens or anticysticercal antibodies in the CSF. The ELISA method may have a sensitivity of up to 87% and a specificity as high as 95% for the detection of anticysticercal antibodies in the CSF. A serum enzyme-linked immuno-electrotransfer blot (EITB) assay for antibodies to *T. solium* glycoprotein antigens is the most reliable serological method for diagnosis.[8] However, positive serology, even a positive EITB assay, may only indicate that an infection of *T. solium* was present somewhere in the body. Serology does not confirm neural infection or indicate whether the organism is viable or dead.

Treatment

Assessment of neurocysticercosis with respect to cyst viability, the status of the immune response to the parasite and the location of the lesions is important for proper therapy. Treatment should be individualized according to the form of neurocysticercosis. It usually includes a combination of symptomatic drugs, cysticidal drugs, surgical resection of the lesions and the placement of ventricular shunts.[10]

Antiparasitic therapy is aimed at achieving a seizure-free status and complete resolution of the lesions. Cysticidal drugs (either albendazole or praziquantel) can destroy viable intracranial cysticerci. Recently, a randomized, blinded, controlled trial using albendazole demonstrated that treatment resulted in a decrease in seizures and enhanced resolution of the cysts in patients with viable intracranial cysts.[11] The improvement could be seen both in clinical terms as well as on neuroimaging.

Although cysticidal drugs are well tolerated and effective against the parasite, there has been a controversy over the past two decades not only over whether cysticidal therapy is beneficial, but also over whether the treatment may be more harmful in some clinical settings.[12] After antiparasitic therapy, there may be an immediate risk of exacerbated seizures and encephalopathy because of acute inflammation of the brain resulting from the release of toxic material from the cysts. The long-term prognosis as far as seizures are concerned may worsen because of an increased incidence of scarring due to local inflammation of the brain. Due to this reason, the debate on the role of antiparasitic therapy continues.

Since the management of neurocysticercosis has been a controversial issue, an international panel was set up to formulate guidelines and methods for management of the disease. There was general agreement that the number of parasites should be an important factor in determining treatment decisions. Although the controversy regarding the role of anthelminthic medications persists, there was a broad consensus that therapy must be individualized and that more controlled therapeutic trials are required. The panel decided to categorize patients as those with a single lesion, those with a few lesions, those with moderate to heavy parasite loads, and those with massive infection. For the sake of clarity, a threshold of five or fewer parasites was chosen to represent cases with a few lesions and a threshold of 100 parasites was chosen to represent massive infection. Since the recommendations for the management of patients with a single lesion and those with a few parasites were the same, the two categories were later merged into one group.

Panel consensus: General concepts[10]

The treatment of neurocysticercosis must be individualized in terms of the number and location of lesions, as well as the viability of the parasites. For example, the growth of a parenchymal cysticercus is not a common event and may be life-threatening. A growing parasite warrants active management, either with antiparasitic drugs or by surgical excision. In patients with intracranial hypertension secondary to neurocysticercosis, the priority is to manage the hypertension before considering any other form of therapy. Antiparasitic drug treatment is never the main priority in the setting of elevated intracranial pressure.

Antiepileptic drugs are the mainstay of therapy for seizures in neurocysticercosis. The management of seizures should be similar to that of secondary seizures due to other causes (remote symptomatic seizures), since they behave like an organic focus that has been present for a long duration. However, after resolution of the parasitic infection as confirmed by neuroimaging studies, most patients who are seizure-free can eventually discontinue antiepileptic drugs. Antiparasitic drugs should not be regarded as an alternative to antiepileptic drug therapy.

Consensus on brain parenchymal cysticercosis

Consensus on viable cysts

There is general agreement that albendazole and praziquantel are effective antiparasitic drugs and can destroy most viable cysts. However, there is some disagreement on how to best manage patients with a few cysts and those with more than a few cysts. On balancing the risks and benefits, the panel reached a consensus that the risk of cyst growth, ventricular invasion or multiple episodes of cyst degeneration, with the corresponding symptomatic periods, outweighs the potential (but theoretical) benefits of milder inflammation and minor scarring by natural evolution. The majority felt that there was no contraindication for the simultaneous use of steroids, but one expert raised the possibility that this might interfere with the clearance of remnants of the parasite. No consensus could be reached on whether to use antiparasitic drugs in patients with massive infections (hundreds of viable cysts), mainly due to the high risk of severe side-effects which may arise after antiparasitic therapy.

Consensus on enhancing lesions

The general agreement is that patients with a single enhancing lesion are likely to do well with antiepileptic drugs, independently of whether antiparasitic therapy is added. Most members of the panel do not routinely use antiparasitic drugs for single enhancing cysticerci. Some felt that since antiparasitic drugs result in faster resolution as seen on radiological studies, they merit routine use, while others felt that antiparasitic drugs should be used in select cases, i.e. those in which antiepileptic therapy cannot be adequately monitored and the risk of an adverse outcome due to seizures is high. Conversely, in the case of patients with massive infections (cysticerci encephalitis), there was agreement that antiparasitic drugs should not be used as they may exacerbate the inflammatory reaction in the brain parenchyma. There was, however, no consensus on whether to use antiparasitic drugs in these patients after the resolution of cerebral oedema.

Consensus on calcified lesions

There was a consensus that antiparasitic agents do not have a role to play in patients with only calcified lesions because the cysts are already dead. The presence of contrast enhancement and oedema around the calcified lesions in the brain led to a discussion on whether anti-inflammatory medication can play a role in patients with calcified lesions, but there are no data from controlled trials on this aspect for final conclusion.

Views on extraparenchymal cysticercosis

Extraparenchymal neurocysticercosis is usually associated with a grave prognosis and the consensus was that it should be managed aggressively. When hydrocephalus or intracranial hypertension is present, its management should be the first priority. The panel felt that patients with cysts located in the ventricular system should be treated surgically, preferably by neuroendoscopic resection. The location of the cysts and the presence of ependymitis need to be assessed before planning the surgical intervention. Antiparasitic therapy should be withheld in these cases due to the possibility of acute blockage of the CSF.

It is agreed that cysticercosis of the basal cisterns should be treated with antiparasitic drugs. This agreement was reached considering the limitations of surgical resection, the poor prognosis using the diversion procedure alone, and the results of the case series that used shunting plus antiparasitic drugs.[13,14] The optimal duration of antiparasitic treatment for such lesions is not known, but it was felt that therapy should be sustained for a longer period than in the case of parenchymal lesions. Subarachnoid cysticercosis should always be managed with corticosteroids as an adjunct to antiparasitic therapy. Giant cysts in the subarachnoid space usually respond well to corticosteroids along with antiparasitic drugs.[13]

Spinal disease

There is a general consensus that surgery is the best form of treatment for spinal disease. Although there are anecdotal reports of good results with antiparasitic drugs for the treatment of spinal cysts, as in the case of brain parenchymal lesions, there are inadequate controlled studies demonstrating better outcomes in patients treated with anthelminthic drugs.

Antiparasitic drugs

It is far from clear whether antiparasitic medication is clinically beneficial for most patients. Shortly after the initial publication of studies that demonstrated the cysticidal efficacy of praziquantel and albendazole, it was observed that many lesions and clinical manifestations of neurocysticercosis resolve completely without antiparasitic drugs.[12] Moreover, most of the pathological effects and clinical features of the disease result from the immune and inflammatory response of the host, and not from the presence of a living parasite.[12] Following antiparasitic therapy, there is usually a period of clinical worsening, although praziquantel and albendazole are well tolerated drugs. There is controversy not only over whether cysticidal therapy is beneficial, but also over whether it may be more harmful than beneficial in some clinical settings.[12]

Which is better—albendazole or praziquantel?

Praziquantel is an isoquinolone derivative which produces spastic paralysis of the parasitic musculature and destroys the scolex. A 15-day course of treatment at a dosage of 50 mg/kg/day can result in the disappearance of 60%–70% of brain parenchymal cysticerci.[12] Albendazole is an imidazole, which inhibits the uptake of glucose by the parasitic membranes, thus causing energy depletion. It can destroy 75%–90% of brain parenchymal cysts and has been proved superior to praziquantel in several trials comparing the cysticidal efficacy of the two drugs. The other advantages of albendazole are its efficacy against meningeal, subarachnoid and ventricular cysticerci, and its comparatively low cost. Further, the serum level of praziquantel decreases when steroids are administrated simultaneously, but this is not the case with albendazole. The use of praziquantel may also cause a drop in the serum levels of phenytoin and carbamazepine.

Controversial issues

An inflammatory reaction and oedema invariably occur 5–7 days after the commencement of anthelminthic medication,[12,13] whereas many untreated patients never develop clinical disease. In human beings, the pathogenesis of the disease seems to result from parasite degeneration and death, which is why anthelminthic medications often produce new symptoms or illness, or worsen the existing symptoms.[12,15,16] In the past few decades, several authors have argued against the benefit of using antiparasitic drugs for patients of neurocysticercosis[12,14,15] on the basis of the results of their studies. In a systematic database review it was pointed out that there are no data to conclusively prove a clinical benefit with antiparasitic therapy alone.[16,17]

Recently, a randomized controlled study[1] was published on the role of antiparasitic therapy in altering the course of seizure disorders and in the resolution of lesions in 300 patients with neurocysticercosis (150 patients received albendazole, steroids and anticonvulsant drugs and the other 150 patients received only anticonvulsant drugs and placebo) with more than one lesion (all parenchymal). The patients were followed up for more than 5 years. The study showed that albendazole, steroids and anticonvulsant agents did not confer greater beneficial effects in the final outcome of seizure control and resolution of leisons than those treated with anticonvulsant drugs and placebo. It was also found that treatment with albendazole may cause problems or adverse effects, such as increased frequency of seizures, encephalopathy and the need for recurrent hospital admission during the early part of treatment. Further, albendazole therapy was associated with a higher incidence of calcification of the lesions.[1] However, in other trials using antiparasitic treatment to reduce the rate of seizures due to cerebral cysticercosis, a significant reduction was observed in the rate of seizures with generalization and a non-significant decrease in the rate of partial seizures during the follow-up period, among patients receiving albendazole compared with those receiving placebo.

The controversy continues on whether the use of antiparasitic agents can be useful in the long-term control of epileptic seizures in patients with neurocysticercosis and whether they should be used in any form of the disease. In the stage of calcification or in the encephalitic stage, it is probably best to steer clear of antiparasitic medication. The risks and benefits must be kept in mind while selecting the treatment option. The patient's economic situation is another important factor, considering that in many regions of the world where neurocysticercosis is endemic, even follow-up neuroimaging studies are mostly not performed due to economic constraints. Further, the patient may not have access to modern surgical techniques. The required standard of healthcare may not be available, but we should try to provide the best options for which research programmes should be instituted on the management of neurocysticercosis, particularly in developing countries.

Future guidelines for research

The following measures may be considered for the safe treatment of neurocysticercosis and its prevention.

- The support of international health organizations is required so that multicentre trials can be conducted.
- There is a need to set up multidisciplinary, well-equipped treatment centres.
- Research should be conducted on basic patho-physiological aspects to understand the survival, growth and degeneration of the parasite, nature and characteristics of the inflammatory reaction, genesis of seizures and epilepsy, and mechanism of anthelminthic action. This might help us discover safer, specific and more effective therapies.
- There is a need to develop non-invasive neuroimaging techniques to detect the nature and degree of inflammation, location of the cysts, and status of the larval cestodes and neuroexcitation.

Though neurocysticercosis is a major neurological problem all over the world, particularly in developing countries, its aetiopathogenesis has not been studied adequately. We do not know enough about the treatment outcomes and the burdens associated with chronic disabling neurological symptoms. Due to the rise in global migration, clinicians in the developed world are also having to tackle cases of neurocysticercosis and the problems associated with treating the disease and its consequences. Thus, we need to immediately implement the four points mentioned above on a global scale, which can be done best through collaboration between national and international health organizations.

References

1. Das K, Mondal GP, Banerjee M, *et al.* Role of antiparasitic therapy for seizures and resolution of lesions in neurocysticercosis patients: An 8-year randomized study. *J Clin Neurosci* 2007;**14**:1172–7.
2. Ong S, Talan DA, Moran GJ, *et al.* Neurocysticercosis in radiographically imaged seizure patients in US emergency departments. *Emerg Infect Dis* 2002;**86**:608–13.
3. Eddi C, Nari A, Amanfu W, *et al. Taenia solium* cysticercosis/taeniosis. Potential linkage with FAO activities; FAO support possibilities. *Acta Trop* 2003;**87**:145–8.
4. Caprio A, Escobar A, Houser WA, *et al.* Cysticercosis and epilepsy: A critical review. *Epilepsia* 1998;**39**:1025–40.
5. White DC. Neurocysticercosis. Current treatment options. *J Infect Dis* 2000;**2**:78–87.
6. Garcia HH, Del Brutto OH. Imaging findings in neurocysticercosis. *Acta Trop* 2003;**87**:71–8.
7. Del Brutto OH, Wadia NH, Dumas M, *et al.* Proposed diagnostic criteria for human cysticercosis and neurocysticercosis. *J Clin Neurosci* 1996;**142**:1–6.
8. Hector HG, Del Brutto OH, Nash TE, *et al.* New concepts in the diagnosis and management of neurocysticercosis (*Taenia solium*). *Am J Trop Med Hyg* 2005;**72**:3–9.
9. Del Brutto OH, Rajshekhar V, White AC Jr, *et al.* Proposed diagnostic criteria for neurocysticercosis. *Neurology* 2001;**57**:177–83.
10. Garcia HH, Evans CAW, Nash TE, *et al.* Current consensus guidelines for treatment of neurocysticercosis. *Clin Microbiol Rev* 2002;**15**:747–56.
11. Garcia HH, Pretel EJ, Gelman RH, *et al.* A trial of

antiparasitic treatment to reduce the rate of seizures due to cerebral cysticercosis. *N Engl J Med* 2004;**350:** 249–58.

12. Riley T, White AC. Management of neurocysticercosis. *CNS Drugs* 2003;**17:**577–91.

13. Del Brutto OH. Albendazole therapy for subarachnoid cystercerci. Clinical and neuroimaging analysis of 17 patients. *J Neurol Neurosurg Psychiatr* 1997;**62:**659–61.

14. Proano JV, Madrazo I. Medical treatment for neurocysticercosis characterized by giant subarachnoid cysts. *N Engl J Med* 2001;**345:**879–85.

15. Bettencourt PR, Garcia CM. High dose praziquantel for neurocysticercosis: Efficacy and tolerability. *Eur Neurol* 1990;**30:**229–39.

16. Salinas R, Prasad K. Drugs for treating neurocysticercosis. Available in the Cochrane Library (data based on Disk and CD ROM). The Cochrane Collaboration Issue 2, Oxford: Oxford Update Software 2002.

5

Bacterial meningitis

M.M. MEHNDIRATTA, A. BATLA, P. MEHNDIRATTA

Acute bacterial meningitis results from rapidly developing inflammation of the pia–arachnoid and cerebrospinal fluid (CSF) in response to bacterial infection. Although antibiotics and vaccination have altered the natural course of meningitis, significant mortality and morbidity are attributed to this disease.

Epidemiology

Bacterial meningitis has an annual incidence of 4–6 cases per 100,000 adults (defined as patients >16 years of age); *Streptococcus pneumoniae* and *Neisseria meningitidis* are responsible for 80% of all cases.[1,2]

Aetiology and pathogenesis

The bacteria commonly associated with meningitis and the age group in which these usually cause the disease are given in Table 1. *N. meningitidis* and *S. pneumoniae* are normally present in the external environment and may even reside in a person's nose and upper respiratory system without causing harm. They spread through droplets from person to person.

In certain predisposing conditions (Table 2), these bacteria cause invasion of blood stream and seeding of the meninges. The bacteria breach the blood–brain barrier either through this invasion (most commonly) or, in conditions such as fractures and parameningeal infections including sinusitis and otitis. The inflamed pia–arachnoid is congested and infiltrated with leucocytes, which are usually neutrophils in the early stages and are replaced by lymphocytes over a period of 7 days. This distribution of cells is reflected in the CSF picture and the initial neutrophilic predominance in pyogenic meningitis is replaced by lymphocytic predominance in the later stages and in partially treated bacterial meningitis. The

Table 1. Aetiological agents of meningitis in various age groups

Age	Common bacterial pathogens
0–4 weeks	*Streptococcus agalactiae, Escherichia coli, Listeria monocytogenes, Klebsiella pneumoniae, Enterococcus* sp., *Salmonella* sp.
4–12 weeks	*S. agalactiae, E. coli, L. monocytogenes, Haemophilus influenzae, Streptococcus pneumoniae, Neisseria meningitidis*
3 months–18 years	*H. influenzae, N. meningitidis, S. pneumoniae*
18–50 years	*S. pneumoniae, N. meningitidis*
>50 years	*S. pneumoniae, N. meningitidis, L. monocytogenes*, aerobic Gram-negative bacilli

Table 2. Predisposing factors and the causative organisms of meningitis

Predisposing factor	Common bacterial pathogens
Immunocompromised state	*S. pneumoniae, N. meningitidis, L. monocytogenes*, aerobic Gram-negative bacilli (including *Pseudomonas aeruginosa*)
Basilar skull fracture	*S. pneumoniae, H. influenzae*, group A haemolytic streptococci
Head trauma, post-neurosurgery	*Staphylococcus aureus, Staphylococcus epidermidis*, aerobic Gram-negative bacilli (including *P. aeruginosa*)
Cerebrospinal fluid shunt	*S. epidermidis, S. aureus*, aerobic Gram-negative bacilli (including *P. aeruginosa*), *Propionebacterium acnes*

exudation of these cells in the subarachnoid space forms a thin film of pus which may later organize and form adhesions leading to complications by implicating various structures in the subarachnoid space and cranial nerve sheaths, and by interfering with the CSF flow. The longer the duration of illness, the more likely are complications.

Clinical features

Early symptoms of acute bacterial meningitis are fever, headache and stiff neck. This classical triad is seen in 44%–85% of patients.[3,4] However, almost all patients present with at least two of four symptoms—headache, fever, neck stiffness and altered mental status (as defined by a score <14 on the Glasgow Coma Scale).[1]

Nausea, vomiting, myalgia and photophobia are common. Unlike adults, infants younger than one year or the elderly may not develop a stiff neck. All stages of coma may be seen and alteration of sensorium in the clinical setting of fever and headache merits an early lumbar puncture (LP) to rule out meningitis (Table 3). Seizures occur in 40% of cases. Focal deficits such as III, VI and VII nerve palsies due to direct infection are seen in a few cases. Bilateral VI nerve palsy is a false localizing sign and suggests increased intracranial pressure rather than nerve damage. In children up to two years of age, acute bacterial meningitis usually causes a fever, feeding problems, vomiting, irritability, seizures

Table 3. Indications for brain imaging before lumbar puncture

Absolute indication

- New-onset seizures
- Papilloedema
- Signs of the presence of a space-occupying lesion
- Evolving signs of brain tissue shift

Relative indication

- An immunocompromised state
- Moderate-to-severe impairment of consciousness[9,10]

and high-pitched crying. The fontanelles may bulge suggesting increased intracranial tension.

Infection with *N. meningitidis* affects many organs. When severe, it produces diarrhoea, vomiting, internal bleeding, low blood pressure, shock and death. A skin rash (usually red and purple spots) may develop because of inflammation and bleeding in the small blood vessels throughout the body, including those under the skin. These effects can develop rapidly and are called the Waterhouse–Friderichsen syndrome. Pneumococci are associated with increased chances of seizure and focal deficits and *H. influenza* with a coexisting infection of the ear or sinuses.

Investigations

The best diagnostic test in cases of suspected meningitis is a CSF examination. It is advisable to

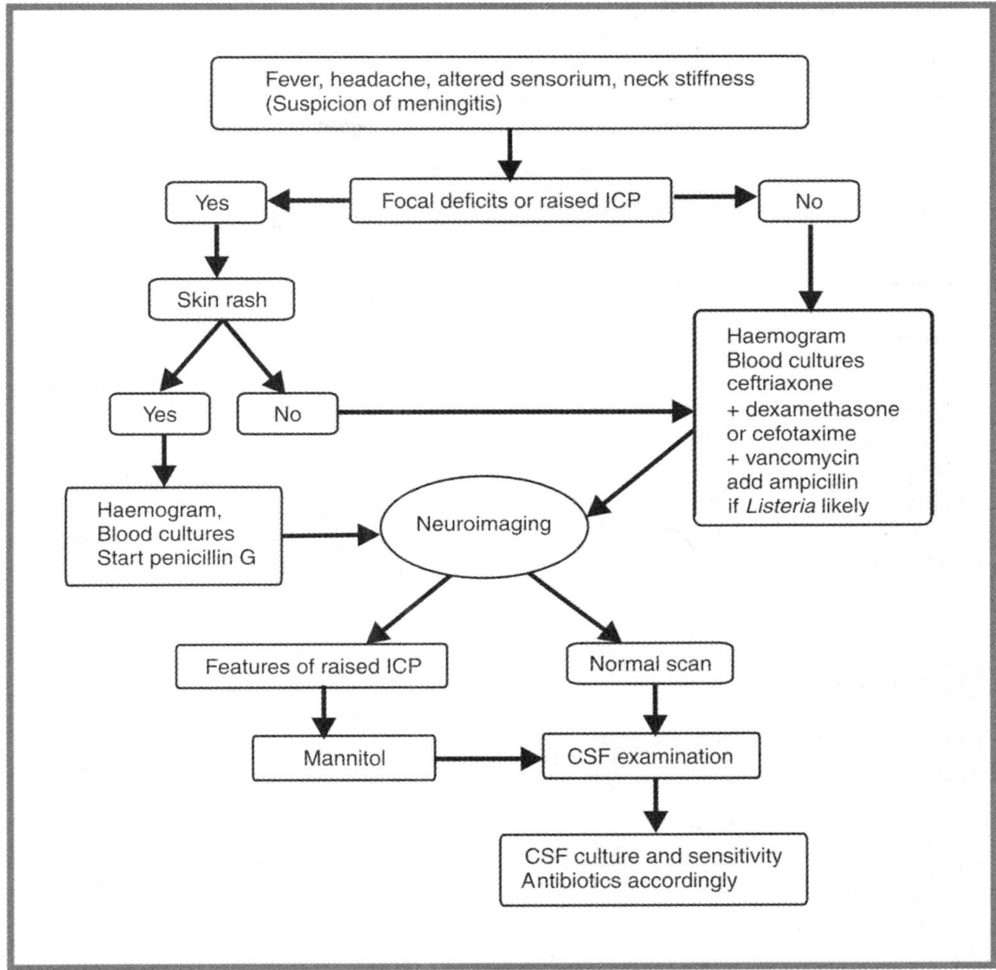

Fig. 1. Approach to a patient with suspected bacterial meningitis

examine the fundus for papilloedema and search for other signs of increased intracranial pressure (ICP). It is recommended that brain imaging be done to rule out increased ICP or mass lesions before LP to prevent the serious complication of brainstem herniation, which is potentially fatal. The schema of approach to a patient (Fig. 1) emphasizes that treatment should not be delayed even if LP is delayed or contraindicated. CSF findings include (Table 4) pleocytosis (100–10,000 white cells per mm³), elevated protein levels (>50 mg/dl [0.5 g/L]), and decreased CSF glucose levels (<40% of simultaneously measured serum glucose).[1,4–8] There is usually a predominance of neutrophils (range: 80%–95%) in the CSF, but a predominance of lymphocytes can also occur.[1,4–8] Normal or marginally elevated CSF white cell counts occur in 5%–10% of patients and are associated with an adverse outcome.[1] Gram-staining of the CSF permits rapid identification of the causative organism (sensitivity 60%–90%, specificity ≥97%).[1,8] The yield of CSF cultures does not alter for at least 12 hours after the first shot of antibiotics; so

Table 4. Differential diagnosis of meningitis by CSF examination

CSF characteristic	Bacterial meningitis	Viral meningitis	TBM	Fungal
Opening pressure	Elevated (>180 mm H_2O)	Normal or slightly elevated	Elevated (>180 mm H_2O)	Elevated (>180 mm H_2O)
White blood cell count	Increased (often >1000/mm³), neutrophil predominance	Increased (10–2000/mm³) lymphocyte predominance	Increased (50–5000/mm³), lymphocyte predominance	Increased (50–5000/mm³), lymphocyte predominance
Glucose level	Decreased (<40 mg/dl)	Normal (>45 mg/dl)	Decreased (<40 mg/dl)	Decreased (<40 mg/dl)
Protein level	Increased (often >100 mg/dl)	Normal or increased	Increased	Normal or increased
Gram/AFB/fungal stain results	Stainable organisms present in 50%–80% of untreated patients	No stainable organisms	AFB seen	Yeast cells seen on India-ink staining
Bacterial culture	Positive	Negative	Negative	Negative

Table 5. Management of bacterial meningitis in adults in the neurology ICU

Raised ICP monitoring and management

- Intracranial pressure monitoring in patients with a high risk of brain herniation
- Intermittent administration of osmotic diuretics (mannitol [25%] or hypertonic [3%] saline) to maintain an ICP of <15 mmHg and a cerebral perfusion pressure of >60 mmHg
- Consider ventriculostomy in patients with acute hydrocephalus, initiate repeated LP, lumbar drain.
- Electroencephalographic monitoring in patients with a history of seizures and fluctuating sensorium (consider non-convulsive status)

Respiratory care

- Intubate or provide non-invasive ventilation in patients with worsening consciousness (clinical and laboratory indicators for intubation include poor cough and pooling secretions, a respiratory rate >35 per minute, arterial oxygen saturation <90% or arterial partial pressure of oxygen <60 mmHg and arterial partial pressure of carbon dioxide >60 mmHg).
- Maintain ventilatory support with mechanical ventilation (usually pressure support or synchronized intermittent mandatory ventilation [SIMV]).

Circulatory care

In patients with septic shock, administer low doses of corticosteroids (if there is a poor response on corticotrophin testing indicating adrenocorticoid insufficiency, corticosteroids should be continued). Initiate inotropic agents (dopamine or milrinone) to maintain blood pressure (mean arterial pressure 70–100 mmHg). Initiate crystalloids or albumin (5%) to maintain adequate fluid balance.

Gastrointestinal care

- Initiate nasogastric tube feeding of a standard nutrition formula.
- Initiate ulcer prophylaxis with proton-pump inhibitors.

Other supportive care

- Prophylaxis against deep venous thrombosis with low molecular-weight heparin (LMWH).
- Maintain normoglycaemic state (serum glucose level <150 mg/dl), with the use of sliding-scale regimens of insulin or continuous intravenous administration of insulin.
- In patients with a body temperature of >40 °C, use antipyretic agents.

Table 6. Treatment of bacterial meningitis

Situation	Preferred antibiotic*
Empirically	
0–12 weeks	Third-generation cephalosporin + ampicillin + dexamethasone (2 days)
3 months–50 years	Third-generation cephalosporin + vancomycin (+ ampicillin)
>50 years	Third-generation cephalosporin + vancomycin + ampicillin
On the basis of CSF Gram-stain results	
Gram-positive cocci	Ceftriaxone (or cefotaxime) + vancomycin
Gram-positive bacilli	Ampicillin + gentamicin
Gram-negative cocci	Penicillin G
Gram-negative bacilli	Ceftazidime
On the basis of culture results	
S. pneumoniae	
Penicillin MIC <0.06 microgram/ml	Penicillin G or ceftriaxone or cefotaxime
Penicillin MIC >0.1 microgram/ml	Ceftriaxone or cefotaxime + vancomycin (if susceptibility to broad-spectrum cephalosporins is reduced)
N. meningitidis	Penicillin G
H. influenzae	Cefotaxime or ceftriaxone
L. monocytogenes	Ampicillin + gentamicin
Group B streptococcus	Penicillin G

antibiotics must be started at the earliest. Blood cultures and the blood picture not only supplement the diagnosis of a bacterial aetiology but may guide antibiotic therapy in case the CSF culture is negative or if an LP was not done due to contraindications.

The characteristic findings during CSF examination are highlighted in Table 5. The opening pressure of the CSF is increased and should be measured while performing the LP. The CSF is turbid and has very high protein content and cell counts. With treatment, the cells show a lymphocyte predominance as opposed to the initial polymorphic predominance. A polymerase chain reaction (PCR) is useful in special situations such as meningococcal epidemics and may be positive in the blood. Latex agglutination test is useful for *H. influenzae* and *S. pneumoniae*.

Lumbar puncture in meningitis

Lumbar puncture is mandatory in any patient in whom bacterial meningitis is suspected. Neuroimaging—either cranial computed tomography (CT) or magnetic resonance imaging (MRI)—to detect brain shift is recommended as a precaution in selected patients before LP.[9,10] It is important to keep in mind the heterogeneity of patients with clinically suspected bacterial meningitis.

Management

The treatment should be started as guided in Fig. 1. If meningococcus is suspected based on rash, the patient must immediately receive parenteral benzyl penicillin (2.4 g i.v. 6-hourly) even before admission, if feasible. There is increasing evidence for the first-line use of vancomycin as resistant *S. pneumoniae* infections are becoming common (Table 6). Ceftriaxone or other third-generation cephalosporins remain the mainstay of treatment and vancomycin is added if resistant *S. pneumoniae* is suspected. Suspicion or confirmation of *Listeria* mandates the addition of ampicillin to the antibiotic regimen. Special situations such as post-head injury and neurosurgery mandate the addition of ceftazidime to cover Gram-negative bacilli. The best antibiotic is the one that shows sensitivity in cultures of the CSF and this should guide the treatment once reports become available.

Delay in treatment

Delay in the initiation of antimicrobial therapy can result in poor outcomes. In most cases delay is due to the performance of cranial imaging before diagnostic LP and the transfer of patients to another hospital. It is thus necessary that if imaging is performed before LP, therapy should be initiated before the patient is sent for neuroimaging. In patients who have not undergone prior imaging and in whom disease progression is apparent, therapy should be started directly after LP, as well as in all patients with a cloudy CSF (suggesting the diagnosis of bacterial meningitis).[11,12] The opening pressure of the CSF is elevated in most patients with bacterial meningitis.

Role of dexamethasone

A quantitative review of steroid use in adults with meningitis included the results of five clinical trials.[13] Treatment with corticosteroids was associated with a significant reduction in mortality and neurological sequelae. In the subgroup of patients with meningococcal meningitis, mortality (relative risk, 0.9; 95% confidence interval [CI]: 0.3–2.1) and neurological sequelae (relative risk, 0.5; 95% CI: 0.1–1.7) were both reduced, although the results were not statistically significant.

There are no controlled studies of the effects of corticosteroid therapy in a substantial number of patients with both meningitis and septic shock, and therefore corticosteroid therapy

cannot be unequivocally recommended for such patients, although the use of low doses (hydrocortisone, 50 mg every 6 hours and fludrocortisone, 50 µg daily) seems reasonable.[14] Starting corticosteroids before or with the first dose of parenteral antimicrobial therapy appears to be more effective than starting corticosteroids after the first dose of antimicrobial therapy.[15]

Cognitive decline after meningitis

Adult survivors of bacterial meningitis are at risk for cognitive impairment, which consists mainly of cognitive slowness.[16] The loss of cognitive speed is stable over time after bacterial meningitis; however, there is a significant improvement in subjective physical impairment in the years after bacterial meningitis. The use of dexamethasone is not associated with cognitive impairment.

Special issues in agent-specific management

Meningococcal meningitis

N. meningitidis infection may manifest as fever and bacteraemia without sepsis, meningococcaemia without meningitis, or meningitis without meningococcaemia. There has been a consistent response to beta-lactams although they fail to eradicate nasopharyngeal carriage of *N. meningitidis*. Chloramphenicol is used in allergic individuals. Rifampicin (age 3–12 months 5 mg/kg 12-hourly, >1 year 10 mg/kg 12-hourly, adults 600 mg 12-hourly) has been recommended for contacts of the index case to prevent spread. Ciprofloxacin 500 mg as single dose is an alternative. Epidemics are common and vaccination during this period may help to limit the mortality, although a vaccine against the most common serotype B is not available.

Waterhouse–Friderichsen syndrome

Waterhouse–Friderichsen syndrome (WFS) is massive, usually bilateral, haemorrhage into the adrenal glands caused by fulminant meningococcaemia. WFS is characterized by overwhelming bacterial infection, rapidly progressive hypotension leading to shock, disseminated intravascular coagulation (DIC) with widespread purpura, particularly of the skin, and rapidly developing adrenocortical insufficiency associated with massive bilateral adrenal haemorrhage. Once diagnosed, meningococcaemia must be managed as an emergency and care of blood pressure and ventilation prevents most deaths in the early period. Renal failure, haemorrhagic diathesis, acute respiratory distress syndrome and multi-organ failure are all known to be the terminal events in these patients.

H. influenzae meningitis

This type usually spreads from the ear or nose. The prevalence of this infection has reduced after routine HiB vaccination. Although still high in India, the infection is common in young children and often leads to complications such as loss of hearing. Dexamethasone i.v. for 2 days at the beginning of treatment has been accepted as standard therapy in children >4 weeks to reduce sequelae.

Pneumococcal meningitis

This type of infection is the most prevalent form of meningitis worldwide in young people. This infection is associated with more seizures, focal deficits and sequelae. Steroids are indicated, especially in young children. The CSF may have few cells but protein is markedly elevated and clumps of pneumococci may be seen on microscopy. With institution of treatment, cell counts may rise to >2000/mm^3 leading to misinterpretation of resistance on repeat CSF examination. Vancomycin is increasingly being recommended at all centres in view of the emerging resistance to beta-lactams. Vaccination is available and should be given to splenectomized patients and patients with sickle cell disease, or chronic illnesses.

Listeria monocytogenes meningitis

Listerial infection is common in the extremes of ages. Meningitis in seen in only one-third of people infected with listeriosis. Ampicillin plus gentamicin is recommended as beta-lactams are known to be ineffective. Co-trinoxazole may be used in allergic people. *Listeria* is also associated with focal cerebritis and rhombencephalitis, usually without meningitis, and presents with focal deficits, headache, fever, clouded sensorium and seizures. This form requires prolonged treatment (6 weeks).

Partially treated bacterial meningitis

In countries such as India the treatment of meningitis is often inadequate and patients may present after a few days of treatment. The CSF in these cases may give a wrong impression of chronic meningitis such as tuberculous meningitis (TBM). The lymphocytic predominance should not cast a doubt if a history of antibiotic use and long duration is available. However, an intensive search for the causative organism is required to settle the diagnosis.

Outcome

Community-acquired meningitis caused by *S. pneumoniae* has high case-fatality rates (19%–37%).[1,4–8] In up to 30% of survivors, long-term neurological sequelae develop, including hearing loss and other focal neurological deficits.[1,4–8] The mortality and morbidity for meningococcal meningitis are lower than those for pneumococcal meningitis, with case fatality rates of 3%–13% and morbidity rates of 3%–7%.[1,4–6] The strongest risk factors for an unfavourable outcome are the presence of systemic compromise, impaired consciousness, low white-cell count in the CSF and infection with *S. pneumoniae*.[1] All cohort studies were performed before dexamethasone was routinely administered; now that routine dexamethasone therapy has been implemented, complications and sequelae are expected to decline.[1,13]

References

1. van de Beek D, de Gans J, Spanjaard L, *et al*. Clinical features and prognostic factors in adults with bacterial meningitis. *N Engl J Med* 2004;**351:** 1849–59. [Erratum, *N Engl J Med* 2005;**352:**950]
2. Schuchat A, Robinson K, Wenger JD, *et al*. Bacterial meningitis in the United States in 1995. *N Engl J Med* 1997;**337:** 970–6.
3. Attia J, Hatala R, Cook DJ, *et al*. The rational clinical examination: Does this adult patient have acute meningitis? *JAMA* 1999;**282:**175–81.
4. Dodge PR, Swartz MN. Bacterial meningitis—a review of selected aspects. II. Special neurologic problems, postmeningitic complications and clinico-pathological correlations. *N Engl J Med* 1965;**272:** 954–60.
5. Durand ML, Calderwood SB, Weber DJ, *et al*. Acute bacterial meningitis in adults: A review of 493 episodes. *N Engl J Med* 1993;**328:**21–8.
6. Sigurdardottir B, Bjornsson OM, Jonsdottir KE, *et al*. Acute bacterial meningitis in adults: A 20-year overview. *Arch Intern Med* 1997;**157:**425–30.
7. Hussein AS, Shafran SD. Acute bacterial meningitis in adults: A 12-year review. *Medicine (Baltimore)* 2000;**79:**360–8.
8. Tunkel AR. Bacterial meningitis. Philadelphia: Lippincott Williams and Wilkins, 2001.
9. van Crevel H, Hijdra A, de Gans J. Lumbar puncture and the risk of herniation: When should we first perform CT? *J Neurol* 2002;**249:**129–37.
10. Hasbun R, Abrahams J, Jekel J, *et al*. Computed tomography of the head before lumbar puncture in adults with suspected meningitis. *N Engl J Med* 2001; **345:**1727–33.
11. Spanos A, Harrell FE Jr, Durack DT. Differential diagnosis of acute meningitis: An analysis of the predictive value of initial observations. *JAMA* 1989; **262:**2700–7.
12. Schuurman T, de Boer RF, Kooistra-Smid AM, *et al*. Prospective study of use of PCR amplification and sequencing of 16S ribosomal DNA from cerebrospinal fluid for diagnosis of bacterial meningitis in a clinical setting. *J Clin Microbiol* 2004; **42:**734–40.
13. van de Beek D, de Gans J, McIntyre P, *et al*. Steroids in adults with bacterial meningitis: A systematic review. *Lancet Infect Dis* 2004;**4:**139–43.
14. Annane D, Sebille V, Charpentier C, *et al*. Effect of treatment with low doses of hydrocortisone and fludrocortisone on mortality in patients with septic shock. *JAMA* 2002;**288:**862–71.
15. van de Beek D, de Gans J, McIntyre P, *et al*. Corticosteroids in acute bacterial meningitis. *Cochrane Database Syst Rev* 2003;**3:**CD004305.
16. Hoogman M, van de Beek D, Weisfelt M, *et al*. Cognitive outcome in adults after bacterial meningitis. *J Neurol Neurosurg Psychiatry* 2007;**78:**1092–6.

6

Japanese encephalitis: An overview

U.K. MISRA, J. KALITA

Summary

Japanese encephalitis (JE) is a mosquito-borne disease produced by a neurotropic RNA virus of the flaviviridae family. The JE virus (JEV) is transmitted naturally between wild and domestic birds and pigs by *Culex* mosquitoes (*Culex tritaeniorhynchus*) which breed in ponds and stagnant water. Humans are dead-end hosts because of a short and low titre of viraemia. Only a minority of infected persons develop encephalitis. In the northern region of India, JE manifests as post-monsoon epidemic whereas in southern areas it occurs sporadically throughout the year. JE is prevalent in Southeast Asia and the Indian subcontinent and over 50,000 cases are reported annually, of which 10,000 die. Of the survivors, 50% develop serious neurological sequelae. The clinical picture is characterized by a febrile prodrome. The encephalitis phase is associated with a high frequency of seizures in children, anterior horn cell involvement resulting in a polio-like illness and movement disorders, which include parkinsonian features and various types of dystonia. CT scan or MRI reveals thalamic, basal ganglia, midbrain, pons and medulla involvement which are highly suggestive of JE in endemic areas. The diagnosis is based on IgM ELISA in the cerebrospinal fluid (CSF) which has sensitivity of >75%.

JE has no specific therapy and management focuses on control of seizures, reducing intracranial pressure, general nursing care and rehabilitation. Prevention is achieved by vaccination, avoiding mosquito bite and vector control.

Introduction

JE is one of the most common causes of viral encephalitis worldwide with estimated 50,000 cases and 15,000 deaths annually.[1] About one-third of the patients die and nearly half the survivors have disabling neurological sequelae. JE is prevalent in China, Southeast Asia and the Indian subcontinent. Because of deforestation and changing agricultural practices, JE is spreading at an alarming rate affecting children and young adults in these areas.

Epidemic encephalitis was first reported in Japan in the 1870s. The term Japanese B encephalitis was originally used to differentiate it from the summer epidemics caused by Von Economo's encephalitis lithergica (type A encephalitis). In 1933, a virus was transferred from the brain of a fatal case of encephalitis to a monkey and the prototype of Nakayama strain of JE was isolated from the brain of a fatal case in 1935. JEV is a RNA virus that belongs to the flaviviridae family.

Epidemiology

JEV is transmitted by Culex mosquitoes and occurs primarily in East and Southeast Asia and the Pacific Rim. The neurotropic flavivirus are found all over the world with common virological and epidemiological features. All flaviviruses are derived from a common ancestor about 10,000–20,000 years back. The examples of neurotropic mosquito-borne arboviruses include Murray valley encephalitis in Australia, St Louis encephalitis virus in North America, West Nile encephalitis virus in Africa, Middle East and recently in North America and Europe.

Enzootic cycle

JEV is transmitted between wild and domestic birds and pigs by Culex mosquitoes; the most important mosquito causing human infection is *Culex tritaeniorhynchus* which breeds in stagnant water, e.g. paddy field or water ponds. The animals which develop high viraemia are important in the natural cycle and amplifying JEV in the environment. Birds may be responsible for spreading the virus to new geographical areas. Pigs are the most important amplifying natural host for transmission of JEV to humans because they are close to humans, have prolonged and high viraemia and produce many offspring, thereby continuously supporting previously un-infected new hosts. The virus does not produce encephalitis in the natural hosts although abortion does occur in pigs.

Human disease

In post-monsoon period, the mosquito density increases significantly resulting in high infection rate of pigs; and human infection soon follows. Humans get infected inadvertently when they encroach the JE transmission cycle. Humans are considered dead-end hosts because they normally do not have sufficiently high and prolonged viraemia to transmit the virus further. Most cases of JEV infection occur in rural or suburban areas. In rural Asia, JEV mainly affects children. About 10% of susceptible population is infected each year.[2] However, most infections in humans are asymptomatic or result in a non-specific flu-like illness. The estimates of symptomatic to asymptomatic cases range from 1 in 25 to 1 in 1000.[3,4] In northern Thailand, the incidence of JE has been estimated to be 40 per 100,000 for ages 5–25 years, which declines to almost 0 for those >35 years.[5] The incidence is also lower for <3 years of age, thus reflecting behavioural factors such as playing outside after the dusk.

When epidemics occur in new areas, e.g. Sri Lanka, India, Nepal, adults are also affected.[6] The susceptibility of immunologically naïve adults was also evident by infection of US army personnel in Japan, Korea and Vietnam. The rate of infection was higher in these troops than in local population which may be due to prior flavivirus infection of native population resulting in partial protection or difference in genetic susceptibility of the troops.

Two epidemiological patterns of JE are recognized. In northern areas (North Vietnam, North Thailand, Korea, Japan, Taiwan, China, Nepal and North India), large epidemics occur in the summer months whereas in southern areas (South Vietnam, South Thailand, Indonesia, Malaysia, the Philippines, Sri Lanka and South India), JE occurs in an endemic fashion and cases are reported throughout the year in sporadic fashion with a post-monsoon peak.[7] The reasons for these epidemiological patterns are attributed to different genotypes of JEV leading to difference in neurovirulence.[8]

In the past 50 years, the geographical area of JE has increased, which may be attributed to the improvement in diagnostic and reporting system; however, there seems to be relentless spread of JE. In China, the first case of JE was reported in 1935 and the JEV was first isolated 5 years later. Today, there are 10,000–20,000 cases reported annually.[7] In 1949, a large epidemic was reported from South Korea. In northern Vietnam, JE epidemics were first reported in 1965 and currently 1000–3000 cases occur annually. In Chang Mai, North Thailand, JE was first reported in 1969 and currently 1500–2500 cases occur annually. JE was first recognized in south India in 1955, and was restricted to southern India till the 1970s. Large outbreaks (2000–7000/year) are reported from eastern and north-eastern states of India. Involvement of both adults and children in Indian outbreaks strongly suggests that JE virus was introduced for the first time in this region. In the late 1970s, first reports of JE came from Bangladesh, Burma and Nepal (up to 500 cases/year) and in 1985, Sri Lanka experienced its first epidemic.

The reasons for spread of JE are incompletely understood and include factors such as changing agricultural practices and increasing irrigation, which in turn allows mosquito breeding, and animal husbandry which in turn provides the host animals. Local religion and culture also influences, for example, the lower prevalence of JE in Indonesia compared to neighboring Bali is attributed to lack of pigs in the predominantly Muslim population of Indonesia. In developed countries such as Japan, Taiwan and Korea the incidence of JE has declined because of mass vaccination of children, pesticide spraying, change in pig farming practice, separation of housing from farming, air conditioning and lack of mosquito breeding ponds.

JE virus

At least 5 genotypes of the JEV occur in Asia which is roughly related to the geographical area of isolation. Complete nucleotide sequence of JEV has been published and includes 5'3' untranslated region and a single open reading frame encoding genes for 3 structural proteins, capsid (C), precursor to membrane protein (PrM), envelope protein (E) and 7 non-structrual proteins. E gene sequence of flavivirus is related to virulence in animal model and a single

aminoacid substitution is sufficient to cause loss of neurovirulence or invasiveness.[9]

Clinical features

Patients present with non-specific febrile illness associated with coryza, diarrhoea, headache, vomiting and altered sensorium which may be preceded by convulsion. In older children and adults abnormal behaviour may be the only presentation and some of these patients were diagnosed as war neurosis in a Korean study.[10]

Some patients recover spontaneously (abortive encephalitis) whereas others may present with meningitis without any evidence of encephalitis. Convulsions occur in 10%–85% of patients with JE and are more common.[11–13] Generalized tonic–clonic seizures are more common than focal (partial). Our study revealed seizures in 30 out of 65 JE patients—generalized tonic–clonic in 17 and partial in 13. Seizure was single in 11, two episodes in 8 and multiple in 11 patients. Status epilepticus occurred in 2 patients.[12] Multiple or prolonged seizures and status epilepticus are associated with poor outcome. Subtle seizures causing twitching of fingers, eye or mouth deviation, nystagmus, excessive salivation have also been reported.[14]

Movement disorders

Mask-like face, rigidity, tremor, hypokinesia, simulating parkinsonian syndrome are common in JE and are noted as the patient comes out of deep coma. These are transient and have a declining course. These features are reported in 70%–80% of American soldiers and 20%–40% of Indian children.[11,15,16] Some patients have additional dystonia which may be of various types—axial, limb and orofacial, and sometimes it can be markedly severe simulating status dystonicus. In a study markedly severe dystonia was found in 5 out of 50 patients with JE; the dystonic spasms lasted for 2–3 min, and up to 20–30 spasms occurred daily and were associated with tachycardia, hypertension, fever, exhaustion and interfered with feeding and breathing necessitating intensive care. This dystonia was refractory to treatment and significantly reduced by 2–6 months.[17] Patients with dystonia had poorer outcome compared to those with parkinsonian features alone.[18]

Acute flaccid paralysis

Acute flaccid paralysis has been reported in 5%–20% of cases.[19,20] Focal weakness in JE patients may simulate poliomyelitis, which may affect one or more limbs. Though we have seen this in patients with encephalitis and it may manifest with focal reflex loss, partial or complete weakness; however, Solomon *et al.* have noted it in patients without any evidence of encephalitis and with normal consciousness, and 30% of their patients subsequently developed encephalitis.[21] On electrodiagnostic study, nerve conductions are normal, there are positive sharp waves and fibrillations with neurogenic potentials. The EMG changes regress over a period of time and recovery is associated with reinnervation. These findings are consistent with anterior horn cell involvement.[15] On spinal MRI, T2 signal changes have been reported in JE.[22] On autopsy study, anterior horn cell involvement simulating poliomyelitis has been reported in JE.[23]

Investigations

CSF opening pressure is increased in 50% of patients. High pressure (>250 mm) is associated with poor outcome.[14] Typically, there is moderate pleocytosis 10–100/mm^3 with predominant lymphocytes though polymorphs may predominate in the early stage.

CT scan shows hypodense area in thalamus, basal ganglia, midbrain, pons and medulla. MRI is more sensitive than CT scan typically demonstrating more extensive lesions in the above-mentioned areas.[24] Thalamic lesions may be of mixed intensity in T1, and T2 sequence suggesting haemorrhagic change. The imaging studies are helpful in differentiating JE from herpes simplex encephalitis (HSE) where changes are typically in frontotemporal areas.[12]

EEG in JE reveals non-specific changes. Three patterns of EEG changes have been reported and include diffuse slowing of theta to delta range (24/27), spike wave discharges (3/27) and alpha coma (3/27).[25] EEG may help in differentiating JE from HSE, in which the changes are typically frontotemporal.

Diagnosis

Efforts to isolate JEV from clinical samples are usually unsuccessful because of low viral titres and production of neutralizing antibodies though sometimes JEV can be isolated from CSF. IgG and IgM capture enzyme-linked immuno-sorbant assays (ELISA) has become a standard diagnosis test for JE.[26] After a few days of illness, IgM antibodies have a sensitivity of >95% for infections of the central nervous system (CNS).

Pathophysiology

On autopsy the leptomeninges are normal or hazy. The brain parenchyma is congested with focal petechiae or haemorrhages in the gray matter. When the patient survives more than 7 days, patchy necrotic areas are seen. White matter is normal. In some patients gray matter of spinal cord reveals confluent discoloration resembling poliomyelitis. Thalamus, basal ganglia and midbrain are heavily affected providing anatomical basis for tremor, and dystonia which are common in JE. Invasion of neurons by JEV is followed by perivascular cuffing infiltration of T-cells and macrophages into the parenchyma and phagocytosis of infected cells.[23,27,28] T-cells in the brain of fatal cases studied by monoclonal antibodies are CD8+ and CD4+, localized in perivascular cuff. Both cell types are found in the CSF in acute infection though the predominant type is CD4+. In patients who die rapidly, there may be no histopathological signs of inflammation but immunohistochemical studies show viral antigen in morphologically normal neurons.[29] This may explain the normal CSF findings in patients in whom JE proves fatal.

Immunology

Interferon and interferon inducers are active against JEV in mice and monkeys[30,31] and endogenous interferon alpha has been detected in plasma and CSF of humans with JE.[32] In addition, both humoral and cellular immune responses occur in infection with JEV. Other factors which affect the blood–brain barrier are implicated in the pathogenesis of JE. Neurocysticercosis or head trauma may facilitate the entry of JEV into the brain. The humoral immune response in JE has been well characterized. When the disease is due to primary infection (JEV is the first flavivirus to infect), rapid and strong immune IgM response occurs in serum and CSF within a few days of infection and by day 7 most patients have raised IgM titres.[33] Attempts to isolate virus generally fail, but in the absence of IgM response virus can be isolated and is associated with a fatal outcome.[34] Antibodies to JEV probably protect the host by restricting viral proliferation during the viraemic phase before virus cross blood–brain barrier. It may also restrict damage during established encephalitis by neutralizing extracellular virus and facilitating lysis of infected cells by antibody-dependent T-cellular cytotoxicity.

In surviving patients, immunoglobulin class switching occurs and within 30 days most have IgG in serum and CSF. Asymptomatic infection of patients with JEV is associated with raised IgM in serum, but not in CSF. In patients with secondary infection (those who have been infected by a different flavivirus, e.g. dengue or yellow fever vaccination), there is anamnestic response to falvivirus group of common antigen, which is characterized by an early rise in IgG with a subsequent slow rise in IgM.

Cellular immunity

The CNS seems to contribute to prevention of disease during acute infection by restricting viral replication before CNS is invaded. In humans infected with St Louis encephalitis, HIV increases the risk of developing encephalitis co-infection. By analogy, other viral infections including influenza, HIV, EBV and dengue, T-cell functions might be important in the control and possibly clearance of JEV. Preliminary experimental data are in agreement with this—T lymphocytes were characterized in 10 convalescent JE and 10 vaccines, and JEV-specific T-cell proliferation including CD4+ and CD8+ were present in both groups.[35,36]

Management

Treatment of JEV is supportive and involves controlling convulsions and intracranial pressure if these are present. Corticosteroids have not shown any benefit.[13] Careful nursing care and rehabilitation programmes are important. Various drugs such as isoquinolone, ribavirin, monoclonal antibodies, interferon-α have been reported effective in experimental models,[37,38] but clinical trials failed to show benefit.[14]

Prevention

Prevention of JE is important in the absence of effective antiviral drugs. The prevention of JE has been tried at various levels—vector control, reservoir level and vaccination. Interrupting the enzootic cycle by control of breeding of Culex mosquito and insecticide spraying have been found to be ineffective.[39] Control of JE is linked to broader economic and environmental issues.

Prevention of mosquito bite

Prevention of mosquito bite by minimizing outdoor exposure at dusk and dawn; wearing clothes with minimal skin exposure and using insect repellant containing NN diethyl-3-methyl-benzamide and sleeping in bed nets may be short-term solutions, but these measures are not practical in endemic areas on a long-term basis.

Prevention in humans is possible by JE vaccination. Formalin inactivated JE vaccine was produced in Russia, Japan and USA by Albert Sabin to protect American troops in Asia during World War II. A similar formalin inactivated vaccine has been manufactured in Japan since 1954 by Osaka University and is available internationally by the name Biken. Similar vaccines are prepared in India, Japan, Korea, Taiwan, Thailand and Vietnam. The efficacy of JE has been shown in double-blind randomized tetanus toxoid controlled trials in Taiwan and Thailand involving more than 300,000 children.[40] Three doses of vaccine are required in western people to provide prophylactic antibody level. It is given at 0, 7 and 30 days with a booster dose at 1 year. In Asian subjects, 2 doses may be sufficient because of prior or subsequent infection to JEV or other flavivirus (West Nile or dengue). A booster vaccination is recommended at 1–2 years for those with continued exposure.

JE vaccine is associated with moderate frequency of local and mild systemic side-effects such as local tenderness, redness and swelling as have been reported in 20% of vaccinated individuals. Fever, headache, malaise and chills have been reported in 10%. There has been concern about neurological side-effects because the vaccine is derived from mouse brain. However, the amount of mouse brain myelin basic protein is negligible. There was no neurological event among 44,000 Thai children receiving vaccine.[40]

A surveillance study in Japan on JE vaccines, during 1965–1973, disclosed neurological events (encephalitis, encephalomyelitis, seizures, peripheral neuropathy) at a rate of 1–2.3/million recipients, which is less than that reported for other virus vaccines. Since 1989 in Europe, America and Australia, a new pattern of reaction has been observed which includes urticaria, itching and angioneurotic oedema on the face. Many of these reactions occurred several days after vaccination. The rate of reaction was 2–10/1000 vaccines and was more likely in those with history of urticaria.[41] No vaccine constituents have been identified as being responsible for this apparently new adverse reaction, though allergy to gelatin stabilizer has been suggested.

Live attenuated vaccine (SA 14-14-2) was released in China in 1998. It is produced by passing the virus though weanling mice and then culturing on hamster kidney cells. This vaccine is considered safe and immunogenic. It has been administered to over 100 million children in China. It is immunogenic at shorter dosage intervals of 1 and 2.5 months. The effectiveness of one dose is 80% and two doses is 97%.[42]

Targets for vaccination

JE vaccine is recommended for native and expatriate residents of endemic areas, laboratory workers potentially exposed to virus and travellers spending 30 days or more in endemic areas.[2] For shorter visits, vaccine is recommended only if there will be excessive outdoor activity in rural areas or if visiting during an epidemic. However, two recent cases of JE in short-term (<2 weeks) visitors to Bali support the view that all travellers to JE endemic should be vaccinated.[43,44] In spite of vaccination, it may be difficult to eradicate JE in endemic areas because it has an enzootic cycle in addition to human.

References

1. Tsai TF. Factors in the changing epidemiology of Japanese encephalitis and West Nile fever. In: Saluzzo JF, Dodet B (eds). *Factors in the emergence of arbovirus diseases.* Paris: Elsevier; 1997;179–89.
2. Inactivated Japanese encephalitis virus vaccine.

Recommendations of the Advisory Committee on Immunization Practises (ACIP). *MMWR* 1993;**42**: 1–14.

3. Halstead SB, Grosz CR. Subclinical Japanese encephalitis. I. Infection of Americans with limited residence in Korea. *Am J Hyg* 1962;**75**:190–201.

4. Huang CH. Studies of Japanese encephalitis in China. *Adv Virus Res* 1982;**27**:71–101.

5. Grossman RA, Edelman R, Chiewanich P, *et al.* Study of Japanese encephalitis virus in Chaingmai Valley, Thailand. II Human clinical infections. *Am J Epidemiol* 1973;**98**:121–32.

6. Umenai T, Krzysko R, Bektimorov TA, *et al.* Japanese encephalitis: Current worldwide status. *Bull World Health Organ* 1985;**63**:625–31.

7. Vaughn DW, Hoke CH. The epidemiology of Japanese encephalitis: Prospects for prevention. *Epidemiol Rev* 1992;**14**:197–221.

8. Chen WR, Tesh RB, Ricco-Hesse R. Genetic variation of Japanese encephalitis virus in nature. *J Gen Virol* 1990;**71**:2915–22.

9. Cecilia D, Gould EA. Nucleotide changes responsible for loss of neuroinvasiveness in Japanese encephalitis virus neutralisation-resistant mice. *Virology* 1991;**181**:70–7.

10. Lincoln AF, Silvertson SE. Acute phase of Japanese B encephalitis. Two hundred and one cases in American soldiers, Korea 1950. *JAMA* 1952;**150**: 268–73.

11. Kumar R, Mathur A, Kumar A, *et al.* Clinical features and prognostic indicators of Japanese encephalitis in children in Lucknow (India). *Indian J Med Res* 1990;**91**:321–7.

12. Misra UK, Kalita J. A comparative study of Japanese and Herpes simplex encephalitis. *Electromyogr Clin Neurophysiol* 1998;**38**:41–6.

13. Hoke CH, Vaughn DW, Nisalak A, *et al.* Effect of high dose dexamethasone on the outcome of acute encephalitis due to Japanese encephalitis virus. *J Infect Dis* 1992;**165**:631–7.

14. Solomon T, Dung NM, Kneen R, *et al.* Seizures and raised intracranial pressure in Vietnamese patients with Japanese encephalitis. *Brain* 2002;**125**:1084–93.

15. Misra UK, Kalita J. Movement disorders in Japanese encephalitis. *J Neurol* 1997;**244**:299–303.

16. Kalita J, Misra UK, Pandey S, *et al.* A comparison of clinical and radiological findings in adults and children with Japanese encephalitis. *Arch Neurol* 2003;**60**:1760–4.

17. Kalita J, Misra UK. Markedly severe dystonia in Japanese encephalitis. *Mov Disord* 2000;**15**:1168–72.

18. Misra UK, Kalita J. Prognosis of Japanese encephalitis patients with dystonia compared to those with parkinsonian features only. *Postgrad Med J* 2002;**78**: 238–41.

19. Dickerson RB, Newton JR, Hansen JE. Diagnosis and immediate prognosis of Japanese B encephalitis. *Am J Med* 1952;**12**:277–88.

20. Kumar R, Agarwal SP, Waklu I, *et al.* Japanese encephalitis: An encephalomyelitis. *Indian Pediatr* 1991;**23**:1525–33.

21. Solomon T, Kneen R, Dung NM, *et al.* Poliomyelitis-like illness due to Japanese encephalitis virus. *Lancet* 1998;**351**:1094–7.

22. Kumar S, Misra UK, Kalita J, *et al.* MRI in Japanese encephalitis. *Neuroradiology* 1997;**39**:180–4.

23. Zimmerman HM. Pathology of Japanese encephalitis. *Am J Pathol* 1946;**22**:965–1000.

24. Kalita J, Misra UK. Comparison of CT scan and MRI findings in the diagnosis of Japanese encephalitis. *J Neurol Sci* 2000;**174**:3–8.

25. Kalita J, Misra UK. EEG in Japanese encephalitis: A clinicoradiological correlation. *Electroencephalogr Clin Neurophysiol* 1998;**106**:238–43.

26. Bundo K, Igarashi A. Antibody-capture ELISA for detection of immunoglobulin M antibodies in sera from Japanese encephalitis and dengue hemorrhagic fever patients. *J Virol Methods* 1985;**11**:15–22.

27. Shankar SK, Vasudev Rao T, Mruthyunjayanna BP, *et al.* Autopsy study of brain during an epidemic of Japanese encephalitis in Karnataka. *Indian J Med Res* 1983;**78**:431–40.

28. Johnson RT, Burke DS, Elwell M, *et al.* Japanese encephalitis: Immunocytochemical studies of viral antigen and inflammatory cells in fatal cases. *Ann Neurol* 1985;**18**:567–73.

29. Li ZS, Hong SF, Gong NL. Immunohistochemical study of Japanese B encephalitis. *Chin Med J (Engl)* 1988;**101**:768–71.

30. Liu J-L. Protective effect of interferon on mice experimentally infected with Japanese encephalitis virus. *Chinese Journal of Microbiology* 1972;**5**:1–9.

31. Ghosh SN, Goverdhan MK, Sathe PS, *et al.* Protective effect of 6-MFA, a fungal interferon inducer against Japanese encephalitis virus in bonnet macaques. *Indian J Med Res* 1990;**91**:408–13.

32. Burke DS, Morrill JC. Levels of interferon in the plasma and cerebrospinal fluid of patients with acute Japanese encephalitis. *J Infect Dis* 1987;**155**:797–9.

33. Burke DS, Nisalak A, Ussery MA, *et al.* Kinetics of

IgM and IgG responses to Japanese encephalitis virus in human serum and cerebro-spinal fluid. *J Infect Dis* 1985;**151**:1093–9.

34. Leake CJ, Burke DS, Nisalak A, *et al.* Isolation of Japanese encephalitis virus from clinical specimens using a continuous mosquito cell line. *Am J Trop Med Hyg* 1986;**35**:1045–50.

35. Konishi E, Mason PW, Innis BI, *et al.* Japanese encephalitis virus specific proliferative responses of human peripheral blood T lymphocytes. *Am J Trop Med Hyg* 1995;**53**:278–83.

36. Aihara H, Takasaki T, Matsutani T, *et al.* Establishment and characterization of Japanese encephalitis virus-specific, human CD4+ T-cell clones: Flavivirus cross-reactivity, protein recognition and cytotoxic activity. *J Virol* 1998;**72**: 8032–6.

37. Takegami T, Simamura E, Hirai K-I, *et al.* Inhibitory effect of furanonaphthoquinone derivatives on the replication of Japanese encephalitis virus. *Antiviral Res* 1998;**37**:37–45.

38. Kimura-Kuroda J, Yasui K. Protection of mice against Japanese encephalitis virus by passive adminis-tration with monoclonal antibodies. *J Immunol* 1988;**15**:3606–10.

39. Innis BL. Japanese encephalitis. In: Porterfield JS (ed). *Exotic viral infections.* London: Chapman and Hall, 1995:147–74.

40. Hoke CH, Nisalak A, Sangawhipa N, *et al.* Protection against Japanese encephalitis by inactiva-ted vaccines. *N Engl J Med* 1988;**319**:608–14.

41. Plesner AM, Ronne T. Allergic mucocutaneous reactions to Japanese encephalitis vaccine. *Vaccine* 1997;**15**:1239–43.

42. Liu ZL, Hennessy S, Strom BL, *et al.* Short-term safety of live attenuated Japanese encephalitis vaccine (SA14-14-2): Results of a randomized trial with 26,239 subjects. *J Infect Dis* 1997;**176**:1366–9.

43. Tsai TF, Yu YX. Japanese encephalitis vaccines. In: Plotkin SA, Mortimer EAJ (eds). *Vaccines.* Philadelphia: WB Saunders, 1994:671–13.

44. Gambel JM, DeFraites RF, Hoke Jr CH, *et al.* Japanese encephalitis vaccine: Persistence of anti-body up to 3 years after a three dose primary series. *J Infect Dis* 1995;**171**:1074.

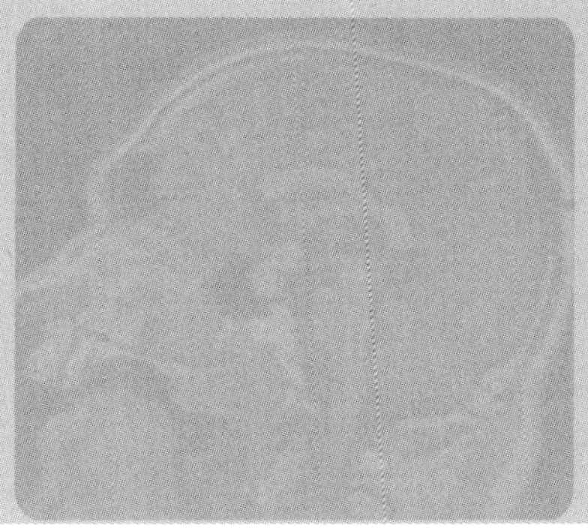

Parkinson disease

7

Current treatment options in Parkinson disease

A.V. SRINIVAS

By the year 2040, neurodegenerative diseases are expected to surpass cancer as the second most common cause of death in the elderly. One of the most common neurodegenerative disorders is Parkinson disease (PD), with over 4 million victims worldwide. Ageing has been implicated as an important risk factor for PD, with the majority of cases occurring in people >60 years of age. Now that our population is experiencing an extended lifespan, the prevalence of PD is likely to increase substantially. It is estimated that one in forty persons will develop this disease.

James Parkinson described PD in 1817 as a clinical syndrome presenting with bradykinesia, tremor and a slow, shuffling gait with postural instability. Rigidity was described later, but is included as a key clinical feature in the current diagnosis of PD. PD accounts for approximately 80% of cases of parkinsonism.[1]

Definition

The characteristic tetrad is known as TRAP

- Resting tremor
- Cogwheel rigidity
- Bradykinesia/akinesia
- Postural reflexes

Of this tetrad, only resting tremor is truly suggestive of PD, an early sign that may remain prominent even in the late stages.[2] The other signs occur in varying degrees in other forms of parkinsonism.

Natural history

The pathological changes of PD may appear as much as 3 decades before the appearance of clinical signs. The onset is so gradual and insidious that patients can rarely pinpoint the first symptom(s). Early symptoms may be so mild that a clinical diagnosis is impossible.[3,4]

Evidence indicates that the progression of PD may be rapid in the preclinical stage as well as during the first years of the disease, with subsequent slowing of process.[5] Correlation of the progressive disability with the biological and pathological changes in PD and the compensating mechanisms are illustrated in Fig. 1.

In this profile of clinical, biochemical and pathological changes in PD, the brain's compensating mechanisms are seen to be an increase in the synthesis of dopamine receptors and turnover of surviving the necrosis (SN) reflected by an increase in the homovanilic acid (HVA)/dopamine (DA) ratio.

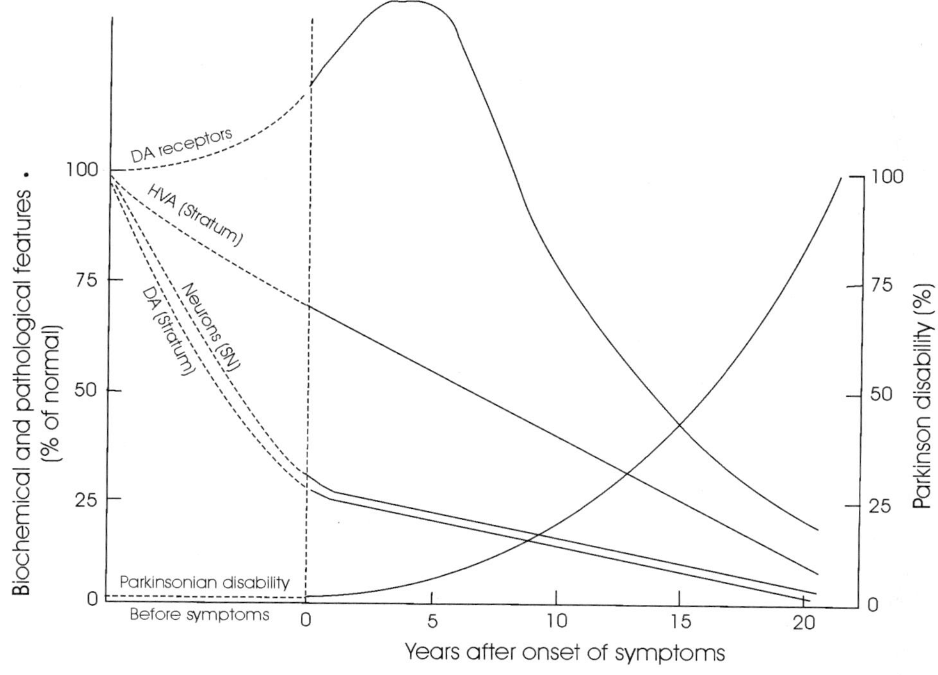

Fig. 1. Progressive changes in Parkinson disease

Before the introduction of levodopa, PD caused severe disability in 16% of patients within 5 years of onset, in 37% of patients over the next 5 years, and in 42% of those surviving 15 years.

- Preclinical PD
  —disease onset

- Early PD
  —symptom onset
  —diagnosis
  —beginning of symptomatic treatment

- Advanced PD
  —onset of motor fluctuations
  —onset of levodopa-resistant symptoms
  —freezing
  —falling
  —death

Recent advances in the treatment of early PD[6]

Initial therapy

It is given during the honeymoon period, i.e. the first 3–6 years (Fig. 2). After confirming the diagnosis, consider if the patient has disability sufficient enough to warrant dopamine replacement. New patients have a range of drugs available for use (Table 1).

Neupro patch

Rotigotine, a member of the dopamine agonist class of drugs, is delivered continuously through the skin (transdermal) using a silicone-based patch that is replaced every 24 hours. A dopamine

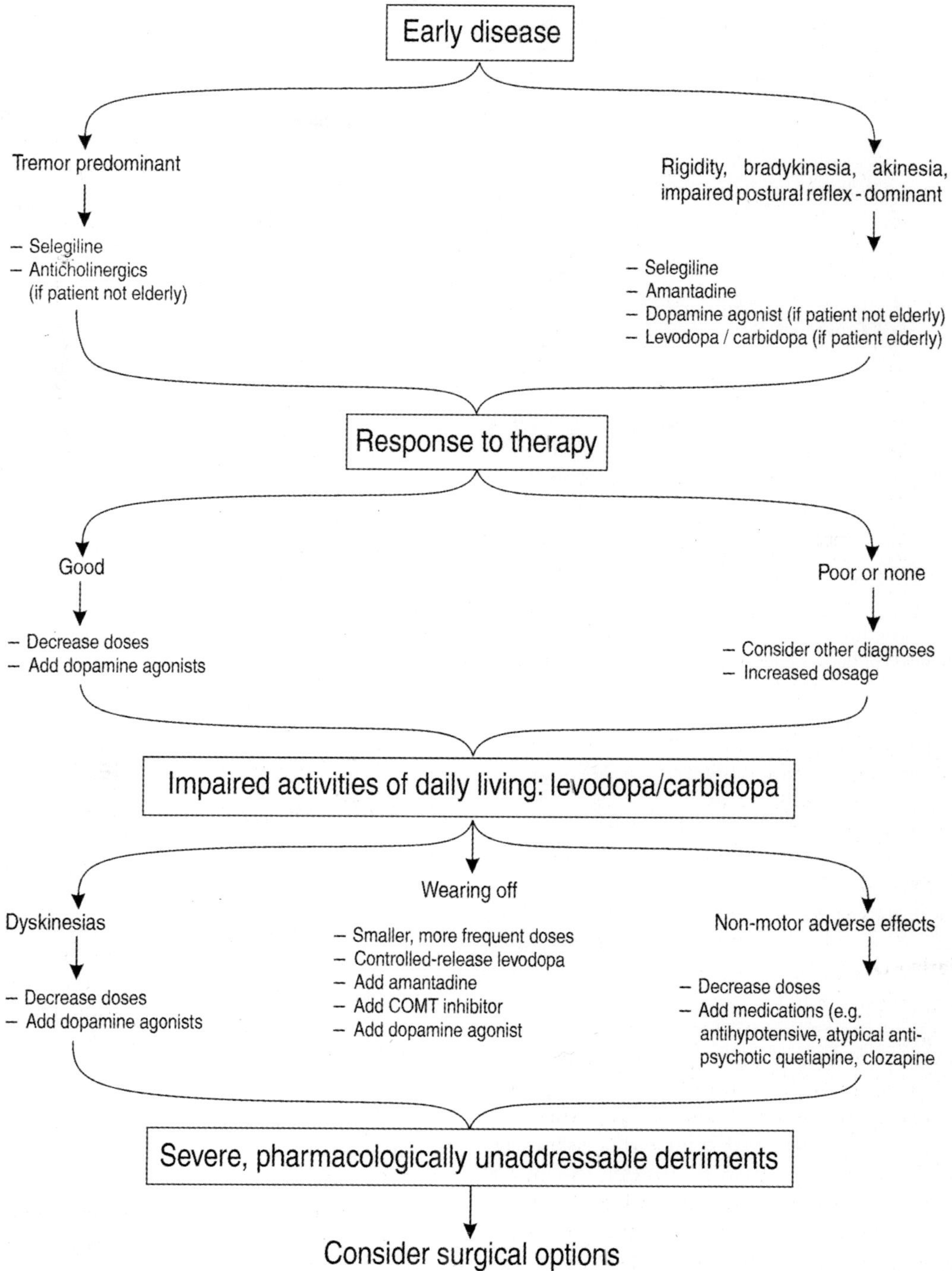

Fig. 2. Treatment options in Parkinson disease

Table 1. Drugs for initial therapy in Parkinson disease

Name of drug	Group and mechanism	Dose (mg/day)	Side-effects	Remarks
Selegiline	MAOB inhibitor	5–15 od	Insomnia, nausea, hypotension	No direct neuroprotective effect. Interaction with meperidine and SSRIs
Amantadine	NMDA receptor antagonist	100–300	Livedo reticularis, hallucinations	Reduces dyskinesias in advanced PD
Trihexyphenidyl, Benztropine, Ethopropazine	Anticholinergics	2 tds 0.5 bd 50–100 tds	Aggravate confusion, poor tolerance in old age, dry mouth, urinary retention	
Bromocriptine Pergolide Ropinirole Pramipexole Cabergoline	DOPA agonists	2.5–5 bd 0.05–0.5 tds 0.25–3 tds 0.125–0.75 tds twice a week	Hypotension, hallucination, leg oedema, confusion, erythromelalgia Somnolence, pulmonary and retroperitoneal fibrosis	Pergolide has severe cardiac side-effects and has been recently withdrawn by FDA in the USA[7]
Levodopa/carbidopa (4:1)	DOPA preparations	50–100 mg levodopa tds Maximum 300–600/day	Nausea, hypotension, constipation, confusion, hallucinations	Easy to use, better tolerated, superior efficacy
Coenzyme Q10	Neuroprotective	1200/day		Supposed to retard dopamine cell loss; needs larger studies

agonist works by activating the dopamine receptors in the body, mimicking the effect of the neurotransmitter dopamine.

The effectiveness of Neupro was demonstrated in one fixed-dose response study and two flexible-dose studies. The parallel group studies were randomized, double-blinded, and placebo-controlled, and involved 1154 patients with early PD who were not taking other medications for PD.

The most common side-effects for Neupro included skin reactions at the patch site, dizziness, nausea, vomiting, drowsiness and insomnia, most of which are typical of this class of drugs. Other potential safety concerns include sudden onset of sleep while engaged in routine activities such as driving or operating machinery (sleep attacks), hallucinations and decreased blood pressure on standing up (postural hypotension).

Treatment of advanced PD

Motor problems/Motor fluctuations

The presence of motor fluctuations decreases the quality of life of patients with PD and contributes to the direct and indirect economic burden of the disease, reducing occupational productivity and increasing the cost of medical care (Table 2).

Possible mechanisms of levodopa-related motor fluctuations are as follows:[8]

- Peripheral pharmacokinetics
  —Delayed gastric emptying
  —Protein competition

- Central pharmacokinetics
  —Variations in striatal levodopa levels (reduced storage)
  —Damage to dopaminergic neurons by toxic

Table 2. Treatment of motor complications of Parkinson disease[7]

Motor response	Management
Wearing-off	• More frequent dosing of levodopa • Catechol-O-methyltransferase (COMT) inhibitor • Dopamine inhibitor • Controlled-release levodopa
Off period dystonia	• Controlled-release levodopa • Dopamine agonist • COMT inhibitor • Dietary adjustments
On–off	• Liquid levodopa • Dopamine agonist • Clozapine
Drug failure	• Domperidone (when available) • Liquid levodopa (individual dose) • Apomorphine
Peak-dose dyskinesia/ dystonia	• Reduce each dose of levodopa • Use dopamine agonist • Add anticholinergic • Amantadine

byproducts of dopamine metabolism

• Central pharmacodynamics
  —Alleged dopamine receptors
  —Altered dopamine receptor sensitivity profile

Freezing

Considered to be a type of akinesia, freezing takes many forms. Patients may have difficulty with starting to walk (start hesitation); they may suddenly 'freeze' in doorways, while crossing the street, and on turning. The problem may occur at any time, is worsened by stress, any may result in falls.

Freezing may occur during either 'on' or 'off' states. 'On' freezing is poorly understood, and although 'off' freezing is a manifestation of PD, unlike the other characteristics signs, it does not respond readily to levodopa.

Gait disturbance

Postural instability is one of the cardinal features of relatively advanced PD. This symptom does not respond to levodopa.

A focused approach to gait disorders is needed. Hesitation when starting to walk (start hesitation) and the temporary inability to move (freezing) can sometimes be overcome by issuing verbal commands ('ready, set, go').

Patients with postural instability may take a few involuntary steps backward. Since these patients have a tendency to fall, their shoes should have leather, not rubber soles and heel lifts to help tilt them forward.

Other motor abnormalities

• Severe burning pain (such as a fresh sunburn), misdiagnosed as fibrositis, and relieved by carbidopa/levodopa
• Restless legs, accompanied by kicking and shaking which occur at regular intervals at the end of each carbidopa/levodopa dose; symptoms resolve with a change is the CR form.

Non-motor problems

Dementia

The dementia associated with PD is estimated to affect at least 20% of patients, with a higher prevalence in older patients; it is rare in those with young-onset disease.

Dementia is associated with a poorer prognosis for survival in patients with PD. These patients respond poorly levodopa and experience frequent side-effects.

Before treating PD-related dementia, it is crucial to eliminate all reversible causes of dementia, such as:

• Vitamin B_{12} deficiency
• Hypothyroidism
• Neurosyphilis
• Normal-pressure hydrocephalus
• Mass lesions.

Depression

An estimated 40%–60% of patients with PD experience depression, which appears to be related to the duration of the disease. Whether depression is related to the loss of frontal dopaminergic projections or serotonin deficiency or is a psychological response to PD has not yet been resolved.[9] However, depression is clearly related to the 'off' periods of levodopa response and lifts with improved control of motor symptoms.

Treatment
- Antidepressant use
  - Stimulating antidepressants if apathy is major feature
  - Sedating antidepressants if sleep disturbance is a major feature.

Apathy

In a survey from Norway on psychiatric features of PD, it was found that apathy was a significant feature affecting these patients. Although apathy is often confused with depression, it is likely to be a separate symptom. The most important aspect is to realize that the patient is not 'lazy' but that there is a neurological basis underlying this phenomenon.

Treatment
- Increase activity
- Caffeine
- Modafinil

Hallucinations and psychosis

Psychiatric adverse effects are much more likely to occur in patients with predisposing characteristics such as:

- Dementia
- Advanced age
- Pre-morbid psychiatric illness
- Exposure to high daily doses of levodopa[10]

Visual hallucinations are the most common clinical feature of drug-induced psychosis and occur in approximately 30% of treated patients. Possible precipitating events include

- Urinary and pulmonary infections
- Metabolic encephalopathy
- Cerebrovascular events

Treatment
- Reduce or stop
  - Adjunctive medications (e.g. amantadine, anticholinergics)
  - Dopamine agonist
  - COMT inhibitor
- Reduce dosage of levodopa
- Clozapine
- Quetiapine

Sleep disorders

The earliest sleep problem is sleep fragmentation. Sleep problems include difficulty initiating sleep, daytime somnolence, restless legs syndrome (RLS), rapid eye movement (REM) behaviour disorders (RBD), sleep apnoea (atypical parkinsonism), nightmares, hallucinations, dyskinesias, nocturnal vocalization, or dementia-altered sleep–wake cycle.

Sleep fragmentation
- Controlled-release carbidopa/levodopa
- Sedating antidepressant
- Clonazepam

Nocturnal vocalization/vivid dreams; RBD
- Reduce dopaminergic medications near bedtime
- Clonazepam

Orthostatic hypotension

Many patients with PD suffer from orthostatic hypotension, caused either by the disease itself or by the medications used to treat it.[11] A number of pharmacological agents are directed at increasing the blood pressure (BP). They include the mineralocorticoids. The mineralocorticoids are likely to take several weeks to become effective. A suggested dosing schedule of fludrocortisone (Florinef) is 0.2 mg/day, increased to 0.4 mg/day. Another appropriate option is the α_1-adrenergic receptor agonist midodrine (ProAmatine).

Dosage and administration of midodrine are:

- Starting dose: 2.5 mg at breakfast and lunch.
- Increase by 2.5 mg increments daily, with maximum 10 mg tid.
- Can be given at 3-hour intervals if needed but not more frequently.

Gastrointestinal problems

Nausea is a recognized, relatively common side-effect of all dopaminergic agents. Taking carbidopa, levodopa with food is sometimes helpful. Should nausea remain a problem, a peripheral dopamine-blocking agent such as domperidone, which does not cross the blood–brain barrier, is extremely effective in reducing both nausea and postural hypotension.

Constipation due to autonomic dysfunction leadin to impaired gut motility is common in PD. Constipation continues to be one of the most frequent autonomic-related complaints throughout the disease process.

- High-fibre diet, hydration, and an exercise programme and regularly scheduled toilet habits are encouraged.
- Anticholinergics and narcotic-containing compounds should be avoided.
- Bulk agents and laxatives can be prescribed. The stool softeners bran, psyllium and docusate (up to 400 mg/day) are effective within 1–3 days.
- Enemas may be effective in difficult cases.

Advanced PD—Non-pharmacological approach to associated disorders

Swallowing problems and sialorrhoea

These disorders may develop at any stage of PD and can be thoroughly evaluated by a speech therapist. Symptoms may include:

- Choking
- Coughing
- Drooling
- Holding.

Motor problems contributing to these difficulties include

- Decreased tongue mobility
- Decreased elevation of the larynx
- Impaired swallowing reflex
- Diminished pharyngeal peristalsis.

Patients may fail to swallow saliva automatically resulting in pooling in the mouth and throat. Saliva build-up may also contribute to muffled speech. Careful attention to the process of swallowing may help in improving sialorrhoea and related problems. Patients should be advised to consciously swallow saliva frequently. Holding the head upright helps to prevent pooling and enhance the swallowing mechanism. Finally, a conscious effort to swallow saliva must be made before speaking.

Patients should eat slowly, taking only small amounts of food with each bite. Food should be chewed thoroughly and swallowed before the next bite is taken.

Dental care

A number of medications, including anticholinergics and antidepressants commonly prescribed for patients with PD, cause xerostomia by suppressing the production of saliva, thus reducing its antibacterial and cleansing actions, resulting in an increased risk of coronal and root surface caries periodontal disease, and tongue erosion.

Denture retention depends to a large extent on appropriate muscle function. Tremors or dyskinesias affecting the tongue may dislodge a mandibular denture, and rigid and uncontrolled facial muscles may prevent the maxillary denture from maintaining a good retentive seal. The increased tendency for tooth decay in patients with PD is now thought to be the result of xerostomia and the decreased ability to perform regular oral hygiene. New varieties of electric and sonic toothbrushes facilitate dental care for patients with PD. Dilute fluoride rinses can be used daily as a 1-minute rinse to protect the teeth.

Nutritional disturbances

Patients often have trouble preparing food, and eating or swallowing. In frustration, they may consume a very restricted diet, a problem enhanced by co-existing depression or dementia.

Specific dietary considerations for patients with PD include:

- Patients with motor fluctuations may find that the medication is more effective if taken 30 minutes before meals.
- Patients with severe fluctuations may eliminate protein during the day to avoid this competition. All protein needs are then provided at dinner.

Seborrhoeic dermatitis

The cause of seborrhoeic dermatitis and the reasons for its association with PD are unknown. Although patients with PD tend to have long-term problems with seborrhoeic dermatitis, levodopa tends to resolve the condition or decrease its severity.

The condition can usually be treated by using

- Ketoconazole shampoo
- Shampoos and lotions containing selenium
- Shampoos, lotions and creams containing pyrithione zinc.

Sexuality

In males, erectile dysfunction is most commonly described. In women, it was found that they have anxiety, inhibition and other concerns. In a recent open-label study, 10 men had improved sexual function with the use of sildenafil, 50 mg per encounter. No significant side-effects were reported after 8 encounters. Levodopa may induce feelings of well-being and in some patients it results in a significant but generally short-lived increase in sexuality. Hypersexuality has also been described with dopaminergic therapy. Treatment of hypersexuality includes counselling, lowering of the dose of medication and the possible use of an atypical antipsychotic agent.

Cardiopulmonary impairment

- The patient's flexed posture can lead to kyphosis and cause a reduction in pulmonary capacity and a restrictive lung disease pattern.
- Breathing exercises, postural re-education and trunk exercises may be helpful.
- Institute a general conditioning programme to increase the patient's endurance.
- If pulmonary function progressively worsens, assisted coughing techniques, and incentive spirometry therapy intervention may be required.

Surgical intervention

Surgical management of PD has been of increased interest over the past few years. Three main techniques currently in use include destructive therapy (lesioning), deep brain chronic stimulation and transplantation.[12,13]

Destructive therapy

- Lesioning options include thalamotomy and pallidotomy.
- Ventral intermediate nucleus thalamotomy is effective at relieving tremor, but its effects on the other clinical manifestations of PD seem to be less significant and more variable. Thalamotomy usually is reserved for a relatively small percentage of patients with predominantly drug-resistant tremor.
- At present, pallidotomy is the surgical procedure most commonly used for advanced

PD. Surgery employs lesioning to disrupt the abnormal activity in the globus pallidus to disinhibit the motor thalamus and cortical motor areas, thereby improving motor functioning. Candidates for pallidotomy include patients who are disabled despite optimal medical management and who have responded to levodopa (L-dopa) therapy in the past but have developed complications from long-term L-dopa treatment. Rigidity, tremor and bradykinesia all seem to respond to pallidotomy.

Deep brain stimulation[12,14]

- Chronic deep brain stimulation seems to have emerged as an alternative to lesioning in patients with PD.
- Stimulation has the advantages of safety, reversibility and adaptability (i.e. stimulation parameters can be adjusted as the clinical features change over time).
- Stimulation sites include the ventral lateral thalamic nuclei (performed to decrease tremor with a good response in 80%–85% of patients), the globus pallidus (for bradykinesia, gait, speech, drug-induced dyskinesias), and the subthalamic nucleus (for bradykinesia, rigidity, tremor, gait/posture). A recent study of 6 male patients showed improved motor rating scores, and reduced timing and spatial errors following deep brain stimulation of the internal globus pallidus.

Transplantation

- Although stimulation and lesioning can improve symptoms, neither corrects the underlying pathology of the disease, which is a lack of dopamine from loss of neurons in the substantia nigra. Transplantation therapy offers the possibility of replacing these lost neurons.[13]
- Clinical trials have examined the use of 3 types of transplants—autologous adrenal medulla transplants, foetal mesencephalon grafts and xenografts.

- Adrenal medulla transplants are not in widespread use because of the high morbidity and mortality from adrenalectomy.
- Foetal mesencephalon grafts have shown promising early results. Trials continue, but ethical concerns, insufficient tissue and procedural difficulties make it unlikely that the procedure will become commonplace.
- The most common xenograft used is the foetal pig mesencephalon. A trial is currently under way to determine the efficacy of this procedure.

Rehabilitation

Non-pharmacological therapy, especially psychological support, is of incalculable value from the diagnosis through the course of PD. Patients derive benefit from the knowledge that the disease is an area of active research and that increasingly effective medications and other interventions are on the horizon.

The comprehensive management of PD patients is a team effort involving a variety of therapeutic interventions and therapists, including the:

- Primary physician
- Neurologist
- Family members
- Physical, occupational, speech therapists.

The diagnosis and management plan of PD and related movement disorders are largely handled by neurologists, family or primary physicians. They are often the first to suspect the diagnosis and refer patients to specialists, and are likely to provide coordination of therapy thereafter.

References

1. Jancovic J. The extra pyramidal disorders. In: Bennet JC, Plum F (eds). *Cecil text book of medicine*. 20th ed. Philadelphia, Pa: WB Saunders Co 1996:2042–6.

2. Adams RD Victor. *Principles of neurology.* 7th ed. New York: McGraw-Hill; 2001:1067–78.

3. Goldman SM Tanner. Etiology of Parkinson's disease. In: Jancovic J, Tolosa E (eds). *Parkinson's disease and movement disorders.* 3rd ed. Baltimore Md: Lippincott Williams and Wilkins; 1998:133–58.

4. Stoessl JA. Etiology of Parkinson's disease. *Can J Neurol Sci* 1999;**26** (Suppl 2):5–12.

5. Poewee WH, Wenning GK. The natural history of PD. *Neurology* 1996;**47**:S146–S152.

6. Golbe LI, Sage JI. Medical treatment of Parkinson's disease. In: Kurlan R (ed). *Treatment of movement disorders.* Philadelphia, PA: JB Lippencott; 1995:1–56.

7. FDA takes pergolide off US market (4/4/2007). (Available at URL: http://www.fda.gov/cder/drug/advisory/pergolide.htm)

8. Grau AJ. *Neurology* 1997;**49** (5 Suppl 4):S47–51.

9. Poewe W, Luginger E. Depression in PD. *Neurology* 2001;**52**:S2–S6.

10. Waters CH. Managing late complications of PD. *Neurology* 1997;**49**:S49–57.

11. Waters CH. Management of patients with complicated PD. Syllabus course 127 American Neurology Annual meeting Seattle, Wash, 1955: 33–42.

12. Lopiano L, Rizzone M, Bergamasco B, *et al.* Deep brain stimulation of the subthalamic nucleus in PD: An analysis of the exclusion causes. *J Neurol Sci* 2002;**195**:167–70.

13. Hallett M, Litvan I, the Task Force on Surgery for Parkinson's Disease. Evaluation of surgery for Parkinson's disease. A report of the therapeutics and techno4logy assessment subcommittee of the American Academy of Neurology. The Task Force on Surgery for Parkinson's disease. *Neurology* 1999; **53**:1910–21.

14. Schuurman PR, Bosch DA, Bossuyt PM, *et al.* A comparison of continuous thalamic stimulation and thalamotomy for suppression of severe tremor. *N Engl J Med* 2000;**342**:461–8.

8

Subthalamic nucleus stimulation: Long-term results

PARESH K. DOSHI

Levodopa is the standard treatment for Parkinson disease (PD) but causes long-term motor complications despite other pharmacological interventions.[1] In 1998, Professor Benabid reported the first series of patients with PD who were treated with bilateral stimulation of the subthalamic nucleus (STN)[2] had improvement in motor function while off medication one year after surgery. Besides off-period improvements, they reported an associated improvement in on-medication dyskinesia and off-medication dystonia.[3,4] We started performing STN stimulation in 1998 and reported our early follow-up in 2003.[5] Our results reflected improvements similar to that seen by the Grenoble group.

Recent literature has been published on the long-term outcome of this therapy.[6–8] We report here the results of a 4-year prospective cohort study of 26 patients with advanced PD, treated in our centre with bilateral stimulation of STN.[9]

Selection of patients

Patients with advanced PD were considered for surgical option. The common guidelines followed were based on Core Assessment Program for Neurosurgical Interventions and Transplantation in PD (CAPSIT-PD).[10]

The most important selection criterion was the diagnosis of PD. Many diseases may mimic PD in the initial stage and these need to be carefully excluded. One of the ways to ensure this was not to consider surgery in patients with <5 years of disease duration. The second criterion was responsiveness to levodopa. Patients should show a minimum 33% improvement in their off-period motor scores after levodopa. Patients should have the ability to tolerate awake surgery as certain patients, especially older patients, may get confused during surgery. Another aspect of patient selection involved the expectations out of surgery. Patient and their partners were adequately counselled about the surgical outcome. We explained to them that the patient would experience 70%–80% on-period and their off-periods would not be as disabling. However, the quality of on-period was not likely to change, i.e. if they had difficulties in speech or gait during on-period, they may not improve. We did not consider age to be a contraindication for surgery. If the patient was physically fit and cognitively sound enough to undergo surgery we gave him the benefit of surgical treatment. Recently, there have been reports of offering surgery to patients early in their disease with encouraging outcome.[11] We have adopted a philosophy of offering surgical option to all those patients who cannot achieve their desired quality of life by best medical management.

Surgery

We located STN on a T2W MRI. To rule out inaccuracies of MRI distortion, a CT scan was performed to cross-check the target localization. Initially, physiological localization was performed by macrostimulation. However, later, we incorporated micro-electrode recording for physiological localization. All patients underwent quadripolar electrodes (DBS 3389, Medtronic) implantation. All surgeries were bilateral. The implantable pulse generator (IPG) was implanted under general anaesthesia the next day. Stimulation settings and medication were progressively adjusted over 8–10 days.

Assessments

Patients were evaluated preoperatively and postoperatively at 1, 2 and 4 years with use of the Unified Parkinson's Disease Rating Scale (UPDRS). They were evaluated in off-medication (12 hours off-medication) and on-medication states. The Schwab and England scale of global activities of daily living and Hohn and Yahr staging was also performed. Video recordings were done in both these states. Mini mental scale evaluation (MMSE) was performed to rule out major cognitive deficits. The primary outcome measures were the scores, total scores and part III scores (motor examination) of the UPDRS. Additional evaluation of Schwab and England ADL and levodopa requirement was also performed. Stimulation parameters at 2 years and 4 years were also compared.

Results

We evaluated patients in off-medication and on-medication status with the stimulator in on condition at 2 years[12] and 4 years of follow-up. A total of 30 patients were evaluated at 2 years and 26 patients were evaluated at 4 years.

Off-medication evaluation

With stimulation in the off-medication state, the total score of the UPDRS improved from a baseline (average score 95) by 58% and 54% at 2 and 4 years, respectively. Similarly, the scores of part III of the UPDRS improved from the baseline value (average score 63.53) by 59% at one year and 54% at 4 years. The scores on the Schwab and England scale, which measures activities of daily living, range 0–100% (with 100% indicating normal function). The scores dramatically improved postoperatively in the off-medication condition, by 72% and 65%, respec-tively at 2 years and 4 years respectively. Off-period dystonia and pain disappeared in all patients immediately after surgery. However, in some patients it reappeared at long-term follow-up. Speech improved in some patients and deteriorated in others. The score for speech improved only during the first year and then progressively worsened, returning to the baseline score at 4 years.

On-medication evaluation

Motor function and activities of daily living in the on-medication state did not improve after STN stimulation. Between the second and fourth year, there were no significant changes in individual scores for tremor and rigidity, but scores for akinesia, speech, postural stability and freezing of gait worsened (p<0.001 for each comparison), resulting in a worsening of the total score for motor function (p<0.001) and the total score for activities of daily living (p<0.001), as assessed on the UPDRS. Activities of daily living as assessed by the Schwab and England scale were unchanged. Compared with base line, the severity of the disability related to dyskinesia decreased by 65%, and the duration of dyskinesia by 77%. Levodopa requirements also decreased by approximately 40%.

The stimulation parameters as evaluated at 1 and 2 years were 2.5 V±0.81 and 2.9 V±0.82, indicating that the current requirement remains stable over time.

We compared 7 patients >70 years with similarly matched younger patients. The average off-period total UPDRS score before surgery was 102 which improved to 44 at 2 years of follow-up. Similarly, the average requirement of levodopa decreased from 950 mg of LEDD to 530 mg of LEDD. This improvement was comparable to that seen in the younger age group.[13]

Adverse events

There were no deaths. The frequency of haematomas in our entire series has been <2%. In two patients who developed haematoma, one patient had uncontrolled hypertension (bled 12 hours after surgery) and the other had valvular heart disease, in whom it occurred on the third day following anticoagulant treatment.

There were 5 cases of infection, requiring explantation of IPG in four and complete system in one patient. Three electrode placements were not optimal, necessitating revision in one of the patient. Apart from this, there was no long-term morbidity. Two patients developed multiple system atrophy, and in them the improvements were lost following progress of the underlying disease. During the first 3 months after surgery, all patients gained weight (mean 4 kg; maximum 10 kg). Patients on average gained another kilogram within the first year; thereafter, their weight was stable. The improvements over baseline were sustained 4 years after surgery. Tremor and rigidity improved substantially at 1 year and remained stable at 4 years. Akinesia also improved at one year, but this improvement was not completely sustained over time. Painful off-period dystonia disappeared at 4 years in most patients. Four years after surgery, most patients were independent in their activities of daily living when assessed off-medication.

Discussion

The average preoperative UPDRS scores of our patients were higher than that reported in other published literature.[2,6,7-8] This can be attributed to delayed patient referral, hesitancy in undergoing surgical treatment, financial constraints, accessibility to surgical facility, etc. However, the improvement in percentage terms was comparable to that achieved by others.

On-period dyskinesias and the severity of the associated disability substantially decreased at 2 years and remained stable at 4 years. However, on-medication motor signs of PD did not improve after surgery; akinesia, speech, postural stability and freezing of gait all worsened by 4 years. This decline was reflected in a mild deterioration in the scores for activities of daily living in the on-medication state, despite the ongoing reduction in the duration and severity of dyskinesia. The deterioration when the patients were on medication in axial symptoms, including speech, postural stability and freezing of gait, is characteristic of the natural history of PD[6] and has been attributed to the increasing severity of cerebral non-dopaminergic lesions.[7] The effect of levodopa on akinesia, rigidity and tremor tends to remain stable over time,[7] whereas gait, postural stability and dysarthria worsen and become less responsive to levodopa. We reduced the dose of dopaminergic medication during the first 6 months and found it to remain stable up to 4 years. The same was true for the current requirements. They too remained stable over time, barring some individuals who needed increase in their stimulation parameters. We can therefore postulate that tolerance, as seen in thalamic stimulation, does not develop in STN stimulation.

Psychiatric problems, including depression or mania, have been reported by several groups in patients treated with stimulation of the subthalamic nucleus.[14-17] These complications may be related to preexisting psychiatric illness, surgery-related stress, changes in medication, alterations in social life that are associated with improvements in motor function and the mismatch between the final outcome of treatment and the patient's expectations. Changes in the limbic circuit may also contribute to psychiatric problems.[18] We encountered depression in 3 patients following surgery.[16] We attribute it mainly to side-effects related to the stimulation. Hypomania is another psychiatric complication that is known to occur following STN stimulation, though in majority of the cases mania improves following surgery. Frank hypomania or mania was not observed, but hypersexuality was encountered in 2 patients following STN stimulation despite good clinical improvement. We postulate this to stimulation of the limbic part of the subthalamic nucleus, symptoms akin to dopamine dysregulation syndrome or increased dopaminergic stimulation.[19]

We found immediate postoperative confusion in 10% of our patients. In most of these patients it was transient, but in one patient it persisted for a week. Postoperative confusion was more common in older patients. We have recently altered our approach to these patients and we perform MRI scan 2 days before surgery (use FrameLink software to fuse the MRI with stereotactic CT scan) and restrict to two or three trajectories instead of four or five. This has reduced operative time and incidence of confusion.

Although STN stimulation requires very close follow-up of the patient by a clinician experienced with this approach,[20] once a good balance is achieved between the amount of stimulation and dopaminergic treatment, therapeutic adjustments are infrequent, as shown by the stable treatment settings and the low number of complications beyond the first postoperative year. Our findings show that the efficacy of stimulation of the subthalamic nucleus in reducing off-medication motor symptoms and levodopa-induced dyskinesia in patients with severe PD is largely maintained 4 years after surgery. However, over time there is deterioration in akinesia, axial symptoms and cognitive problems that is consistent with the progression of the underlying disease. This deterioration may be more marked in elderly patients. We believe that the surgical option should be explored earlier rather than later. This has been borne out by the study conducted by Agid[11] and his group. However, this should only be undertaken by an experienced team to ensure good results with minimal morbidity. Patients who already have disabling motor signs resistant to levodopa or who have cognitive deterioration are not good candidates for this treatment.

References

1. Lang AE, Lozano AM. Parkinson's disease. *N Engl J Med* 1998;**339**:1044–53.
2. Limousin P, Krack P, Pollak P, *et al.* Electrical stimulation of the subthalamic nucleus in advanced Parkinson's disease. *N Engl J Med* 1998;**339**:1105–11.
3. Krack P, Limousin P, Benabid AL, *et al.* Chronic stimulation of subthalamic nucleus improves levodopa-induced dyskinesias in Parkinson's disease. *Lancet* 1997;**350**:1676.
4. Krack P, Pollak P, Limousin P, *et al.* From off-period dystonia to peak-dose chorea: The clinical spectrum of varying subthalamic nucleus activity. *Brain* 1999;**122**:1133–46.
5. Doshi PK, Chhaya NA, Bhatt MH. Bilateral subthalamic nucleus stimulation for Parkinson's disease. *Neurol India* 2003;**51**:43–8.
6. Markham CH, Diamond SG. Long-term follow-up of early dopa treatment in Parkinson's disease. *Arch Neurol* 1986;**19**:365–72.
7. Bonnet AM, Loria Y, Saint-Hilaire MH, *et al.* Does long-term aggravation of Parkinson's disease result from non-dopaminergic lesions? *Neurology* 1987;**37**:1539–42.
8. Oh MY, Abosch A, Kim SH, *et al.* Long-term hardware-related complications of deep brain stimulation. *Neurosurgery* 2002;**50**:1268–76.
9. Doshi PK, Chhaya NA, Aggarwal A, *et al.* Chronic bilatreral subthalamic nucleus (STN) deep brain stimulation (DBS) for advanced Parkinson's disease (PD)—a four year follow up. *Mov Disord* 2006;**21**:S682.
10. Defer GL, Widner H, Marie RM, Remy P, Levivier M, and conference participants. Core assessment

program for surgical interventional therapies in Parkinson's disease (CAPSIT-PD). *Mov Disord* 1999; **14:**572–84.

11. Schüpbach WM, Maltête D, Houeto JL, *et al.* Neurosurgery at an earlier stage of Parkinson disease: A randomized, controlled trial. *Neurology* 2007;**68:** 267–71.

12. Chhaya NA, Doshi PK, Vaidya SR, *et al.* Two-year follow-up of bilateral subthalamic nucleus stimulation in Parkinson's disease. *Mov Disord* 2004;**19:**S892.

13. Doshi PK, Chhaya NA, Bhatt MH. To compare clinical improvement in young and old Parkinson's disease after STN DBS. *Mov Disord* 2005;**20:**S128.

14. Houeto JL, Mesnage V, Mallet L, *et al.* Behavioural disorders, Parkinson's disease and subthalamic stimulation. *J Neurol Neurosurg Psychiatry* 2002;**72:** 701–7.

15. Romito LM, Raja M, Daniele A, *et al.* Transient mania with hypersexuality after surgery for high frequency stimulation of the subthalamic nucleus in Parkinson's disease. *Mov Disord* 2002;**17:**1371–4.

16. Doshi PK, Chhaya N, Bhatt MH. Depression leading to attempted suicide after bilateral subthalamic nucleus stimulation for Parkinson's disease. *Mov Disord* 2002;**17:**1084–5.

17. Berney A, Vingerhoets F, Perrin A, *et al.* Effect on mood of subthalamic DBS for Parkinson's disease: A consecutive series of 24 patients. *Neurology* 2002;**59:** 1427–9.

18. Funkiewiez A, Ardouin C, Krack P, *et al.* Acute psychotropic effects of bilateral subthalamic nucleus stimulation and Levodopa in Parkinson's disease. *Mov Disord* 2003;**18:**524–30.

19. Doshi PK, Bhargava P. Hypersexuality following Subthalamic Nucleus Stimulation for Parkinson's disease. *Neurology India.* In Press.

20. Krack P, Fraix V, Mendes A, *et al.* Postoperative management of subthalamic nucleus stimulation for Parkinson's disease. *Mov Disord* 2002;**17**(Suppl 3):S188–S197.

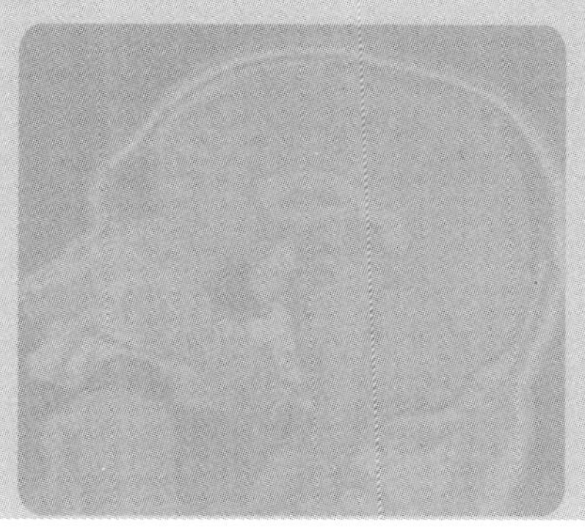

Spine and peripheral nerve surgery

9

Craniovertebral realignment for basilar invagination

ATUL GOEL

The surgical management of congenital cranio-vertebral anomalies is complex due to the relative difficulty in accessing the region, critical relationships of the neurovascular structures and intricate biomechanical issues involved. Basilar invagination forms a prominent component of craniovertebral anomalies. Chiari malformation and syringomyelia are commonly associated with basilar invagination and are the soft tissue components of the dysgenesis. Basilar invagination, a primary developmental anomaly, has been a subject of clinical interest for a long time. Various classical presentations have referred to this issue. Plain radiological and tomographic parameters have been principally used to diagnose basilar invagination for many years.

With the development of high-resolution CT scan and MRI, there has been a renewed interest in the normal anatomy and pathological lesions of the craniovertebral junction. Improved imaging has provided the opportunity to clearly observe the bony abnormality and the distorted neural and vascular relationships. Dynamic MRI and CT scan have helped in evaluating the pathology of basilar invagination, assessing the biomechanics of the joints and formulating a rational surgical strategy. Despite the clarity of imaging, controversy regarding the management of basilar invagination continues. Till date, the natural history has not been clearly elucidated in the literature. The surgical indications for a given approach are still under discussion.

In 1997, we presented a classification system for basilar invagination that divided it into two categories based on the presence or absence of Chiari malformation. This classification helped in improving the understanding of the pathology and pathogenesis of the anomaly, selecting the appropriate surgical treatment and predicting the outcome.[1,2]

With our improved understanding of the subject, we reclassified basilar invagination into two groups, based on parameters that determined an alternative treatment strategy. In group A basilar invagination, there was a 'fixed' atlantoaxial dislocation and the tip of the odontoid process 'invaginated' into the foramen magnum and was above the Chamberlain line,[3] McRae line of the foramen magnum[4] and Wackenheim clival line.[5] The definition of basilar invagination suggested by von Torklus as prolapse of the cervical spine into the base of the skull[6] was suitable for this group of patients. In group B basilar invagination, the alignment of the odontoid process and clivus remained normal despite the presence of basilar invagination and other associated anomalies. In this group, the tip of the odontoid process was above the Chamberlain line but below the McRae and Wackenheim lines. Essentially, in group A basilar invagination, there was an element of instability in the region that was manifested by the tip of the odontoid process distancing itself from the anterior arch of the atlas or the lower end of the clivus. In this group, the atlantoaxial joints were 'active' and the orientation was oblique as shown in the figure (Fig 1, 5b), instead of the normal horizontal orientation. We have found similarities with such a position of the C1–C2 facets with that seen in patients with spondylolisthesis in the subaxial spine. In group B, the atlantoaxial joints were either fused or normally aligned.

We recently studied the treatment of group A basilar invagination, and discussed the feasibility of manipulation and distraction of the facets of the atlas and axis to reduce the basilar invagination and fix the atlantoaxial joint.[7–10] Our current experience with the technique in over 180 cases convinces us that distraction and direct

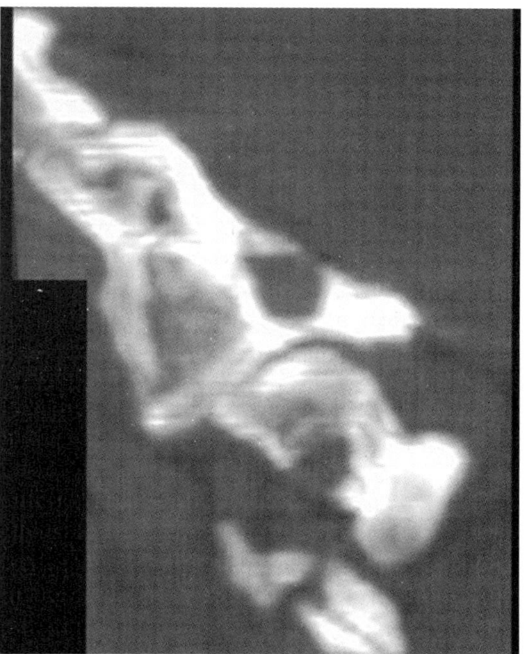

Fig. 1. CT scan showing listhesis of the C1 facet over the C2 facet. This listhesis of C1 over C2 is probably the cause of basilar invagination.

lateral mass fixation of the atlantoaxial joint is the ideal form of treatment in cases with group A basilar invagination, and transoral surgery can be entirely avoided. The technique resulted in realignment of the facets in the horizontal position and results in realignment of the entire craniovertebral junction as well as the rest of the spine.

The majority of patients with group A basilar invagination (104 patients, 58%) had a history of minor to major head injury prior to the onset of the symptoms. Pyramidal symptoms formed a dominant component. Kinaesthetic sensations were affected in 99 patients (55%). Spinothalamic dysfunction was less frequent (65 patients, 36%). Neck pain as a major presenting symptom was seen in 139 patients (77%). Torticollis was present in 74 patients (41%). Analysis of the radiological and clinical features suggested that the symptoms and signs were a result of brainstem compression by the odontoid process.

The radiological findings suggested that the odontoid process resulted in direct compression of the brainstem. Analysis on the basis of the Chamberlain line and on the distance from the odontoid tip to the pontomedullary junction showed that basilar invagination was only mild or moderate in these cases. Modified omega angle measurements suggested that the odontoid process had tilted horizontally rather than rostrally.[1]

Lateral mass atlantoaxial fixation and joint distraction for group A basilar invagination

The standard and most accepted form of treatment for group A basilar invagination is a transoral decompression.[1,7,11] Most authors recommend a posterior occipitocervical fixation following anterior decompression. It appears to us that the atlantoaxial joint in such cases is in an abnormal position as a result of a congenital abnormality of the bones, and progressive worsening of the dislocation is probably second-ary to increasing 'slippage' of the facets of the atlas over those of the axis. Slippage of the atlas over the axis appears to be aggravated by trauma. With our experience in handling the atlantoaxial joint, we have realized that the joint in these cases is not 'fixed' or 'fused', but is mobile and in some cases hypermobile, and this is probably the prime cause for the basilar invagination. A history of trauma preceding the clinical events, the predomi-nant complaint of pain in the neck and improve-ment in neurological symptoms following institution of cervical traction suggests 'vertical' instability of the craniovertebral region.

We had earlier attempted to reduce basilar invagination by performing occipitocervical fixation following cervical traction.[1,11] However, all the four cases treated in this manner subse-quently needed transoral decompression as reduction of the basilar invagination and atlantoaxial dislocation could not be sustained by the implant. Wide removal of the atlantoaxial joint capsule and articular cartilage by drilling, and subsequent distraction of the joint by manual manipulation provided a unique oppor-tunity to reduce the basilar invagination and atlantoaxial dislocation. Maintenance of the joint in a distracted and reduced position with the help of a bone graft with or without the assistance of hydroxyapatite or metal spacers, and subsequent fixation of the joint with the help of interarticular screws and a metal plate provided a biomech-anically firm fixation and sustained distraction. The fixation was seen to be strong enough to sustain vertical, transverse and rotatory strains of the most mobile region of the spine.

Following surgery, alignment of the odontoid process and clivus as well as the entire cranio-vertebral junction improved towards normalcy. The tip of the odontoid process receded in relationship to the Wackenheim clival line, Chamberlain line and McRae line, suggesting reduction in the basilar invagination. The posterior tilt of the odontoid process, as evaluated by modified omega angle, was reduced after the surgery.[1,12] We could obtain varying degrees of reduction of the basilar invagination and atlantoaxial dislocation. The extent of distraction of the joint and subsequent reduction in basilar invagination was more significant in younger than in older patients. In addition to the odontoid process changing its angulation, the angulation of the clivus also returned towards normalcy, suggesting that the entire cranio-vertebral junction and cervical spine were realigned by the procedure.

As a significant number of cases with group A basilar invagination had an occipitalized or assimilated atlas, dissection and exposure of the facet of the fused atlas was significantly more difficult and tedious. Use of an operating micro-scope and neuronavigation techniques helped to enhance the safety of the procedure. All patients had sustained neurological improve-ment to varying degrees, suggesting that the operation had been effective. The extent of neurological improvement observed by us after using the technique described appeared to be far more satisfactory and sustained when compared with the improvement obtained after a transoral surgery and subsequent occipitocervical fixation. All patients with a preoperative torticollis showed improvement of this symptom, although no deliberate differential manipulation of the joints on the two sides was carried out. Resection of the C2 ganglion is necessary to achieve exposure. In our present experience and that reported by us earlier, we have observed that resection of the C2 ganglion results in an area of numbness along the distribution of the nerve.[13,14] However, the area of numbness progressively reduces in size over the years and was not seen to be a disabling feature by any of the patients. All activities related to neck movements were restricted for a three-month period to provide an opportunity for bone fusion in the joint. Stainless steel plates, non-locking screws and custom-made titanium spacers were used. Over time, we have modified the quality and shape of the spacer. Inclusion of spikes on the surface of the spacer has made it stronger and given it more teeth.

Surgical experience and technique of intraoperative joint distraction and reduction of fixed atlantoaxial dislocation

All 180 patients underwent joint manipulation surgery (Figs 2, 4–6). No patient underwent a transoral decompression as a first-stage operation. The basic surgical steps of the joint manipulation surgery are the same as discussed in our papers on lateral mass plate and screw fixation of the atlantoaxial joint.[7–9,13,14] Cervical traction is given prior to induction of anaesthesia and the weights are progressively increased to approximately one-fifth of the total body weight. The patient is placed prone with the head end of the table elevated to about 35 degrees. Use of the operating microscope and neuronavigation assistance facilitate the dissection and add safety to the screw implantation. The atlantoaxial facet joints are widely exposed on both sides after sectioning the large C2 ganglion. In a number of our patients, exposure of the facet of the atlas was markedly difficult as there was assimilation of the atlas resulting in a rostrally located C1 facet. The joint capsule is excised and the articular cartilage is widely removed using a micro drill. The joints on both sides are distracted by means of an intervertebral spreader used in anterior cervical disc surgery. The status of the dislocation and basilar invagination is evaluated by intraoperative radiographic control. Small pieces of cortico-cancellous bone graft harvested from the iliac crest is stuffed into the joint. A specially designed titanium spacer or hydroxyapatite blocks are used in selected cases as a strut graft and stuffed into the joints to provide additional distraction and stability to the joint (Figs 2–6). Plate and screw fixation of the region is subsequently carried out by the interarticular technique. A two-holed stainless steel plate measuring 15–20 mm in length is used. The screws are 2.4–2.6 mm in diameter and 16–22 mm in length. The screws are passed bilaterally through the holes in the plate into the lateral mass of the atlas and axis (Figs 2, 4–6). In cases where due to anatomical limitation or surgical technique the lateral mass

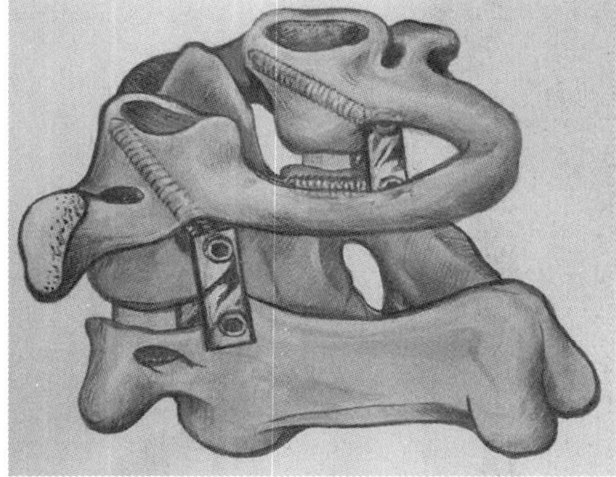

Fig. 2. Plates and screws used for atlantoaxial fixation

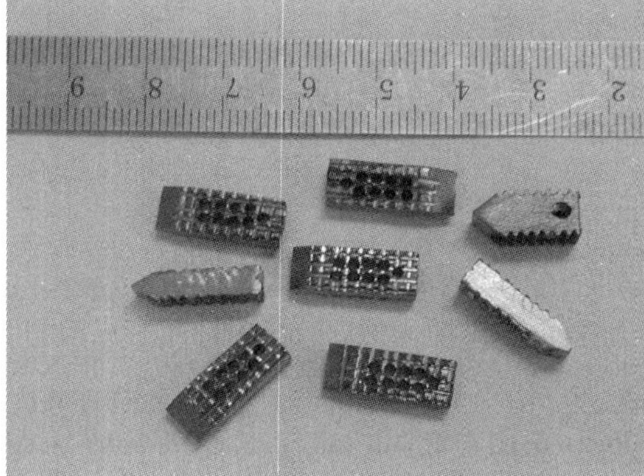

Fig. 3. Variety of titanium spacers used for distraction

plating cannot be completed, a C1–C2 transarticular screw fixation method described by Magerl[15] or an occipitoaxial fixation described by us[11,14] is done (Fig. 2). The point of entry and the direction of the screw for the transarticular fixation are altered to suit the complex local anatomy in these cases and done under direct vision. Additional bone grafts are placed between the posterior elements of C1 and C2 after decorticating the host bone area with a burr. Postoperatively, traction is discontinued and the patient is placed in a four-post hard cervical collar for three months and all physical activities involving the neck are restrained during this period.

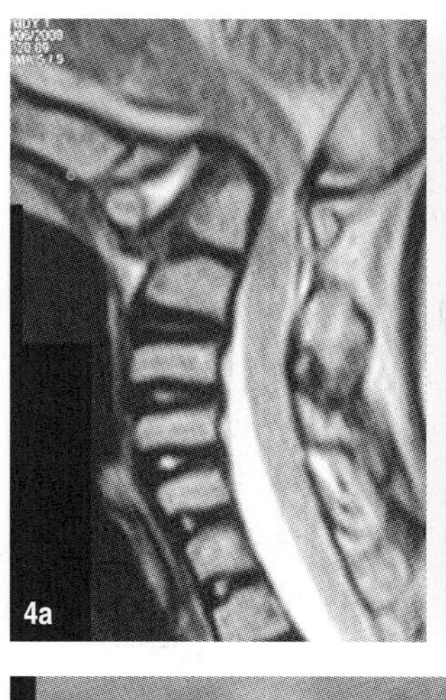

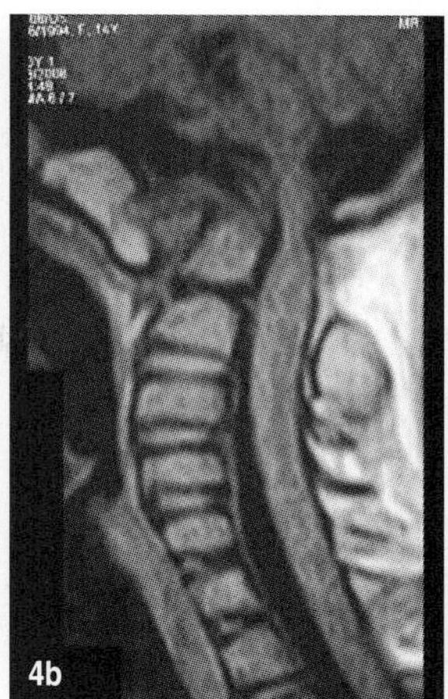

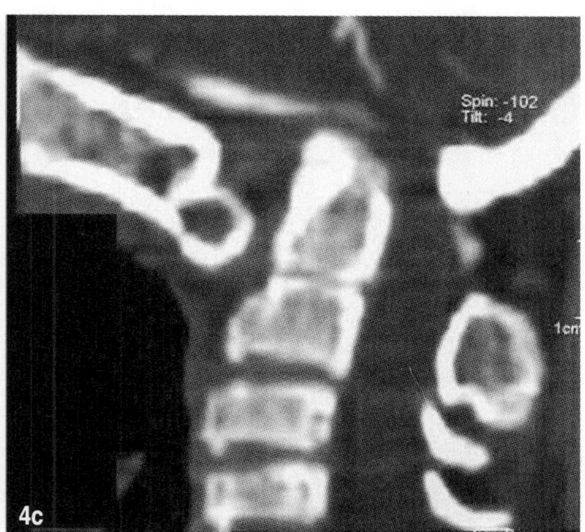

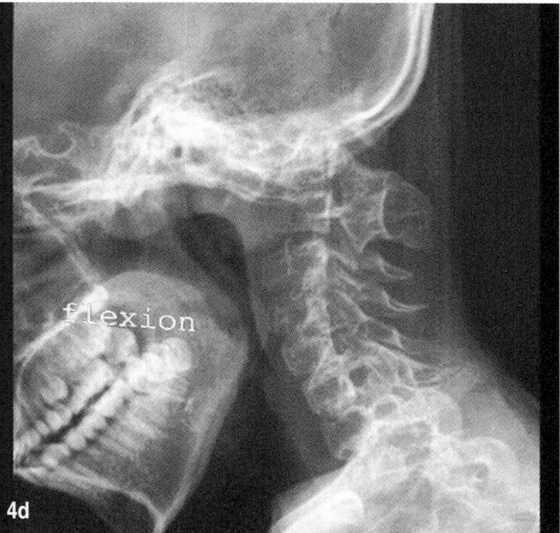

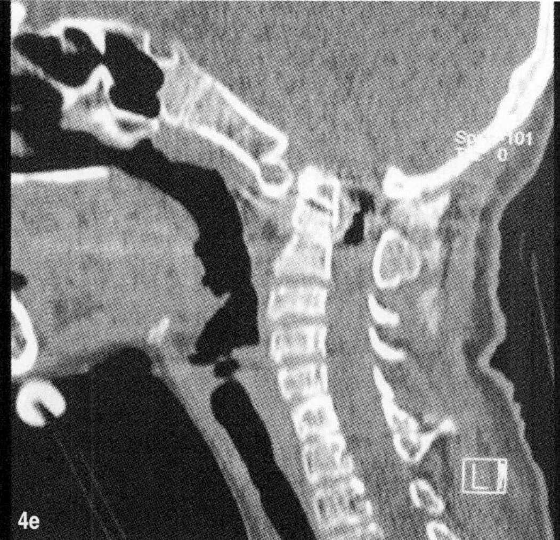

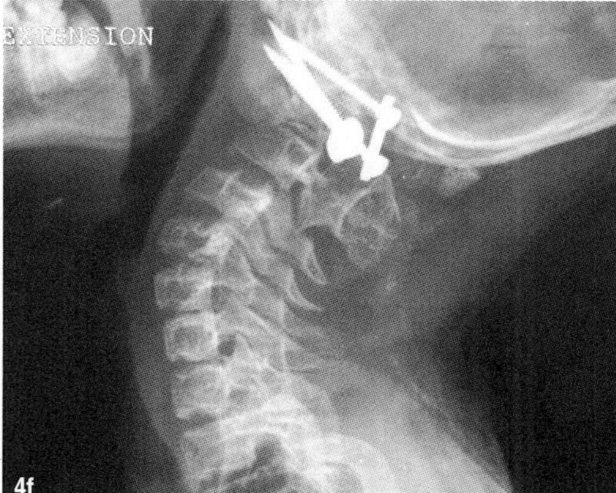

Fig. 4a. T2-weighted MRI of an eleven-year-old girl showing basilar invagination

Fig. 4b. T1-weighted MRI

Fig. 4c. CT scan showing basilar invagination, partial assimilation of the atlas and C2–C3 fusion

Fig. 4d. Lateral X-ray in flexion

Fig. 4e. Postoperative CT scan. Please note the craniovertebral and cervical spinal realignment.

Fig. 4f. Postoperative X-ray with the neck in extension. Please note the recovery in posterior cervical lordosis and neck size.

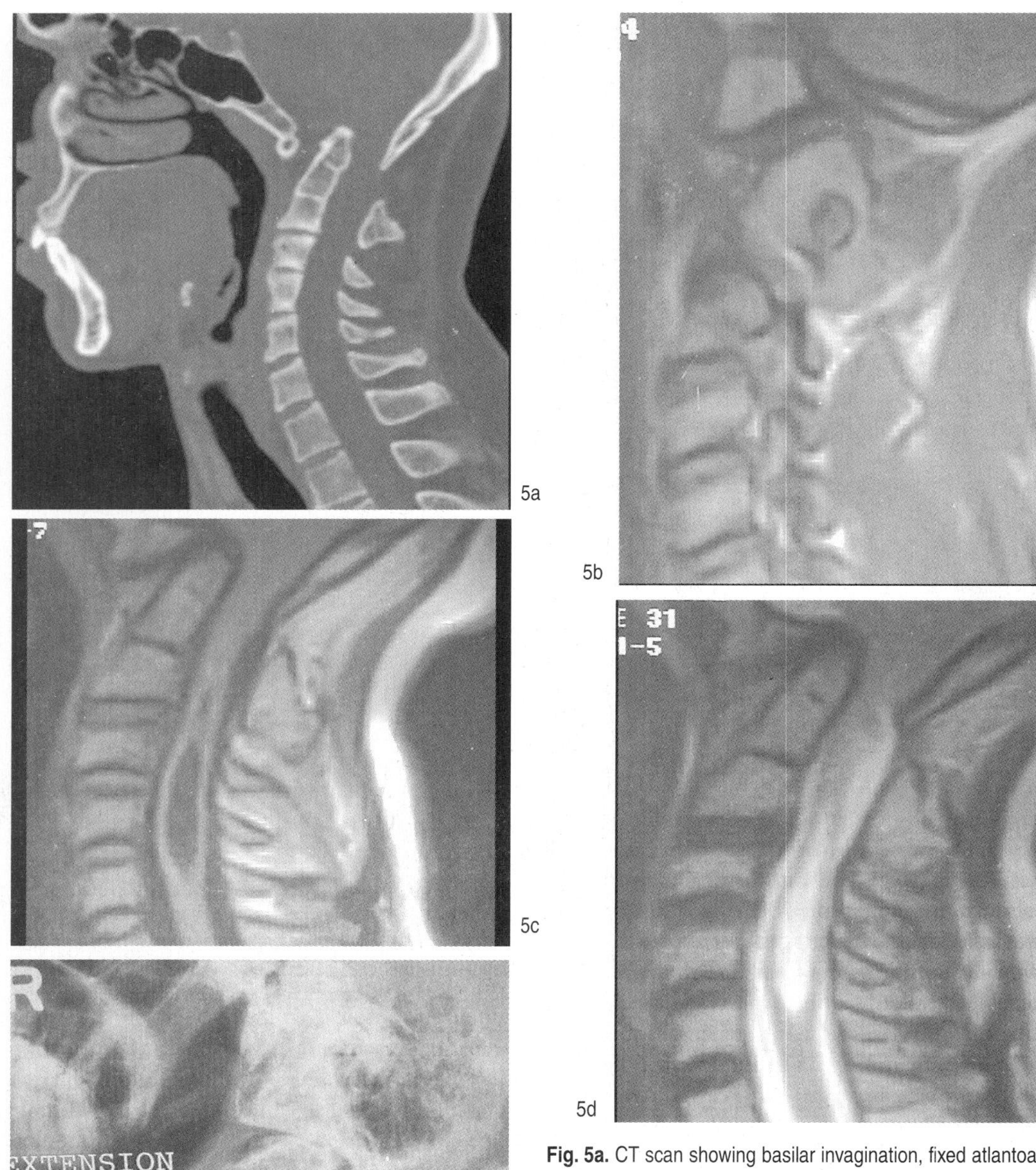

Fig. 5a. CT scan showing basilar invagination, fixed atlantoaxial dislocation and assimilation of the atlas

Fig. 5b. Sagittal CT scan cut through the joint showing the oblique angulation of the facets of the atlantoaxial joint

Fig. 5c. T1-weighted MRI showing basilar invagination, Chiari 1 malformation and syringomyelia

Fig. 5d. T2-weighted MRI

Fig. 5e. X-ray showing the craniovertebral junction

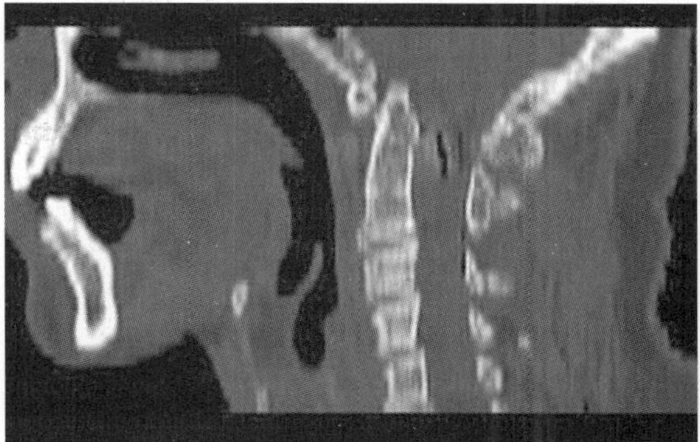

Fig. 5f. Postoperative CT scan showing reduction of basilar invagination

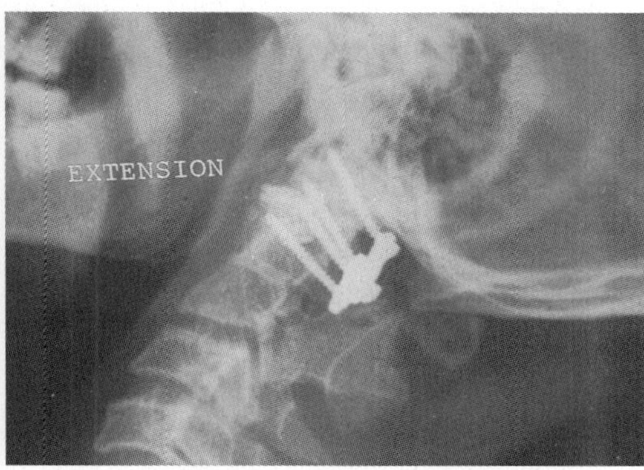

Fig. 5g. Postoperative X-ray showing fixation

Fig. 5f. CT scan cut through the joint showing the realignment of the facets and placement of the spacer within the joint and distraction

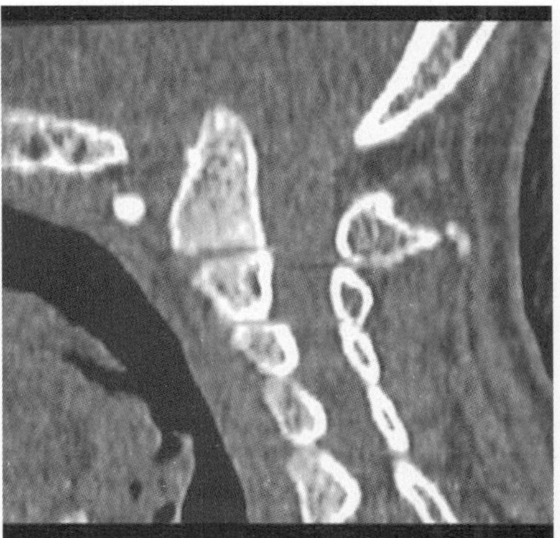

Fig. 6a. Preoperative CT scan showing basilar invagination

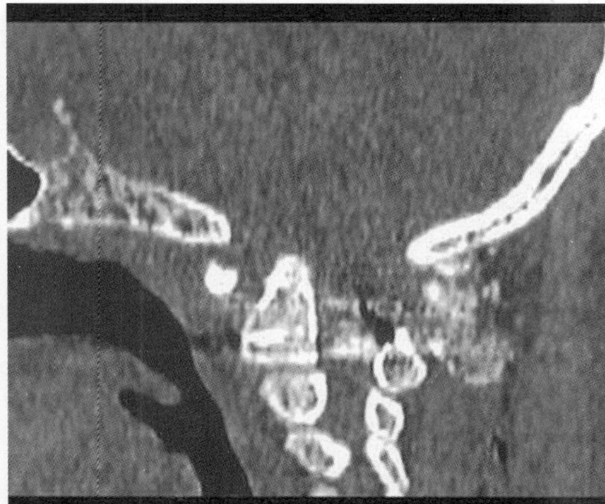

Fig. 6b. Postoperative CT scan showing reduction of the basilar invagination

Surgical issues

Exposure of the atlantoaxial joint in cases with basilar invagination is considerably more difficult and technically challenging when compared with a normally aligned atlantoaxial joint encountered during the treatment of post-traumatic instability. The joint is markedly rostral in location and the microscope needs to be appropriately angled. Due to the bony abnormalities in the region and frequently encountered rotation, orientation can easily be lost. The presence of occipitalization of the atlas can lead to an anomalous course of the vertebral artery over the posterior surface of the facet of the atlas, leading to considerable difficulty in dissection. In cases where there is injury to the vertebral artery during dissection, control of bleeding can become difficult. Temporary clip application and direct suturing of the artery can be attempted. However, in cases where such suturing is not possible, coagulation and sacrifice of the artery appears to be a reasonable and apparently safe option. If there is a suspicion of vertebral artery injury during the screw insertion procedure, the bleeding should be stopped with bone wax and an alternative site for insertion selected. However, screw insertion might even be completed through the same hole. The pedicle of C2 forms an important landmark for dissection and can suggest the location of the vertebral artery. Dissection and subsequent resection of the C2 ganglion should be done under direct vision as, on rare occasions, the vertebral artery can traverse parallel to the course of the ganglion. Appropriate drilling of the bones that hinder exposure can provide a suitable view of the region. Frequently, venous bleeding can be troublesome.

Results of surgery

Clinical neurological improvement varies but, in most cases, it is remarkable and satisfying. Despite the complex and deformed nature of the anomalies encountered in the series, there were no postoperative vascular, neurological or infective complications. In 3 out of 180 operated cases, reduction of the basilar invagination was not entirely satisfactory and a delayed transoral surgery was performed to decompress the region. No patient needed a re-exploration for failure of fixation of the implant. Immediate postoperative and follow-up radiographs confirmed fixation and fusion, and reduction of the basilar invagination. Torticollis improved significantly following surgery in all patients (Fig. 1). No patient complained of numbness in the suboccipital region, but on being asked a leading question, agreed that they had a patch of suboccipital numbness.

Basilar invagination group A associated with syringomyelia: Treatment by lateral mass distraction surgery

We had classified syringomyelia into three groups and suggested a specific treatment protocol on the basis of the possible pathogenetic factors.[16] In this study, we had suggested that syringomyelia is a tertiary response to a primary craniovertebral anomaly in the form of basilar invagination and secondary Chiari 1 malformation, a result of reduction in volume of the posterior cranial fossa. Accordingly, a posterior fossa bony decompression was considered the optimum treatment in this subgroup of patients. We identified cases of syringomyelia where there were associated bony abnormalities of the craniovertebral region, which included 'fixed' atlanto-axial dislocation or those having group A basilar invagination. In some of these cases, there was associated Chiari 1 malformation. This select group of patients was treated by attempts to reduce the atlantoaxial dislocation and basilar invagination, and direct lateral mass plate and screw atlantoaxial fixation according to the techniques described by us.[8] No bony or dural decompression or neural manipulation of any kind was done in these cases.

The complex of basilar invagination, Chiari 1 malformation and syringomyelia is relatively common and there are multiple reports on the subject. Such cases are generally treated by either anterior transoral or posterior foramen magnum bony decompression. The indications and need for opening the dura and manipulating the arachnoid membrane, tonsils and obex, and draining the syrinx cavity are currently under debate. There are no reports in the literature identifying the need for a specific fixation procedure for cases of fixed atlantoaxial dislocation where it is associated with basilar invagination in the presence of syringomyelia.

The majority of patients with Chiari malformation-related syringomyelia without any bony anomaly of the craniovertebral region have hyporeflexia of the upper extremities and spastic lower extremities. The presence of spastic quadriparesis in all our patients suggests that the symptoms were related to compression of the brainstem from the invaginated dens rather than due to syringomyelia. It was observed that the patients were relatively young, neck pain formed a part of the symptom complex, and motor symptoms and ataxia were far more prominent symptoms in cases with the complex of malformations that included group A basilar invagination, Chiari 1 malformation and syringomyelia than in cases with a similar complex but without bony anomalies of the craniovertebral region. It appears that when the angulation of the facets is not as acute or is only marginally affected, the progress of basilar invagination is slow and takes place over several years, providing an opportunity for the syrinx to develop relentlessly.

It was observed that in cases of syringomyelia where there was 'fixed' atlantoaxial dislocation with or without the association of group A basilar invagination and Chiari malformation, an attempt could be made to realign the bones in the craniovertebral junction. Our technique of reduction of fixed atlantoaxial dislocation, and distraction and reduction of basilar invagination could be used effectively in such a situation.[7] As observed by us earlier.[8] It appears that the atlantoaxial joint in such cases is in an abnormal position as a result of a congenital abnormality of the bones, and progressive worsening of the dislocation is probably secondary to increasing 'slippage' of the atlas over the axis. As there was remarkable clinical improvement following reduction of the atlantoaxial dislocation and basilar invagination, it appears that the complex of atlantoaxial dislocation, basilar invagination and syringomyelia are probably secondary to the primary craniovertebral instability. The basilar invagination in group A cases with associated syringomyelia was less severe and symptoms were longer-standing than in cases where there was no syringomyelia. The conduct of surgery and joint manipulation was relatively easier in these cases.

Following surgery, alignment of the odontoid process and clivus, and the entire craniovertebral junction improved towards normalcy. We could reduce the basilar invagination and atlantoaxial dislocation to varying degrees. The atlantoaxial alignments changed towards normalcy and the tip of the odontoid process receded in relationship to the Wackenheim clival line and Chamberlain line, suggesting a reduction in the basilar invagination and atlantoaxial dislocation. The posterior tilt of the odontoid process, as evaluated by modified omega angle, was reduced after the surgery.[1,7] All patients had a sustained neurological improvement to varying degrees, suggesting the effectiveness of the operation. Stainless steel plates, non-locking screws and custom-made spacers were used due to the higher costs of branded material. Due to the type of metal used in the procedure, the effect on syringomyelia could not be confirmed.

Conclusion

With our current experience with the described technique, our results are promising and encourage us to undertake further study on the subject. The procedure is technically demanding and anatomically precise, but if learned adequately and performed successfully, the neurological outcome is extremely gratifying.

References

1. Goel A, Bhatjiwale M, Desai K. Basilar invagination: A study based on 190 surgically treated cases. *J Neurosurg* 1998;**88**:962–8.
2. Chiari H. Ueber Verderbungen des Kleinhirns infolge von Hydrocephalie des Grossihirns. *Dwochenschr* 1891;**17**:1172–5.
3. Chamberlain WE. Basilar impression (platybasia). A bizarre developmental anomaly of the occipital bone and upper cervical spine with striking and misleading neurologic manifestations. *Yale J Biol Med* 1939;**11**:487–96.
4. McRae DL. Bony abnormalities in the region of foramen magnum: Correlation of anatomic and neurologic findings. *Acta Radiol* 1953;**40**:335–54.
5. Thiebaut F, Wackenheim A, Vrousos C. [New median sagittal pneumostratigraphical findings concerning the posterior fossa]. *J Radiol Electrol* 1961;**42**:1–7 (Fre).
6. Von Torklus D, Gehle W. The upper cervical spine: Regional anatomy, pathology, and traumatology. In: *A systematic radiological atlas and textbook.* New York: Grune and Stratton, 1972:1–98.
7. Goel A. Treatment of basilar invagination by atlantoaxial joint distraction and direct lateral mass fixation. *J Neurosurg Spine* 2004;**1**:281–6.
8. Goel A, Sharma P. Craniovertebral junction realignment for the treatment of basilar invagination with syringomyelia: Preliminary report of 12 cases. *Neurol Med Chir (Tokyo)* 2005;**45**:512–18.
9. Goel A, Kulkarni AG, Sharma P. Reduction of fixed atlantoaxial dislocation in 24 cases: Technical note. *J Neurosurg Spine* 2005;**2**:505–9.
10. Goel A. Progressive basilar invagination after trans-oral odontoidectomy: Treatment by facet distraction and craniovertebral realignment. *Spine* 2005;**30**: E551–5.
11. Goel A, Achawal S. Surgical treatment for Arnold Chiari malformation associated with atlantoaxial dislocation. *Br J Neurosurg* 1995;**9**:67–72.
12. Klaus E. Rontgendiagnostik der platybasic und basilar impression. *Fortschr Rontgenstr* 1957;**86**:460–9.
13. Goel A, Desai K, Muzumdar D. Atlantoaxial fixation using plate and screw method: A report of 160 treated patients. *Neurosurgery* 2002;**51**:1351–7.
14. Goel A, Laheri VK. Plate and screw fixation for atlanto-axial dislocation. (Technical report). *Acta Neurochir (Wien)* 1994;**129**:47–53.
15. Grob D, Magerl F. Operative stabilisierung bei fraketuren von C1 und C2. *Orthopade* 1987;**16**:46–54.
16. Goel A, Desai KI. Surgery for syringomyelia: An analysis based on 163 surgical cases. *Acta Neurochir (Wien)* 2000;**142**:293–302.

10

Multisegmental cervical oblique corpectomy

ARI G. CHACKO, ROY T. DANIEL, MATHEW JOSEPH, VIVEK B. JOSEPH

Two main approaches, either anterior or posterior, have been used to treat cervical cord compression due to spondylotic disease or ossified posterior longitudinal ligament (OPLL). Discectomy and central corpectomy with grafting have been widely used through the anterior approach, with or without anterior plating. From the posterior route, a cervical laminectomy, with or without lateral mass screws/rods, has been performed. The choice between the anterior or posterior route depends on the location of the compressive pathology, the curvature of the spine, the presence of instability and the number of pathological levels.

Since 1992, George *et al.* have developed and perfected the technique of oblique corpectomy through a lateral cervical approach as an alternative to central corpectomy.[1]

Since 2001, following a detailed cadaver dissection to familiarize ourselves with the anatomy and with the surgical technique, we have been applying oblique corpectomy in the management of cervical myelopathy due to spondylotic disease or OPLL. In this chapter, we describe the operative procedure and explain the preoperative selection criteria, biomechanical effects and clinical results.

Principle of oblique corpectomy

The technique of oblique corpectomy allows for a wide decompression of the spinal canal through an anterolateral approach, preserving a significant buttress of vertebral body and disc ventrally. This column of body and disc preserves the stability of the spine, obviating the need for a graft, and also preserves spinal motion. These are the two most important advantages that this technique has over the central corpectomy with grafting. On the other hand, the technique is demanding since it implies working in the vicinity of the vertebral artery (VA). It is thus essential to gain a good knowledge of the anatomy of the VA through a study of the preoperative images. The most frequent complication is Horner syndrome since the sympathetic chain lies directly on the longus colli muscle.

Preoperative selection criteria

The most recognized indications for an anterior decompression of the cervical spine are the presence of anterior osteophytic spurs or OPLL, irrespective of the spinal curvature. Cervical laminectomy/laminoplasty is best reserved for long segments of anterior/posterior compression in the presence of a lordotic spine. Preoperative instability is a contraindication to the procedure and can be determined by dynamic X-rays. Cervical kyphosis is not a contraindication if instability has been ruled out by dynamic X-rays. Disseminated idiopathic skeletal hyperostosis associated with both ossified anterior longitudinal ligament (OALL) and OPLL is ideally treated by an oblique corpectomy as the OALL, if asymptomatic, can be left alone with the anterolateral approach.[2]

Operative procedure

Cervical dissection

The patient is placed in a supine position with his head on a ring, extended and turned slightly to the contralateral side, and a small pillow is placed under the shoulders. A longitudinal skin incision is made along the anterior border of the sternocleidomastoid muscle. The length of the incision depends on the number of vertebral levels to be exposed. The platysma is divided along the skin incision and the deep fascia incised. The carotid sheath is retracted medially and dissection continued along the sternomastoid muscle, until a pad of fat is seen lateral to the jugular vein. Above the C3–C4 level, care must be taken to identify the spinal accessory nerve that runs obliquely across the deep surface of the sternomastoid muscle. The fat is incised and using this plane, the entire carotid sheath is retracted to the midline. The transverse processes of the cervical vertebrae are identified with a finger—the C6 transverse process is the lowest that can be palpated. Under the aponeurosis of the longus colli muscle lies the sympathetic chain. The aponeurosis is incised longitudinally and generally the sympathetic chain is retracted medially; but on occasion, when it is situated far laterally, it is retracted laterally. A self-retaining retractor is placed.

Locating the position of the vertebral artery

The next step is to use the image intensifier to confirm the vertebral level before incising the longus colli. To avoid damaging the VA, the longus colli muscle should be divided transversely over the transverse process. The VA lies unprotected between two consecutive vertebrae, but is protected above C6 in the foramen transversarium by the costotransverse bar of the transverse process. Variations in the level at which the VA enters the foramen transversarium can be detected with the help of the preoperative MRI. In 2%–5% of cases, the VA may enter the foramen transversarium at a level higher than C6 and is liable to damage as it may lie superficial to or within the longus colli muscle. The longus colli muscle is cauterized and cut directly on the transverse process at each level of the pathological process. It is then excised from the medial border of the vertebral bodies.

Oblique corpectomy

The initial step is to define the lateral limit of the corpectomy with the help of a microscope and diamond drill. The costotransverse bar is drilled down to the periosteum and this marks the position of the VA. The costotransverse bar joins the vertebral body at the uncovertebral joint. An 8 mm cutting burr is then used to make a vertical trough down to the posterior longitudinal ligament (PLL) at the uncovertebral joint and on either side of the disc space, leaving about 3 mm of cortical bone to protect the VA laterally. The drilling is continued along the entire craniocaudal extent of the corpectomy. The disc material encountered along this vertical trough is usually torn away with the sharp cutting burr. When the posterior cortical bone and PLL are reached, the microscope is repositioned to obtain an oblique view across to the contralateral side of the spinal canal. The operating table may need to be raised to obtain this oblique view. Using a smaller cutting burr, drilling is then continued from the posterior cortical margin to the contralateral side. This ensures that a minimum of ventral vertebral body is removed. It can be difficult to determine when to stop drilling on the contralateral side, as there are no obvious landmarks. A rough idea of the distance to be drilled may be obtained by measuring the distance between the ipsilateral vertebral artery and the junction of the contra-lateral pedicle with the OPLL or posterior cortical margin on the preoperative MRI. The drilling to the contralateral side is best completed before opening the PLL, as the latter can bulge into and obscure the operative field.

Posterior longitudinal ligament resection

The PLL is opened with a sharp hook or a Karlin knife and then excised using Kerrison rongeurs. In OPLL, since the dura may be involved in the ossification process, care should be taken not to be too aggressive while removing the PLL. At the end of the surgery, the spinal cord is well decompressed. Particular attention needs to be paid to the epidural venous plexus while achiev-ing haemostasis and in this regard the use of surgical is beneficial. A tube drain is left *in situ* in the depth of the field on the ventral aspect of the vertebral bodies. The deep fascia is closed with 2-0 absorbable suture, the platysma with 3-0 absorbable suture and the skin with 4-0 subcuticular suture. Postoperatively, the patient is mobilized the same day and allowed to go home after 2–3 days.

Clinical results

Between 2001 and 2005, we operated on 116 patients with myelopathy due to cervical spondylo-tic disease. Their mean age was 50±10.7 years (range 18–82 years); there were 100 men and 16 women. Their preoperative symptomatology and functional Nurick grade are shown in Tables 1 and 2, respectively. Forty-four patients had a single-level corpectomy, 52 had a two-level corpectomy and 20 had a three-level corpectomy. Follow-up was obtained in 68 cases (58%), with a mean follow-up of 18 months. The improve-ment in the Nurick grade is shown in Table 3.

Figure 1 shows the substantial decompression achieved by a three-level oblique corpectomy as seen in the MRI taken on 2 years' follow-up. There was an overall improvement in 52% of the patients, while 45% remained the same. There was an improvement in the Nurick grade of a

Table 1. Clinical presentation in 116 patients

Clinical feature	*n*	(%)
Radicular pain	18	(16)
Paresthesias	95	(82)
Bladder problems	52	(45)
Gait difficulty	116	(100)
Posterior column signs	75	(65)

Table 2. Preoperative Nurick grade in 116 patients

Nurick grade	*n*	(%)
I	2	(1.7)
II	7	(6.0)
III	67	(57.7)
IV	51	(43.9)
V	18	(15.5)

Table 3. Comparison of the Nurick grade preoperatively and postoperatively in 67 patients for whom at least 6 months follow-up was available

Nurick grade	Postoperative				
	I	II	III	IV	V
Preoperative I					
II	2	3		1	
III	2	15	11	1	
IV		4	7	11	
V	1	2	1	1	5

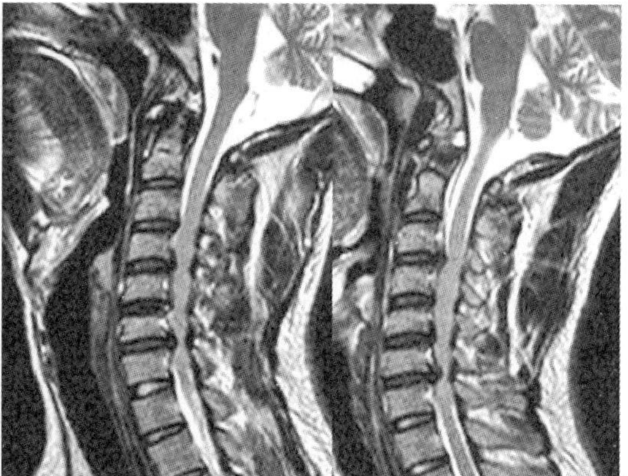

Fig. 1a. Sagittal T2-w MRI of the cervical spine showing multiple anterior indentations of the ventral subarachnoid space with cord compression at the C3–C4; C4–C5; C5–C6 and the C6–C7 levels. Note the posterior compression from the buckling of the ligament flavum at each of these levels.

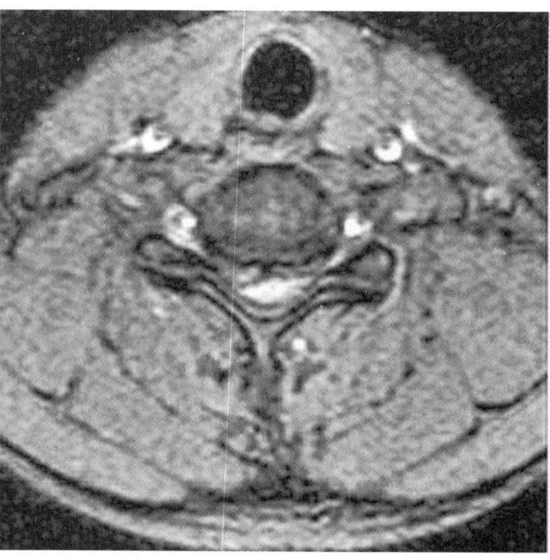

Fig. 1b. Axial T2-w MRI of the cervical spine showing marked compression of the cervical cord primarily from ventrally.

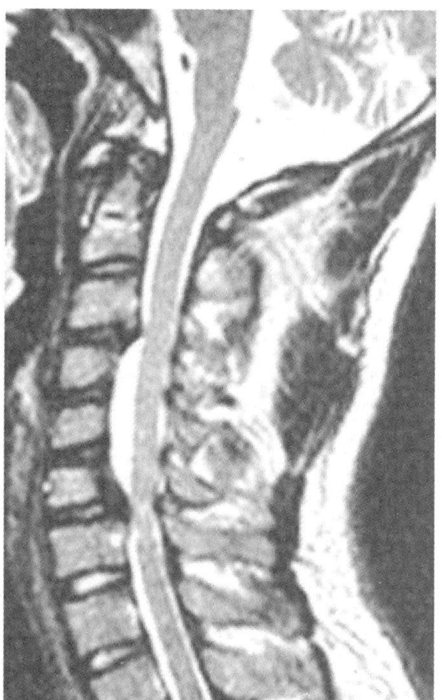

Fig. 1c. 2-year postoperative sagittal T2-w MRI of the same patient following the three-level C4–C5–C6 oblique corpectomy. Note the ventral decompression, preservation of cervical lordosis and reduction of the posterior compression probably due to ventral movement of the cord.

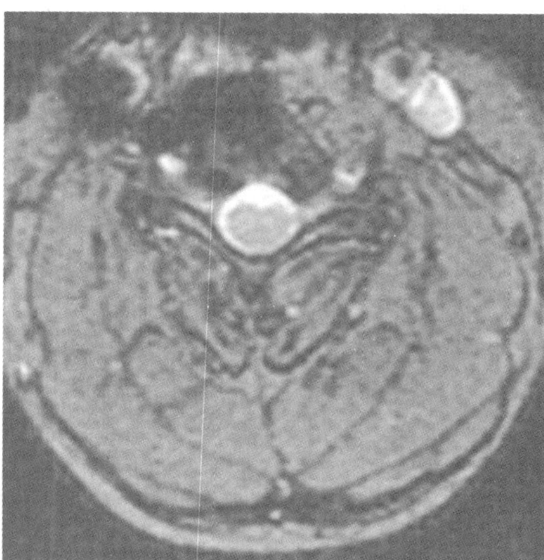

Fig. 1d. Axial T2-w image at the C4–C5 level showing the substantial ventral decompression through the oblique corpectomy.

significant number of patients in grades IV and V. A patient who improved from grade V to grade I had a large extruded soft disc that had migrated behind the body of C5. Two patients had VA injuries in the early part of the series—one was asymptomatic, while the other developed a lateral medullary syndrome. Temporary Horner syndrome was seen in 37% of patients, the majority of whom improved, and permanent Horner syndrome was seen in 9%. Two patients worsened in the immediate postoperative period—one from grade III to grade IV and the other from grade II to grade IV. One of these patients had a wound haematoma that required evacuation, following which he improved to grade III. In the case of 5 patients, the follow-up X-rays showed an asymptomatic kyphosis that did not require any intervention.

Discussion

Cervical spondylotic myelopathy (CSM) is a degenerative disease that results in neck pain, upper and lower limb numbness, paresthesiae and stiffness, gait difficulties and bladder dysfunction. The treatment options for CSM include immobilization of the neck, physiotherapy and surgical decompression of the spinal cord, with or without fusion. A Cochrane review that analysed two trials comparing surgery and conservative therapy for CSM found that surgery was superior in the short term for relief from pain, weakness or sensory loss. However, at one year, there was no difference between the surgically treated group and the conservatively treated group.[3] Conservative treatment for CSM is considered to be effective if it is performed intensively in selected patients and timely surgical intervention is carried out if the symptoms show no change or neurological worsening occurs.[4] Historically, multilevel cervical laminectomies without fusion were the earliest form of surgical treatment to be advocated. The results were often poor and neurological deterioration occurred either immediately or later due to progressive kyphosis.[5] It appears that cervical laminectomy may be considered when the spine is lordotic and the compressive element extends over several segments.[6,7] Some authors have recently revived the use of cervical laminectomy with concurrent fusion, using lateral mass plates[8] and performing skip laminectomies to reduce the extent of bone removal.[9]

Laminoplasty techniques are posterior decompressive procedures that involve widening the canal by elevating the laminae and maintaining their new position with the help of spacers. Since progressive kyphosis can be a problem with these procedures too, various modifications have been described.[10] Central corpectomy provides excellent ventral decompression of the cord, but is inherently destabilizing, requiring bone grafting with or without instrumentation.[11–15] The majority of patients treated by central corpectomy experience clinical improvement ranging from 57%–86%. The others report either static neurological function or deterioration. Even those with a poor grade stand a good chance of improving after central corpectomy, a fact which highlights the importance of offering decompressive surgery to these patients.[13] The factors believed to have an influence on the outcome are age, duration of the symptoms, preoperative functional grade, preoperative spinal curvature and intramedullary changes as seen on the preoperative MRI. Age and the preoperative spinal curvature are probably the most significant factors that predict the outcome.[16] The mortality and morbidity rates vary from 5% to 28%.[11] In the elderly population, respiratory and cardiac complications predominate, while complications related to grafts and implants occur across all ages. Delayed deterioration following improvement has been documented in about 5% of patients.[14] Although fusion-related accelerated degenerative changes, which occur in about 75% of patients at segments adjacent to the fused segment, are asymptomatic in the short-term; they may be clinically relevant at long-term follow-up.[17]

The technique of oblique corpectomy,

introduced by George *et al.*[1] as an alternative to the central corpectomy, has been adopted by other authors, who have confirmed good results.[2,18–20] The main advantage of this technique is that it allows for adequate ventral decompression without the need for bony fusion. Bruneau *et al.*,[21] who restrict the use of the oblique corpectomy to those who have collapsed hard discs and recommend its use for patients with straight or kyphotic spines, reported the results they obtained in their last 100 patients. Improvement was noted in 72% of patients; 28% were unchanged, while none worsened. Instability requiring stabilization was noted in 3 patients. Permanent Horner syndrome was seen in 2%. As for our cohort of patients, they were at least a decade younger than those reported in western series, and we included patients with OPLL and soft, non-collapsed disc spaces.[2] The clinical improvement that we report is slightly less than that reported by others, but a large number of our patients had a poor functional grade pre-operatively.

Rocchi *et al.*[20] published their experience with 48 patients. Clinical improvement was seen in 85% of patients and clinical deterioration in 4%. No instability was seen postoperatively. Kiris *et al.*[18] found that 92.5% of the 40 patients who underwent an oblique corpectomy for CSM showed an improvement at the 6-month follow-up examination, according to the Japanese Orthopaedic Association (JOA) score. The improvement was the most prominent in the lower limbs. At a long-term follow-up of 59 months, there were no signs of instability, postural change or axial pain.

The major difficulties associated with oblique corpectomy are the complications related to operating in the vicinity of the VA and the mobilization of the sympathetic chain which may result in a Horner syndrome.

Conclusion

Cervical spondylotic myelopathy can be managed effectively through conservative methods, such as neck immobilization, posterior decompressive surgeries such as laminectomy or laminoplasty and anterior surgery via a central corpectomy with grafting. Surgeons need to be aware of the advantages and disadvantages of each method. The multilevel oblique corpectomy not only provides sufficient anterior decompression of the spinal canal, but also preserves stability post-operatively without the need for grafting. Since no fusion is performed, normal cervical motion is preserved, including in the operated segments. It may be offered to patients who have CSM with predominant ventral compression and stable spines irrespective of the preoperative spinal alignment. Clinical improvement occurs in the majority of patients. This technique is technically more demanding during the initial learning process.

References

1. George B, Gauthier N, Lot G. Multisegmental cervical spondylotic myelopathy and radiculopathy treated by multilevel oblique corpectomies without fusion. *Neurosurgery* 1999;**44**:81–90.
2. Chacko AG, Daniel RT. Multilevel cervical oblique corpectomy in the treatment of ossified posterior longitudinal ligament in the presence of ossified anterior longitudinal ligament. *Spine* 2007;**32**: E575–E580.
3. Fouyas IP, Statham PF, Sandercock PA. Cochrane review on the role of surgery in cervical spondylotic radiculomyelopathy. *Spine* 2002;**27**:736–47.
4. Yoshimatsu H, Nagata K, Goto H, *et al.* Conservative treatment for cervical spondylotic myelopathy prediction of treatment effects by multivariate analysis. *Spine J* 2001;**1**:269–73.
5. Albert TJ, Vacarro A. Postlaminectomy kyphosis. *Spine* 1998;**23**:2738–45.
6. Kaptain GJ, Simmons NE, Replogle RE, *et al.* Incidence and outcome of kyphotic deformity following laminectomy for cervical spondylotic myelopathy. *J Neurosurg* 2000;**93**:199–204.
7. Jain SK, Salunke PS, Vyas KH, *et al.* Multisegmental cervical ossification of the posterior longitudinal ligament: Anterior vs. posterior approach. *Neurol India* 2005;**53**:283–5; discussion 286.
8. Houten JK, Cooper PR. Laminectomy and posterior

cervical plating for multilevel cervical spondylotic myelopathy and ossification of the posterior longitudinal ligament: Effects on cervical alignment, spinal cord compression, and neurological outcome. *Neurosurgery* 2003;**52**:1081–7.

9. Shiraishi T. Skip laminectomy—a new treatment for cervical spondylotic myelopathy, preserving bilateral muscular attachments to the spinous processes: A preliminary report. *Spine J* 2002;**2**:108–15.

10. Hosono N, Sakaura H, Mukai Y, *et al. En bloc* laminoplasty without dissection of paraspinal muscles. *J Neurosurg Spine* 2005;**3**:29–33.

11. Fessler RG, Steck JC, Giovanini MA. Anterior cervical corpectomy for cervical spondylotic myelopathy. *Neurosurgery* 1998;**43**:257–65; discussion 265–7.

12. Naderi S, Alberstone CD, Rupp FW, *et al.* Cervical spondylotic myelopathy treated with corpectomy: Technique and results in 44 patients. *Neurosurg Focus* 1996;**1**:e5; discussion 1p following e5.

13. Rajshekhar V, Kumar GS. Functional outcome after central corpectomy in poor-grade patients with cervical spondylotic myelopathy or ossified posterior longitudinal ligament. *Neurosurgery* 2005;**56**:1279–84; discussion 1284–5.

14. Saunders RL, Bernini PM, Shirreffs TG (Jr), *et al.* Central corpectomy for cervical spondylotic myelopathy: A consecutive series with long-term follow-up evaluation. *J Neurosurg* 1991;**74**:163–70.

15. Saunders RL, Pikus HJ, Ball P. Four-level cervical corpectomy. *Spine* 1998;**23**:2455–61.

16. Naderi S, Ozgen S, Pamir MN, *et al.* Cervical spondylotic myelopathy: Surgical results and factors affecting prognosis. *Neurosurgery* 1998;**43**:43–9; discussion 49–50.

17. Kulkarni V, Rajshekhar V, Raghuram L. Accelerated spondylotic changes adjacent to the fused segment following central cervical corpectomy: Magnetic resonance imaging study evidence. *J Neurosurg* 2004;**100**:2–6.

18. Kiris T, Kilincer C. Cervical spondylotic myelopathy treated by oblique corpectomy: A prospective study. *Neurosurgery* 2008;**62**:674–82; discussion 674–82.

19. Koc RK, Menku A, Akdemir H, *et al.* Cervical spondylotic myelopathy and radiculopathy treated by oblique corpectomies without fusion. *Neurosurg Rev* 2004;**27**:252–8.

20. Rocchi G, Caroli E, Salvati M, *et al.* Multilevel oblique corpectomy without fusion: Our experience in 48 patients. *Spine* 2005;**30**:1963–9.

21. Bruneau M, Cornelius JF, George B. Multilevel oblique corpectomies: Surgical indications and technique. *Neurosurgery* 2007;**61**:106–12; discussion 112.

11

Cervical arthroplasty: Indications and early results

P.K. SAHOO

Half a century has gone by since the initial description of anterior cervical discectomy by Cloward,[1] Robinson and Smith.[2] In the present era, anterior approaches have become the mainstay of treatment for compression of the cervical spinal cord and nerve roots because of the excellent clinical results of these surgeries.

Previous experience with complete discectomy, without a concomitant fusion, was frequently unsatisfactory. A proportion of the patients developed new neck pain or kyphosis due to the destabilizing decompression.[3] This resulted in the widely accepted practice of routinely fusing the discectomy site. Although fusion may serve to relieve axial neck pain among patients with abnormal cervical biomechanics, in the vast majority of patients, a fusion is necessary only to address the potential for iatrogenic instability from complete disc removal.

Cervical artificial disc replacement is currently an area of intense scientific investigation and there is tremendous enthusiasm about exploring disc replacement as a technique for preventing transitional-level disease and maintaining normal cervical motion. Several studies of clinical experience with cervical disc replacement have been published in this decade and a number of motion-preserving prostheses are now commercially available.

Rationale of cervical disc arthroplasty

Long-term data (spanning up to 10 years) suggest that fusion has significant radiographic and clinical consequences. Hilibrand *et al.*[4] provide perhaps the greatest insight into this problem. These investigators identified the occurrence of symptomatic adjacent-level disease, progressing at an average rate of 2.9% per year, during the first 10 post-fusion years among 374 patients in their study group. Two-thirds of these patients required re-operation. The levels most likely to develop adjacent segment disease were C5–C6 and C6–C7. According to the study of Goffin *et al.*,[5] the rate of adjacent-level radiological degeneration was 92% over a mean period of 8.6 years.

Biomechanical investigations support the clinical observation that fusions are associated with adjacent-level degeneration.[6,7] The disc pressures at the adjacent segments before and after fusion at C5–C6 were measured by Eck *et al.*[8] They found a 73% increase in cranial and 45% increase in caudal disc pressures during flexion, and an increased intervertebral motion, especially rostrally. Another investigation done by Fuller *et al.*[9] found an increase of up to 40% in the adjacent levels.

Although only a small group of patients require surgery for adjacent-level decompensation, it seems worthwhile to prevent adjacent-level disease as far as possible.

In the clinical realm, contemporary experience with long-term evaluation of patients who have undergone anterior cervical discectomy with fusion (ACDF) suggests that symptomatic adjacent segment degeneration occurs at a rate of 2%–3% per year and up to 15% of these patients will require a second operation to treat the transitional levels.[4,10,11] Strategies to tackle these long-term consequences of spinal fusion include (i) limiting the length of surgical fusion, (ii) prophylactic treatment of adjacent discs exhibiting early signs of degeneration, (iii) use of non-destabilizing techniques for decompression, and (iv) cervical disc arthroplasty.

Currently available cervical disc arthroplasty devices

Worldwide, eight types of total disc implants for the cervical spine (Table 1) are available. Investigational Device Exemption (IDE) studies are awaiting the approval of the Food and Drug Administration (FDA), USA at the moment.[12–14]

The Bryan cervical disc

The Bryan disc was conceived and developed by the neurosurgeon, Vincent Bryan, and a mechanical engineer, Alex Kunsler, in 1993. After years of extensive research and development, the first Bryan cervical disc was implanted in January 2000.[15] More than 7000 patients have since been treated with the Bryan disc. Initial studies in Europe and Australia comparing disc replacement with ACDF showed that the treatment options were clinically equivalent at intermediate-term follow up with regard to neurological recovery and symptoms of axial pain. Trials of both single- and two-level implantations have been performed

in Europe. A 2-year follow-up assessment of 49 patients treated with disc replacement showed that 90% had fair to excellent neurological outcomes, similar to the reported historical experiences with ACDF.[16] However, the comparative effects of disc replacement and ACDF on the adjacent motion segments remain undetermined and long-term data on outcomes, collected 5–10 years after the implantation of the prosthesis, will be necessary to demonstrate the putative advantages of disc replacement.

The Bryan cervical disc (Medtronic Sofamor Danek, Memphis, USA) is composed of two titanium alloy shells, with an intervening polyurethane nucleus supplied as a single pre-assemble unit (Fig. 1). The central nucleus is encased within a thin circumferential polyurethane sheath, which connects the two metal shells. The outer aspect of each shell is a porous high-friction surface, composed of 250 µm titanium beads sintered to its surface. These shells abut the machined bony end-plates of the vertebral bodies above and below. The inner aspect of each shell, which is in contact with the polyurethane nucleus, is smooth. A lip on the anterior surface of the shells allows grasping and manipulation of the prosthesis during implantation. The implant comes in five sizes, with diameters of 14 mm, 15 mm, 16 mm, 17 mm and 18 mm, and a set height.

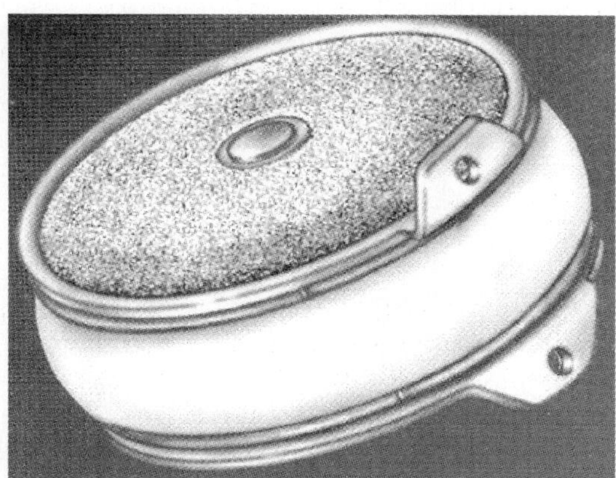

Fig. 1. Bryan™ (Medtronic Sofamor Danek, Memphis, USA) single-piece prosthesis: Metal and polyurethane

Table 1. Features of currently available cervical disc arthroplasty devices

Disc	Bearing surface	Bearing surface material	Centre of rotation shape	Short-term fixation	Issues	US IDE study	Total implanted (worldwide) as of December 2004
Bryan	Metal (Titanium)-on-poly	Torodial	Centre of disc space	Press fit into milled end-plate	Constraint; segmental kyphosis	Complete Fall 2004	7000
Prestige	Metal-on-metal (Titanium carbide)	Oval	Upper vertebral body; posterior	Flanges subsidence	Initial fixation	Summer 2004	500
ProDisc-C	Metal (CoCr)-on-poly	Spherical	Lower vertebral body; posterior	Midline keel issues	Semi-constrained imaging	Started May 2004	800
PCM	Metal (CoCr)-on-poly	Spherical (shallow)	Lower vertebral body	Ridges into UC joints	Initial stability	None	300
Cervicore	Metal (CoCr)-on-poly	Saddle	Variable	Flanges with screws	Same as Bristol (Prestige 1)	Started 2005	Not known
Discover	Metal-on-metal (Titanium carbide)	Spherical	Lower vertebral body	Midline keel issues	Semi-constrained	None	Not known
Cervidisc	Metal-on-ceramic (Zirconium Al_2O_2)	Spherical	Upper vertebral body	Spikes off market	Subsidence	None	52
Mobidisc cervical	Metal (CoCr)-on-poly	Spherical	Lower vertebral body	Keel	Not known	None	Not known

US IDE study: United States Investigational Device Exemption study

Motion occurs at the interface between the smooth inner surfaces of the shell and the polyurethane nucleus. The unit is axially symmetrical in structure and in motion before implantation. The device is designed to provide up to 11 degrees of flexion, extension and lateral bending and 2 mm of translation. In early clinical follow-up studies, 93% of patients at 6 months and 88% of patients at 12 months maintained motion of >2 degrees at the treated level.[5] Motion at 12 months averaged 9±4 degrees after surgery.

At the time of surgery, the internal environment of the disc is filled with saline through a small port in the shells, which is subsequently sealed. A watertight seal is created between the two outer shells by a connecting circumferential sheath, which is secured in place with a titanium-retaining ring. This sheath maintains the internal liquid environment, prevents fibroblast in-growth and also serves to trap any wear debris that may be created with motion. This prosthesis has been in use in India for the past 6 years.

Prestige (Medtronic Sofamor Danek, Memphis, USA)

The Prestige I (Fig. 2) cervical prosthesis (also named Frenchay artificial joint), which is a modified version of the original Cummins prosthesis (1991–1996), was developed in 1998 and is a two-piece prosthesis constructed of stainless steel. It employs a ball-in-groove articulation.

The Prestige II was designed in 1999. The main way in which it differs from its predecessor is its more anatomical end-plate design, which is rougher to improve bony in-growth.[17]

The Prestige ST became available in 2002. The major difference in its design is a 2 mm reduction in the height of each anterior flange. This device is currently in clinical trials by the FDA in the USA. It is available in four different heights (6 mm to 9 mm) and two choices of depth (12 mm and 14 mm). The width is consistent at 17.8 mm.[14,17]

The most recent development is the Prestige STLP (Fig. 3). The major difference between this version and its predecessors is that it allows for multi-level implantation. Fixation is now achieved by a set of rails that are placed on the prosthesis–bone contact surface that eliminates the anterior profile of the device.[17] This prosthesis has been in use in India for the past 2 years.

ProDisc-C (Spine Solution, Paoli, USA)

The ProDisc-C (Fig. 4) is made of two cobalt–chrome metal end-plates and a fixed polyethylene core that provides coupled motion without independent translation when the device is implanted. The ProDisc-C maintains a single centre of rotation in the vertebral bone below the intervertebral space. It comes in six sizes of footprints. Implantation is performed by inserting

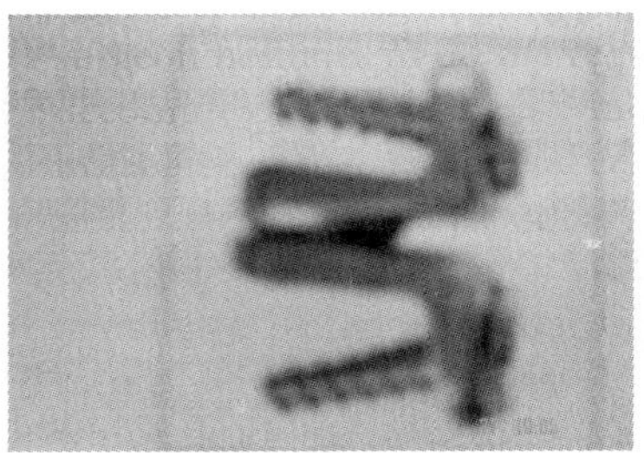

Fig. 2. Prestige I™ (Medtronic Sofamor Danek, Memphis, USA) two-piece prosthesis with metal-on-metal articulating surface

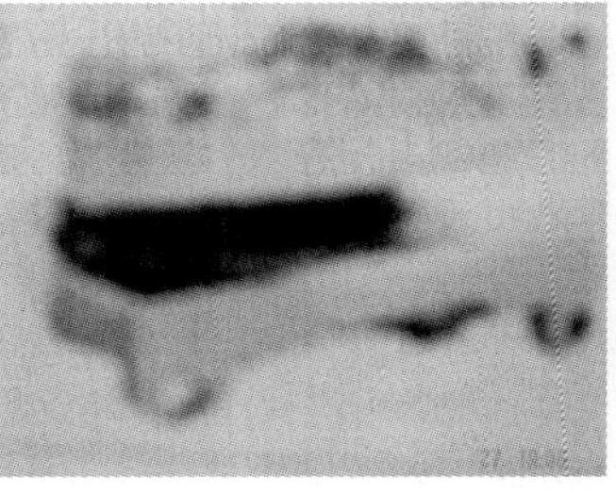

Fig. 3. Prestige STLP™ (Medtronic Sofamor Danek, Memphis, USA) with possibility of multil-evel implantation

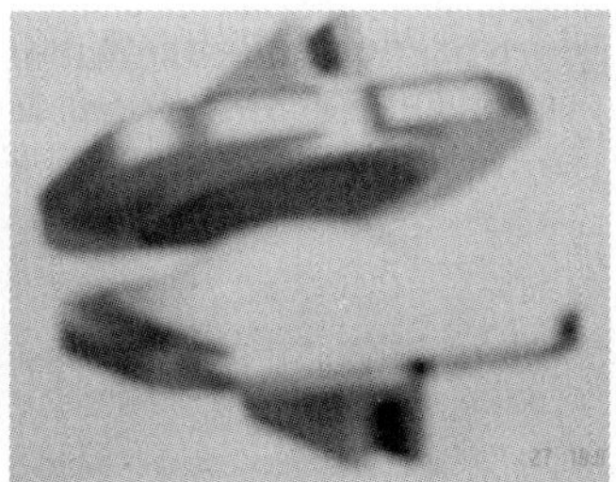

Fig. 4. ProDisc C™ (Spine Solution, Paoli, USA) metal-on-polyethylene semi-constrained design

102 P.K. SAHOO

a keel in a slot of the cranial and caudal vertebral body. The surfaces of the prosthesis towards the bones bear a plasma-spray titanium layer for secondary fixation.[14,18,19] This prosthesis has been in use in India for the past year.

PCM (Cervitech, Roundhill, USA)

The Porous Coated Motion (PCM) (Fig. 5) uses polythene-on-metal and has a uniarticular design, with one centre of rotation maintained below the intervertebral space. The end-plates are manufactured from cobalt–chrome alloy. The outside of the components feature a TiCap coating. Primary stability is assured by a press-fit implantation.[19,20] McAfee[12] published a clinical study of 23 patients, who underwent a total of 32 PCM cervical arthroplasties. At 9 months' follow up, over 70% had an improvement of 15 points or more as compared with the preoperative Ostwestry Neck Disability Index. Over 80% of patients had >20% improvement on VAS. All 32 prostheses demonstrated successful in-growth, with no evidence of loosening. The PCM has not yet been included in any FDA-controlled study.

Discover (DePuy spine, USA)

The Discover cervical disc (Fig. 6) by DePuy spine, USA has a metal-on-metal design with a central polyethylene core. It is available in S, S-XW, M, MXW and large size, and heights of 6 mm, 7 mm, 8 mm and 9 mm. The prosthesis was introduced in India 2 years ago and has been implanted in very few cases.

Cervicore (Spine Core, Summit, USA)

Another disc replacement design using a metal-on-metal joint to imitate normal motion at the cervical disc space is the Cervicore prosthesis (Fig. 7). This has a metal-on-metal design with a saddle-shaped bearing surface. The surface permits the device to maintain a centre of rotation for flexion/extension in the vertebral body below, while simultaneously maintaining a centre of rotation in the bone above for lateral bending.[14]

No clinical data were available on this prosthesis when this review was written. So far, there have been no clinical trials of the device in the USA.

Cervical disc arthroplasty devices: Material considerations

These implants were developed, to a large extent, on the basis of the literature on other joint replacements, which have been under evaluation and in use for decades. At the moment, there are two different disc designs available. One general artificial disc design comprises metal end-plates with an intervening low-friction polymer to allow motion between the polished metal surface and the polymer. The ProDisc-C and the PCM

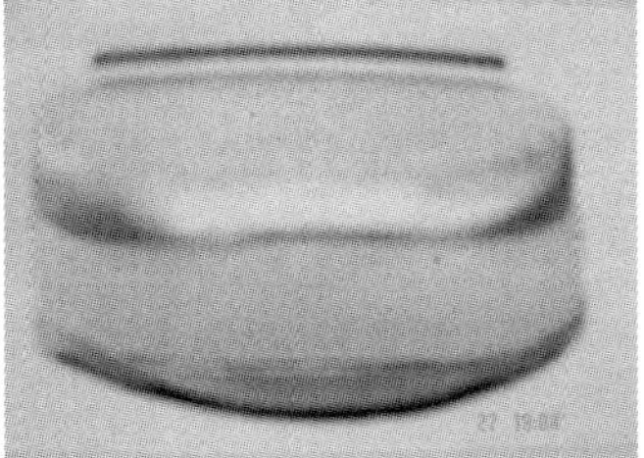

Fig. 5. PCM (Porous coated motion) Cervitech, Roundhilll, USA) polyethylene-on-metal mono-articular design

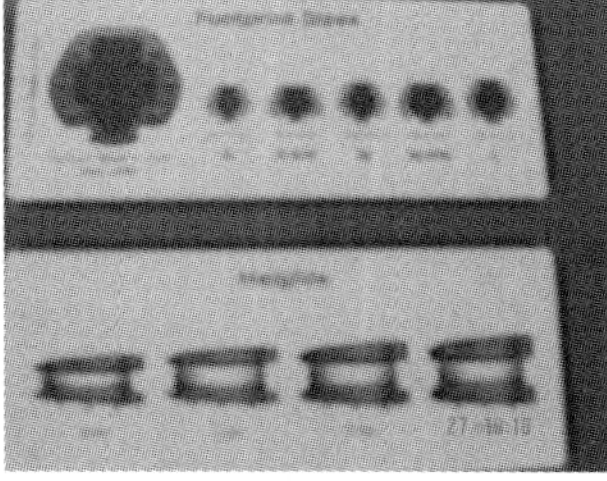

Fig. 6. Discover (DePuy spine USA)

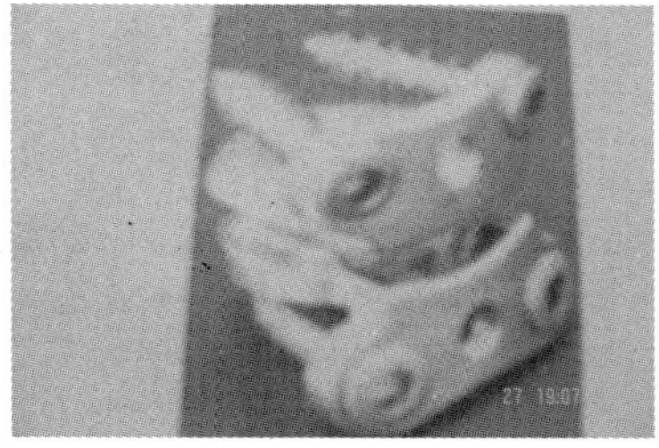

Fig. 7. Cervicore™ (Spine Core, Summit, USA) metal-on-metal design with a saddle-shaped bearing surface

device employ polythene, the use of which is well known in other types of arthroplasty, such as in the hip or in the knee.

The Bryan disc is a metal-on-polyurethane device. The use of a softer polymer is intended to provide not only motion, but also shock absorption.

The other types of disc implants are metal-on-metal joints. The Prestige and Cervicore are representative of these kind of devices.

The problem of aseptic loosening of arthroplasties due to wear debris is well known in the literature.[21,22] Clinical reports and further investigations have found, however, that such wear debris is not a significant problem in patients after total lumbar disc replacement.[19,23–25] This is likely to be the case with cervical spine implants as well, due to lower ranges of motion and loads, as compared with total hip or knee arthroplasties.[21] Nonetheless, it must be considered that the duration of most studies does not cover the expected standing times of total artificial lumbar discs.

Indications of cervical disc arthroplasty

Cervical disc replacement is appropriate for cases of predominantly anterior compression of the cervical spinal cord and/or nerve roots. Implantation of the Bryan disc into a degenerated disc adjacent to a previous fusion has been described and clinical investigation of the usefulness of disc replacement for treating transitional-level disease is currently under way.

Patients with predominantly posterior compression are generally poor candidates for cervical disc replacement. Similarly, when a significant component of the cervical stenosis occurs behind the vertebral body, a cervical corpectomy would be more appropriate. Whether the Bryan cervical disc would be beneficial in the presence of a laminectomy at the same level is unknown and patients with incompetent posterior elements or abnormal cervical motion should not undergo

Table 2. Inclusion/exclusion criteria currently accepted for cervical disc arthroplasty

Inclusion criteria

- Degenerative disc disease requiring surgical treatment at one level (in the FDA trials) to three levels from C3–Th1 for symptoms or signs of cervical radiculopathy and/or myelopathy, with or without axial neck pain
- Failed conservative treatment lasting at least 6 weeks for any one or more of disc herniations with radiculopathy
- Spondylotic radiculopathy
- Disc herniation with myelopathy
- Spondylotic myelopathy
- Compressive lesion must be proven by MRI/CT or myelography
- 18–55 years of age
- Non-discogenic pain sources should be excluded

Exclusion criteria

- Post-laminectomy with kyphotic deformity
- Translational instability
- Ankylosing spondylitis
- Rheumatoid arthritis
- Ossification of the posterior longitudinal ligament or diffuse hyperostosis
- Insulin-requiring diabetes mellitus
- Infection
- Pregnancy
- Metabolic bone diseases

disc replacement. In addition, patients with severe osteoporosis, spinal infection and local neoplastic disease would be poor candidates for disc implantation (Table 2).

Goals of cervical disc replacement

The objective of disc replacement is to replace the worn out disc with a new, functional intervertebral cervical disc prosthesis. When the prosthesis is implanted accurately, it should maintain vertebral body height, foramen height, stability and sagittal shape. It should preserve motion at the operated spinal level, protect the patient from developing adjoining motion segment disc degeneration and prevent recurrent spondylosis. Decompression of neural structures is essential for neurological recovery.

Surgical strategy for cervical disc arthroplasty

Unlike interbody fusion procedures, which require only that the spine be fused into a physiological position, disc replacement requires meticulous attention to technique. Proper implant selection is essential, because the interspace height as well as the radius of motion will be determined by the size of the disc. Proper positioning of the prosthesis is also essential because the location of the disc establishes the centrum of rotation and force movements on the spine. Placement off the midline or in a sagittally unfavourable location can thus lead to abnormal neck biomechanics. In addition, because the Bryan Disc is held in place by a precise friction fit between the convex surface of the prosthesis and the machined bony end-plate, special care must be taken during the implantation procedure. Several steps are required. These are: (i) precise implant selection and patient positioning, (ii) exposure and initial receipt site preparation, (iii) neural decompression, (iv) assembly of the gravity-guided bone milling rig, (v) precise machining of the adjoining end-plates to ensure a proper bone–implant interface, and (vi) implantation of the prosthesis.

Surgical technique for the Bryan cervical disc prosthesis

Pre-operative implant selection and positioning of patient

The proper size of the implant is estimated on the basis of preoperative imaging. Using computed tomographic slices parallel to the disc spaces, the smaller of the two adjacent end plates should be measured (Fig. 8). The footprint is perfectly circular and with the help of preset templates, an implant spanning the anterior and posterior osteophytes should be excluded in the selection process.

The patient is placed in a supine position and the chin should be affixed with tapes to maintain the neck in a neutral position and to avoid deviation from the midline (Fig. 9). The table should be wide enough to fully accommodate the patient's shoulders. Care must be taken to ensure that the coronal plane of the body is balanced and level with the floor. Furthermore, because the milling guides will be secured on the retractor frame attached to the operating table, the patient should be oriented squarely on the table.

A weighted radiopaque goniometer is then

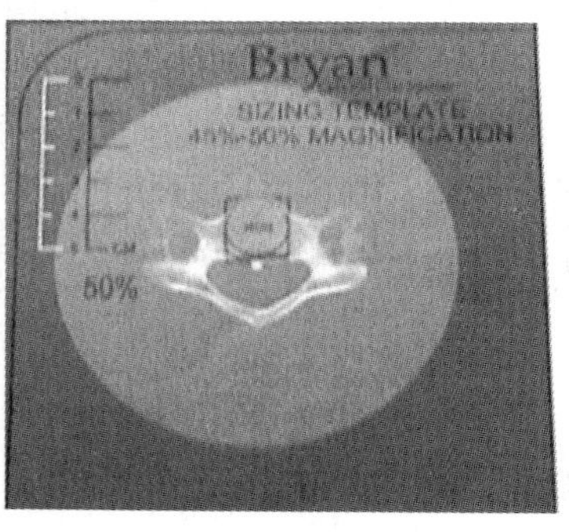
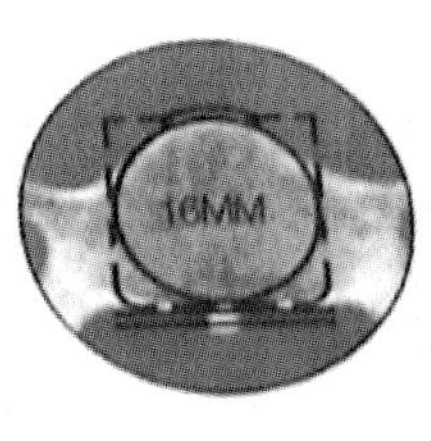

Fig. 8. Preoperative CT image showing implant selection using templates

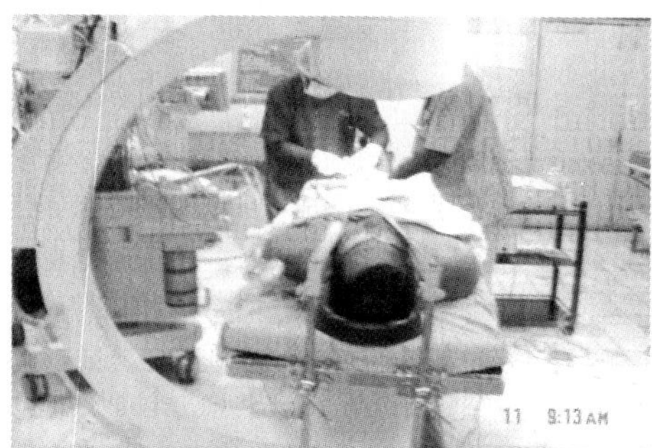

Fig. 9. Patient positioning

attached to the fluoroscopic C-arm and preliminary images are obtained to ensure that the discectomy level can be visualized. An image showing both the goniometer and patient's spine allows the surgeon to determine the plane of the disc space relative to the plane of gravity (Fig. 10). Any subsequent change in the patient's position would require re-imaging with the goniometer. Because the procedure is dependent on intraoperative radiography, the surgeon must be sure that the target disc space level can be visualized on a lateral fluoroscopic C-arm image. Thus, patients with short necks and large shoulders may not be candidates for C6–C7 disc replacement. Care should also be taken to ensure that an anteroposterior X-ray image over the target site can be obtained without obstruction from the metallic components of the operating room table.

Exposure and initial recipient site preparation

A standard ACDF exposure is then performed, with soft tissue retraction achieved by the use of a specially designed Bryan retractor frame, which is affixed to the operating table (Fig. 11). The retractor will require a slightly longer incision than in the case of a typical ACDF and the incision should extend slightly past the midline. Proper positioning of the retractor blades provides a perfectly aligned sagittal corridor to the anterior cervical spine, without lateral deviation. Because

the retractor frame will serve as the support from which all bone milling will occur, it should be attached securely to the bed and positioned carefully in the midline over the anterior neck. The use of superior and inferior retractors is optional. Once adequate exposure is complete, the anterior osteophytes are removed with a drill and Kerrison punch, but the anterior cortex of the vertebral body should be carefully preserved.

Neural decompression

A standard discectomy of the width of the implant should then be performed, preserving the vertebral end-plates. The use of a thin cam distractor can increase the disc space height and ease neural decompression (Fig. 12), which is performed in a standard manner. The cam distractor can be left on the contralateral side of the interspace to maintain distraction, while decompression is accomplished on the ipsilateral side. Two cam sizes are supplied. Progressive dilatation to the larger cam provides intervertebral distraction that is adequate to accommodate the prosthesis. Generous removal of the medial aspect of the uncinate processes is necessary. At this point, careful haemostasis of epidural bleeding should be secured.

The end-plates should be carefully preserved because they will be machined to a preset depth and concavity. Overly aggressive bone removal can create an interspace larger than the height of

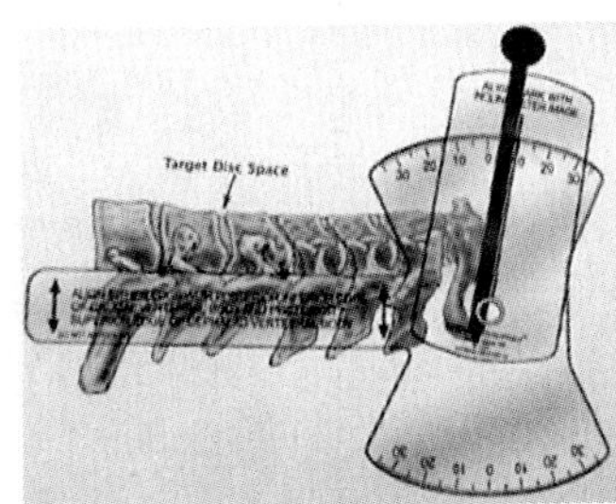

Fig. 10. Diagram showing gravity-weighted goniometer projection onto the lateral image intensifier image to determine the disc angulation

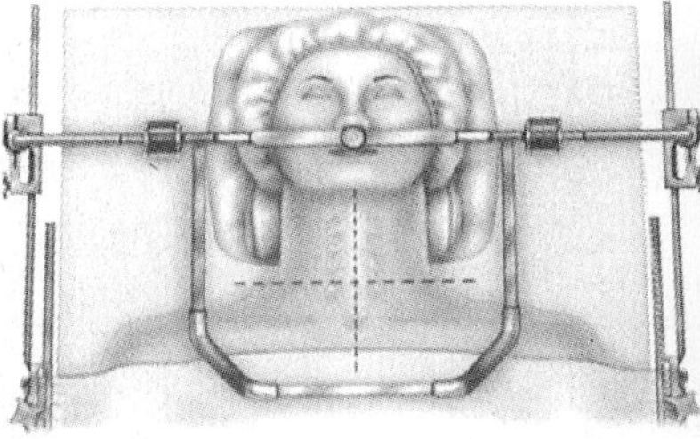

Fig. 11. Diagram showing placement of the bed-based retractor frame

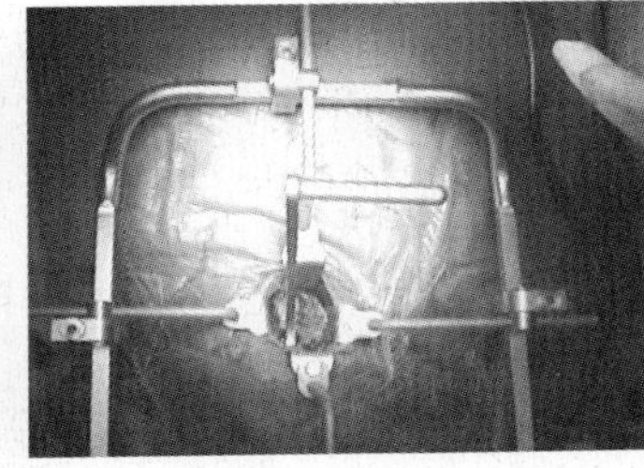

Fig. 12. Sagittal cam distractor

the prosthesis. This would result in a poor fit between the Bryan cervical disc and the adjacent vertebral bodies, and could lead to migration of the implant.

Assembly of the gravity-guided bone-milling rig

After discectomy, the midline of the implant recipient site is determined by the use of a centering device (Fig. 13). The tips of the caliper-like device are placed against the lateral aspects of the decompression on the remainder of the uncinate processes. The midline is then marked on the vertebral bodies, above and below. The sagittal wedge is placed in the discectomy site, and the milling guide is inserted over it and affixed onto the retractor frame. This will serve as a guide for all the subsequent steps.

A protractor is then placed on the milling rig to determine the sagittal inclination of the disc space, a value that should be identical to the inclination angle determined preoperatively by fluoroscopic imaging (Fig. 14). After the inclination has been confirmed, the anchor posts are drilled into the caudal and cranial vertebral bodies to secure the rig rigidly to the spine to facilitate the subsequent steps (Fig. 15).

Precise machining of adjoining end-plates to ensure proper bone–implant interface

The distance from the rig to the anterior and posterior aspects of both vertebral bodies must then be measured and confirmed by the use of lateral fluoroscopy (Fig. 16). A 4 mm cylindrical burr is attached to a high-speed drill and a stop is set on the basis of depth measurements obtained

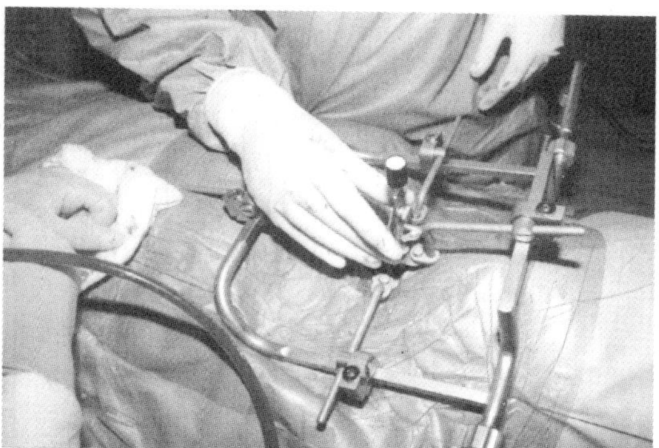

Fig. 13. Transverse centering tool

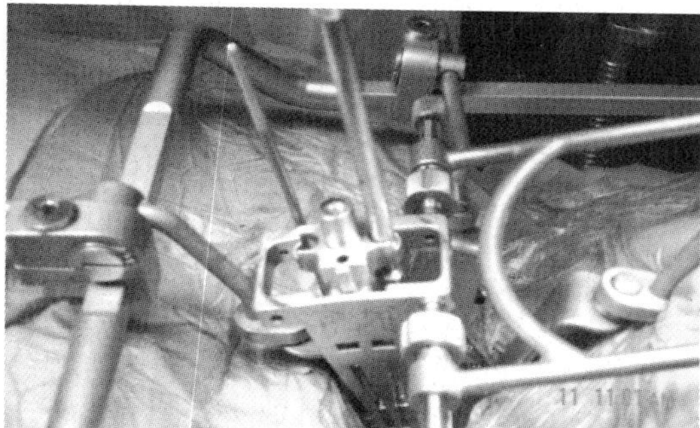

Fig. 15. Anchoring of the posts into the lower vertebral bodies

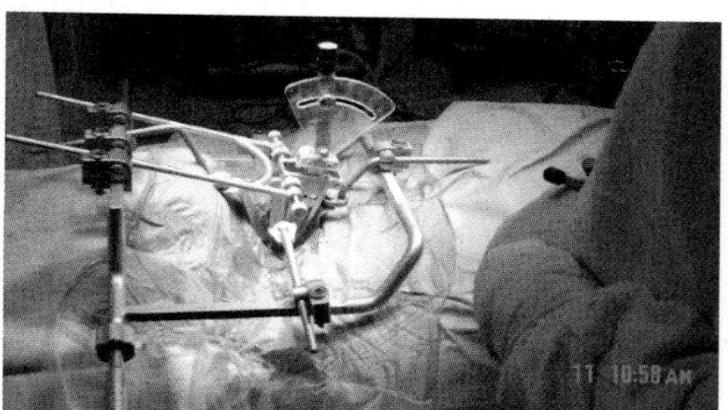

Fig. 14. Placement of protractor confirming the site of the disc space

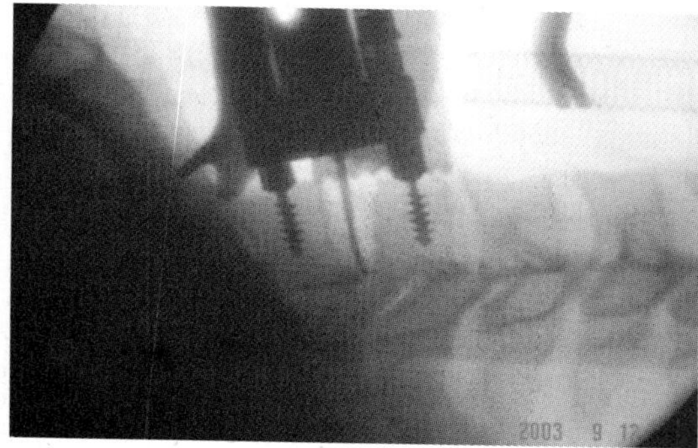

Fig. 16. Measurement of anterior and posterior distance

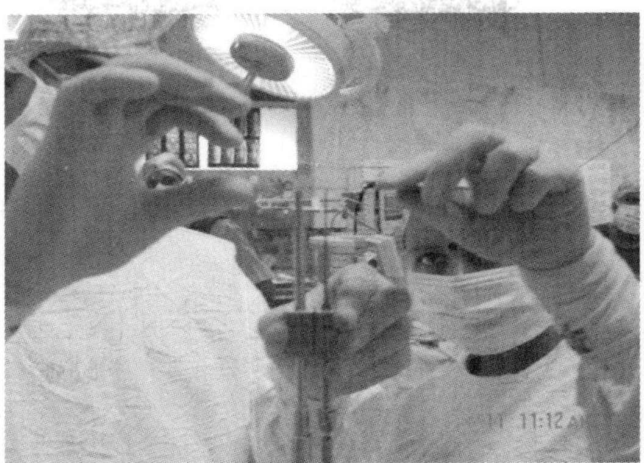

Fig. 17. Setting of burr stop at the appropriate depth

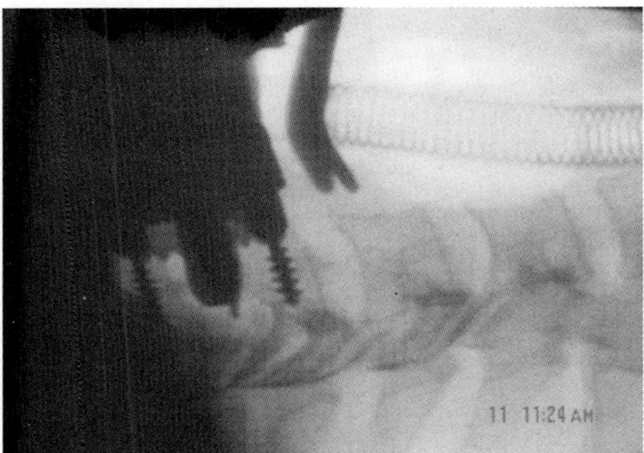

Fig. 19a. Milling of the endplates

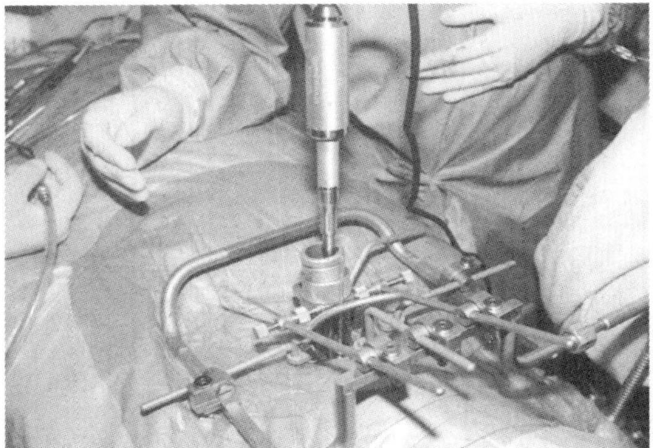

Fig. 18. Burring device

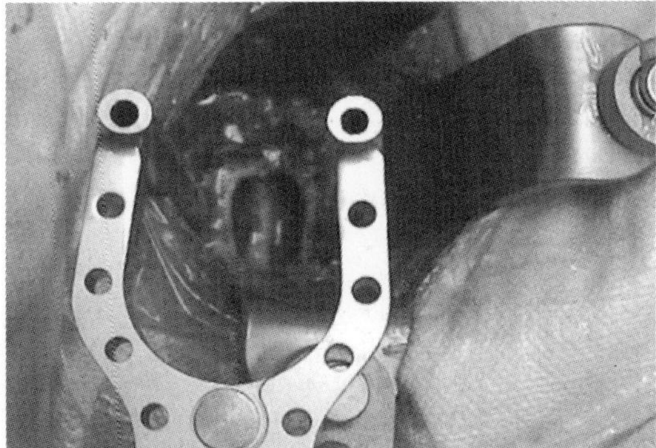

Fig. 19b. Prepared milling end-plates matching the intended implant size

through the posterior aspect of the vertebral bodies (Fig. 17). The placement of the burr in the discectomy site then allows for semi-automated removal of the end-plate in a precise manner. Movement of the burr along a broad preset axial arc, using a windshield wiper motion in both directions laterally burrs the end-plates flat (Fig. 18). Repositioning of the apparatus to a preset distance cranially and caudally increases the amount of bone removed from each vertebral body to accommodate the prosthesis.

A final measurement is taken to confirm the appropriate size of the implant. Both end-plates are then prepared with a dome-shaped milling disc which matches the intended size of the implant (Figs 19a, b). In a manner similar to the use of cylindrical burr, the milling disc is attached to a long hinged arm on the guide that rotates along a sagittal arc. The inferior and superior end-plates are engaged by rotation of the arm in a caudal and cranial direction. This creates concavities in the vertebral bodies that will precisely match the convex titanium alloy shells.

Prosthesis implantation

The milling guide is then detached, leaving the vertebral anchor posts in place. The artificial disc is filled with normal saline, which acts as an internal lubricant. This is done by screwing a seal plug into the centre port of one of the shells, filling the saline through the opposite port and

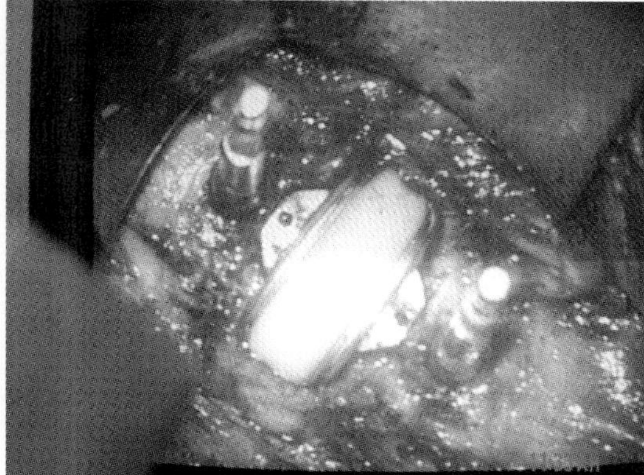

Fig. 20. Implant in position

then sealing this port. The wound is irrigated copiously to wash out any bone dust left behind from the drilling process. A final inspection of the epidural space should be performed to ensure that there adequate neurological decompression and meticulous haemostasis have been obtained.

Distraction across the posts expands the height of the recipient site to allow insertion of the prosthesis. The Bryan disc is attached to an implant holder and inserted into the prepared space (Fig. 20). The distraction posts are then removed. Final AP and lateral fluoroscopic images should be obtained to ensure proper sizing and positioning of the implant. The closure is performed in two layers, as in ACDF. The oesophagus should be inspected for trauma and careful attention should be paid to haemostasis. No cervical collar or neck immobilization is necessary.

Experience with the Bryan cervical disc arthroplasty

A prospective study was carried out at our institution between January 2002 and December 2007 on 110 patients who presented with cervical spondylotic myeloradiculopathy and were implanted with the Bryan prosthetic cervical disc.

On admission, the patients were clinically evaluated and a detailed neurological examination was carried out in all cases. Nurick grading was used to quantify neurological deficits (Table 3). Radiological evaluation, which included AP and lateral radiographs of the cervical spine, as well as MRI, was performed to investigate (i) the level of disc prolapse, (ii) the extent of thecal and nerve root compression, and (iii) cord changes. Computerized tomography was carried out to preoperatively determine the size of the Bryan cervical disc to be used.

The effectiveness of the device was assessed by evaluating the amount of pain, neurological function and range of cervical motion during follow up. Scores for the results regarding the quality of life were calculated according to the modified Odom criteria, both during the postoperative period and subsequently at follow-up of 6 months, 12 months and 24 months. The following categories were used:

- **Excellent:** Improvement of pre-operative symptoms and signs
- **Good:** Minimal persistence of preoperative symptoms, and abnormal findings improved or unchanged

Table 3. Nurick grading for neurological disability

Grade	Features	No. of patients	Single level	Two level
Grade 0	Signs and symptoms of root involvement; no evidence of cord involvement	90	90	—
I	Signs of spinal cord involvement; normal gait	8	4	4
II	Slight difficulty in walking; full-time employment not prevented	8	6	2
III	Difficulty in walking; employment prevented but ambulant without support	2	Nil	2
IV	Able to walk only with help or frame	2	Nil	2
V	Chair-bound; bed-ridden	Nil	Nil	Nil

- **Fair:** Definite relief from some preoperative symptoms, and other symptoms slightly improved or unchanged
- **Poor:** Symptoms and signs unchanged or exacerbated

Lateral and AP radiographs of the cervical spine were taken in the postoperative period and at follow up of 6 months, 12 months and 24 months to assess the range of motion and

position of the device. During the postoperative period, the patients were advised not to use any cervical collar and resume normal activities as soon as the postoperative pain subsided.

Observations

As mentioned earlier, all the patients were operated through the anterior cervical approach, using the specially designed Bryan cervical discectomy apparatus as per the protocol of our institution. Cervical discectomy and arthroplasty were carried out for 16 patients with C4–C5 disc prolapse (Fig. 21), 52 with C5–C6 disc prolapse (Fig. 22), 32 with C6–C7 disc prolapse (Fig. 23), and 5 each with C4–C5, C5–C6 and C6–C7 disc prolapse. Bryan cervical disc size 14 was implanted in 2, size 15 in 42, size 16 in 4, size 17 in 70 and size 18 in 2.

The operative time was 4 hours for the first 5 patients and subsequently, 2 hours for single-level and 3 hours for two-level cervical disc replacement. There were no intraoperative vascular, visceral or neural complications. No intraoperative or postoperative blood transfusion was required. In the immediate postoperative period, one patient with C6–C7 disc replacement developed temporary hoarseness of voice, which improved subsequently over a period of 2 months.

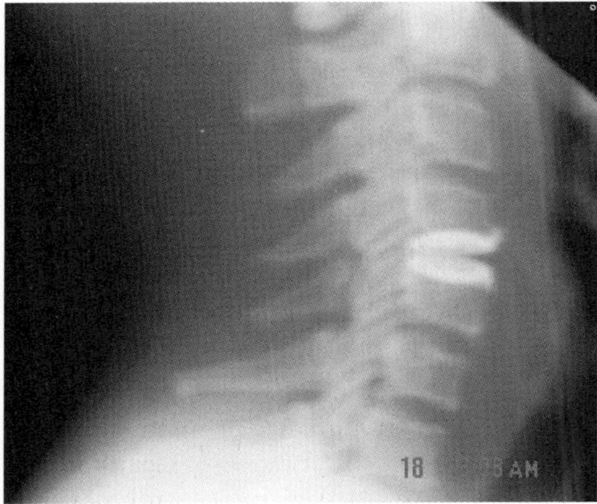

Fig. 21. C4–C5 disc replacement

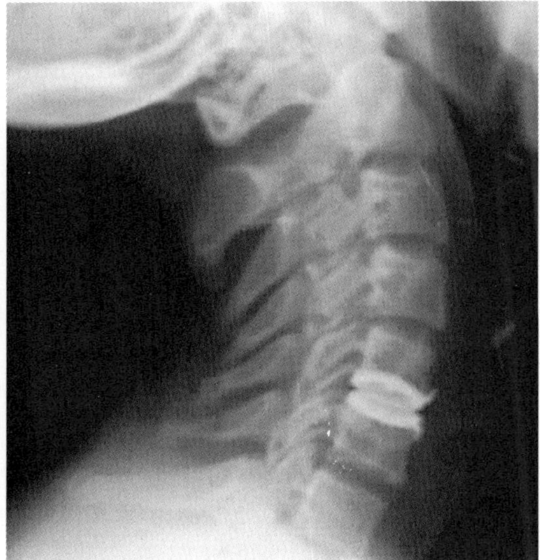

Fig. 22. C5–C6 disc replacement

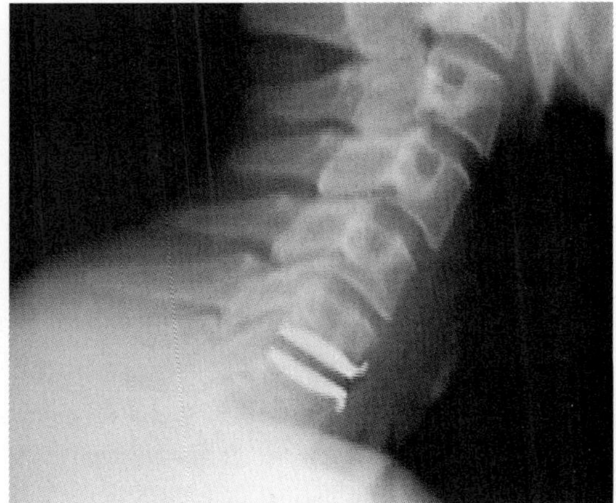

Fig. 23. C6–C7 disc replacement

Results

During the immediate postoperative period and at follow up of 2 months, 6 months, 1 year and 2 years, the results in terms of quality of life were excellent in 92% and good in 8% of cases of single-level disc replacement, as per the Odom criteria. As for two-level disc replacement, the results were excellent in 20% of patients and good in 80%. None of the patients deteriorated postoperatively or during follow up.

Postoperative AP and lateral radiographs of the cervical spine showed that the device was in position (Fig. 24). Radiologically, no migration or displacement of the device was seen in this series in the postoperative period. The device is MRI-compatible but showed minimal artifacts.

Experiences with various cervical disc prostheses

With established cervical spondylotic myelo-radiculopathy, the management option for cervical disc prolapse is surgical decompression. Anterior cervical discectomy and ACDF is the standard surgical approach for cervical spondylotic myeloradiculolpathy due to anterior thecal/nerve root compression.[26]

Initial descriptions of the anterior approach for cervical discectomy always included bony fusion,[27] which was popularized by Smith and Robinson in 1955[28] and Cloward in 1958.[29] This was advocated to prevent the possibility of late kyphosis from disc space collapse or radiculopathy from foraminal narrowing. Arguments in favour of fusion include the maintenance of disc space height, which helps avoid vertebral settling and minimizes the potential for progressive deterioration due to instabilities.[30] The basic principle is that the bone graft between the involved interspaces gives inherent stability and allows fusion to occur even in degenerative situations. Anterior cervical decompression and fusion is now widely accepted as a safe and effective treatment modality for cervical disc

herniation. Studies of this procedure have found it to be reproducible and there is a high level of satisfaction among the patients who have undergone it.[29,31,32] The fusion rate of an anterior graft is affected by several factors, including the type of graft[28] and the surgical technique.[33]

Interbody fusion of the cervical spine

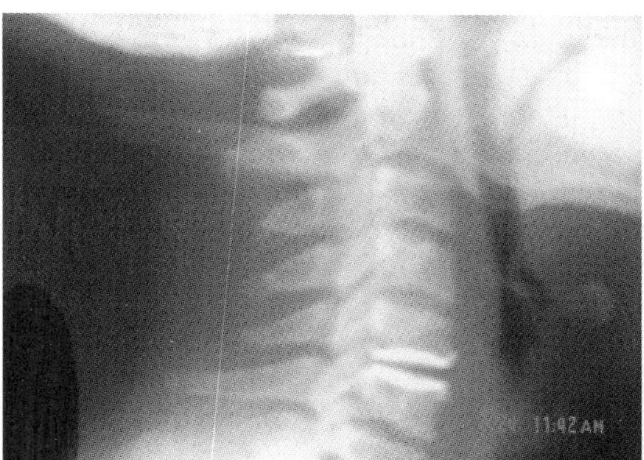

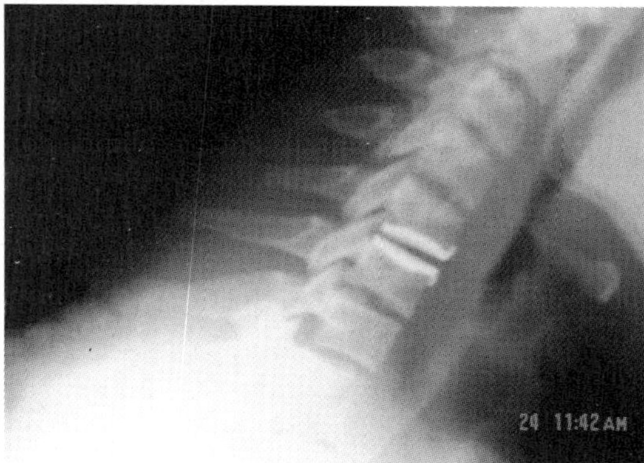

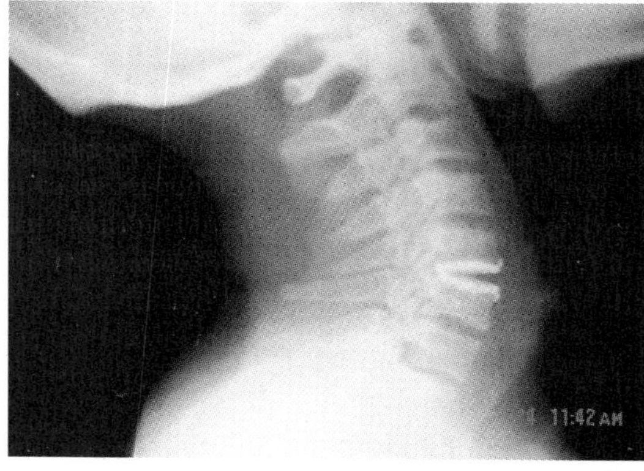

Fig. 24. Follow up C5–C6 cervical disc replacement

following cervical discectomy, besides causing restriction of neck movement, also accelerates degeneration of the adjacent disc levels due to increased stress from fusion.[34–37] Artificial disc replacement is not a new concept, the first attempts having been made in the early 1950s. Considerable advances have been made during the past 15 years, with large numbers of patients, mostly in Europe, having undergone surgery with total disc prostheses.

Proponents of disc prosthesis advance several reasons in favour of disc replacement, such as decompression being followed by immediate relief from pain, preservation of function, frequency of failed fusion, and absence of drawbacks linked to autologous bone harvesting. Arthroplasty offers the benefit of prophylaxis for accelerated spondylosis at the operated level. In addition, by allowing the biomechanical stress factors at adjacent levels, it should theoretically offer a prophylactic benefit at these levels as well. Therefore, cervical disc replacement offers the same benefit offered by decompression and fusion, while simultaneously providing full motion of the neck. The latter protects the adjacent disc levels from the abnormal stress associated with fusion by maintaining physiological motion and kinematics.[38]

In 1998, Gill and co-workers patented the Bristol cervical disc.[39] This device, which is a ball-and-socket type made of stainless steel, is screwed to the anterior sides of the adjacent vertebral bodies. Cummins reported having obtained good results in 20 patients implanted with such a device. The device is still being clinically evaluated.[40]

The Prestige cervical disc replacement is an effective means of reconstructing the cervical spine after anterior discectomy. It preserves normal motion and may decrease the incidence of adjacent segment disease.[17]

McAfee[12] published a clinical study of 23 patients, who underwent a total of 32 PCM cervical arthroplasties. At 9 months' follow up, over 70% had an improvement of 15 points or more as compared to the preoperative Ostwestry Neck Disability Index. Over 80% had greater than 20% improvement on VAS. All 32 prosthesis demonstrated successful ingrowth with no evidence of loosening. The PCM is not yet in FDA-controlled study.

Our institution is the first centre in Asia to carry out single-level and bi-level Bryan cervical disc replacement, which it has been doing since January 2002. In early clinical follow-up studies, 93% of patients at 6 months and 88% of patients at 12 months maintained motion of >2 degrees at the treated level.[5] Motion at 12 months averaged 9±4 degrees. Our study has clearly demonstrated excellent to good clinical results in the case of all 110 patients who received the Bryan total cervical disc prosthesis. There was relief from neck pain and brachialgia, as well as an improvement in the patients' quality of life and functionality. The prosthesis also provided clinical and radiological stability, and a normal range of cervical motion. Similar results have been reported by Goffin *et al.*[38]

The complications associated with the Bryan cervical disc are comparable to those encountered with ACDF in general. In the initial European studies, eight re-interventions were required in 146 subjects. These involved primarily the evaluation of local haematomas, incomplete decompression, or the repair of soft tissue trauma.[16] There were no device failures or explanations required during the study periods. However, if there is evidence of an improper fit during implantation, the prosthesis should be removed and the procedure salvaged with surgical fusion, using partial corpectomies, an interposition graft and plating.

Heterotopic ossification (HO) is a well-known complication of joint replacement. The Bryan disc has satisfactory wear characteristics and does not produce a significant inflammatory response.[41] Leung *et al.*[42] found a strong association between the occurrence of HO and subsequent loss of movement of the implanted cervical artificial disc. According to them, sex and age are two possible risk factors in the development of HO after cervical disc replacement.

Experience with mechanical disc replacements has resulted in unintended fusion at the treated site and poor clinical results.[43] During burring and milling for implantation of the Bryan disc prosthesis, great care should be taken to wash out any bony debris from the milling procedure because these particles can be intensely osteogenic. In addition, we routinely administer non-steroidal anti-inflammatory medications post-operatively for four weeks to prevent HO.

Some authors have found that Bryan disc arthroplasty often leads to segmental kyphosis. However, this can be prevented by using a prosthesis of the proper size.

Discectomy and implantation of the device alleviates neurological symptoms and signs similar to those with anterior cervical discectomy and fusion. Radiographic evidence supports the fact that a normal range of motion is established. The procedure is safe and the patients recover quickly. Restrictive postoperative management is not necessary.

Conclusion

Anterior cervical discectomy and fusion is a reliable procedure, which is associated with excellent clinical and radiological outcomes in 85%–95% of patients.[44,45] It is a procedure with a low peri- and postoperative complication rate.[46–48] It will be difficult to achieve such good results with any other type of cervical disc arthroplasty.

Although perhaps more complicated than a standard ACDF, surgical implantation of the Bryan cervical disc is appealing. The data collected by European studies during the intermediate follow up of one- and two-level disc replacement, as well as by our study, suggest that discectomy followed by disc replacement alleviates neurological symptoms with an efficacy similar to that of ACDF, while preserving normal cervical motion. Longer term follow up of these patient cohorts will be needed to determine how long this prosthesis remains functional and to protect from adjacent segment motion.

Excellent to good clinical results have been clearly demonstrated in our study on 110 patients receiving the Bryan total cervical disc prosthesis, with improved quality of life and functionality. It also provided clinical and radiological stability and a normal range of cervical motion. Similar results have also been reported by others.[38,49,50] So far, cervical disc arthroplasty seems to be a promising technique for cases of cervical disc prolapse. Only with truly scientific studies using patient randomization, pre- and post-surgery outcome analyses by unbiased independent observers, and statistical analysis by independent experts will the real value of these devices be known.

The crucial points which will probably decide the fate of cervical disc arthroplasty are the percentage of spontaneous fusion over time, the limitations of restoring disturbed curvatures, intraoperative technology and, last but not the least, the prices of the implants.

References

1. Cloward R. The anterior approach for removal of ruptured discs. *J Neurol* 1958;**15**:602–16.
2. Robinson R, Smith G. Anterolateral cervical disc removal and interbody fusion for cervical disc syndrome. *Bull Johns Hopkins Hosp* 1955;**96**:223–4.
3. Abd-Alrahman N, Dokmak A, Abou-Madawi A. Anterior cervical discectomy (ACD) versus anterior cervical fusion (ACF). Clinical and radiological outcome study. *Acta Neurochir (Wien)* 1999;**141**: 1089–92.
4. Hilibrand A, Carlson G, Palumbo M, *et al*. Radiculopathy and myelopathy at segments adjacent to the site of a previous anterior cervical arthrodesis. *J Bone Joint Surg Am* 1999;**81**:519–28.
5. Goffin J, Casey A, Kher P, *et al*. Preliminary clinical experience with the Bryan cervical disc prosthesis. *Neurosurgery (United States)* 2002;**51**:840–5; discussion 845–7.
6. Ishihara H, Kanamori M, Kawaguchi Y, *et al*. Adjacent segment disease after anterior cervical interbody fusion. *Spine J (United States)* 2004;**4**: 624–8.
7. Wigfield C, Gill S, Nelson R, *et al*. Influence of an

artificial cervical joint compared with fusion on adjacent-level motion in the treatment of degenerative cervical disc disease. *J Neurosurg Spine* 2002;**96**:17–21.

8. Eck JC, Humphreys SC, Lim TH, *et al.* Biomechanical study on the effect of cervical spine fusion on adjacent-level intradiscal pressure and segmental motion. *Spine (United States)* 2002;**27**: 2431–4.

9. Fuller DA, Kirkpatrick JS, Emery SE, *et al.* A kinematic study of the cervical spine before and after segmental arthrodesis. *Spine* 1998;**23**:1649–56.

10. Clements D, O'Leary P. Anterior cervical discectomy and fusion. *Spine* 1990;**15**:1023–5.

11. Baba H, Furusawa N, Imura S, *et al.* Late radiographic findings after anterior cervical fusion for spondylotic myelopathy. *Spine* 1993;**18**: 2167–73.

12. www.spine-health.com/research/artificialdisc/artdiseso3.html.

13. Anderson PA, Sasso RC, Roulean JP, *et al.* The Bryan cervical disc: Wear properties and early clinical results. *Spine J* 2004;**4**:303S–309S.

14. Singh K. Vaccro AR. Albert TJ. Assessing the potential impact of total disc arthroplasty on surgeon practice patterns in North America. *Spine J* 2004;**4**:195S–201S.

15. Bryan V. Cervical motion segment replacement. *Eur Spine J* 2002; **11** (Suppl 2) S92–S97.

16. Goffin J, Van Calenbergh F, van Loon J, *et al.* Intermediate follow up after treatment of degenerative disc disease by the Bryan cervical disc prosthesis— single level and bi-level. *Spine* 2003;**28**: 2673–8.

17. Traynelis VC. The prestige cervical disc replacement. *Spine J* 2004;**4**:310S–314S.

18. Link HD, McAfee PC, Pimenta L. Choosing a cervical disc replacement. *Spine J* 2004;**4**:294S–302S.

19. Puttlitz CM, Roussean MA. Xu Z, *et al.* Intervertebral disc replacement maintains cervical spine kinetics. *Spine* 2004;**29**:2809–14.

20. www.spine-health.com/research/artificialdisc/artdiseso2.html

21. Willert HG, Buchhorn GH, Hess T. The significance of wear and material fatique in loosening of hip prosthesis. *Orthopade* 1989;**18**:S350–S369.

22. Anderson PA, Rouleau JP, Bryan VE. Wear analysis of the Bryan cervical disc prosthesis. *Spine* 2003; **28**:S186–S194.

23. Anderson PA, Rouleau JP, Toth JM, *et al.* A comparison of simulator-tested and -retrieved cervical disc prostheses. Invited submission from the Joint Section Meeting on Disorders of the Spine and Peripheral Nerves, March 2004. *J Neurosurg Spine (United States)* 2004;**1**:202–10.

24. Mayer HM. *Cervical disk replacement spine art— spine arthroplasty.* Magazine No. 1/2004. Berlin, Heidelberg: Springer-Verlag; 2004.

25. Anderson PA, Sasso RC, Roulean JP, *et al.* The Bryan cervical disc: Wear properties and early clinical results. *Spine J* 2004;**4**:303S–309S.

26. Stephen MR, Vello B. The anterior surgical approach to the cervical spine for intervertebral disc disease. *Neurosurgery* 2004;**54**:1144–9.

27. Bohlman HH, Emery SE, Goodfellow DB, *et al.* Robinson anterior cervical discectomy and arthrodesis for cervical radiculopathy. *J Bone Joint Surg Am* 1993;**75**:1298–307.

28. Emery SE, Boltetsa MJ, Banks MA, *et al.* Robinson anterior cervical fusion: Comparison to standard and modified techniques. *Spine* 1994;**19**:660–3.

29. Emery SE, Fisher JRS, Bohlman HH. Three-level anterior cervical discectomy and fusion: Radiographic and clinical results. *Spine* 1997;**22**: 2622–5.

30. Connolly PJ, Esses SI, Kostuik JP. Anterior cervical fusion: Outcome analysis of patients fused with and without anterior cervical plates. *J Spinal Disord* 1996;**9**:202–6.

31. Isu T, Kanada K, Koboyashi N, *et al.* The surgical technique of anterior cervical fusion using bone grafts obtained from cervical vertebral bodies. *J Neurosurg* 1994;**80**:16–19.

32. Emery SE, Bohlman HH, Boletsa MJ, *et al.* Anterior cervical decompression and arthrodesis for the treatment of cervical spondylotic myelopathy. Two- to seventeen-year follow-up. *J Bone Joint Surg Am* 1998;**80**:941–51.

33. Cauthen JC, Kikard RE, Volger JB, *et al.* Outcome analysis of noninstrumented anterior cervical discectomy and interbody fusion in 348 patients. *Spine* 1998;**23**:188–92.

34. Alan SH, Gregory DC, Mark AP, *et al.* Radiculopathy and myelopathy at segments adjacent to the site of a previous anterior cervical arthrodesis. *J Bone Joint Surg* 1999;**81A**:519–28.

35. Cherubino P, Benazzo F, Borromeo U, *et al.* Degenerative arthritis of the adjacent spinal joint following anterior cervical spinal fusion. Clinico-radiologic and statistical correlations. *Ital J Orthop Traumatol* 1990;**16**:533–43.

36. Matsunaga S, Kabayama S, Yamamoto T, *et al.* Strain on intervertebral discs after anterior cervical decompression and fusion. *Spine* 1999;**24**:670–5.

37. Kulkarni V, Rajshekhar V, Raghuram L. Accelerated spondylotic changes adjacent to the fused segment following central cervical corpectomy: Magnetic resonance imaging study evidence. *J Neurosurg Spine* 2004;**100**:2–6.

38. Goffin J. Initial results with the Bryan cervical disc prosthesis. *J Neurosurg Spine* 2003;**28**:2673–8.

39. Gill SS, Walker C, Van Hoeck J, *et al.* Artificial intervertebral joint permitting translation and rotational motion, United States. Patent 2000; 6113637.

40. Cummins BH, Robertson JT, Gill SG. Surgical experience with an implanted artificial cervical joint. *J Neurosurg* 1998;**88**:943–8.

41. Anderson P, Rouleau JP, Bryan VE, *et al.* Wear analysis of the Bryan cervical disc prosthesis, Focus Issue. *Spine* 2003;**28** (Suppl 20):S186–S194.

42. Casey ATH, Goffin J, Kehr P, *et al.* Clinical significance of heterotopic ossification in cervical disc replacement: A prospective multicenter clinical trial clinical studies. *Neurosurgery* 2005; 759–63.

43. Pointillart V. Cervical disc prosthesis in humans: First failure. *Spine* 2001;**26**:E90–E92.

44. Moreland DB, Asch HL, Clabeaux DE, *et al.* Anterior cervical discectomy and fusion with implantable titanium cage: Initial impressions, patient outcomes and comparison to fusion with allograft. *Spine J* 2004;**4**:184–91.

45. Albert TJ, Eichenbaum MD. Goals of cervical disc replacement. *Spine J* 2004;**4**:292S–293S.

46. Mayer HM, Wieehert K, Korge A, *et al.* Minimally invasive total disc replacements: Surgical technique and preliminary clinical results. *Eur Spine J 202*;**11** (Suppl 2): S124–S130.

47. Tropinano P, Huang RC, Girardi FP, *et al.* Lumbar total disc replacement. Seven to eleven-year follow-up. *J Bone Joint Surg Am* 2005;**87A**:490–6.

48. McAfee PC. The indications for lumbar and cervical disc replacement. *Spine J* 2004;**4**:177S–181S.

49. Bryan VE Jr. Cervical motion segment replacement. *Eur Spine J* 2002;**2** (Suppl 11): S92–S97.

50. Goffin J, Vincent P, Bengent L, *et al.* Two year clinical result from a multicentre study of Bryan cervical disc system. *Spine J* 2004;**4** (Suppl 5):43S–44S.

12

Cervical myelopathy: Neurosurgical treatment

VOLKER SEIFERT, CHRISTIAN ULRICH

Introduction

Cervical myelopathy (CM) is a disease of the spinal cord due to degenerative changes of the cervical spine. Based on the chronological course two types can be distinguished: the acute and chronic myelopathy.[1,2] Whereas acute myelopathy is most frequently a compressive medial or latero-medial disc herniation, chronic CM is based on progressive degenerative changes of the cervical spine with additional vascular and mechanical factors.[1,2] Typical radiological findings in the chronic course of CM are osteochondrotic changes with bony spurs at the base and covering plate, which is also summarized as cervical spondylosis. Intraoperatively, often a combination of soft disc herniation and degenerative osteophytic changes is present that do not always correlate with the clinical or rather chronological course.

Pathology and pathobiomechanics

Although a detailed discussion of complex pathological and pathobiomechanical changes responsible for the development of CM is beyond the scope and intention of this chapter, a brief survey of current concepts is justified. As mentioned above, CM, particularly the chronic course, is due to multifactorial causes.[1,2] The reduced size of the cervical canal, of either congenital or acquired origin, and the development of posterior osteophytes initially induce affection and later on compression of the spinal cord. In addition to the chronic narrowing of the spinal canal, soft disc herniation can cause an acute deterioration. Moreover, calcification and ossification of the posterior longitudinal ligament or hypertrophy of the ligamentum flavum may result in further cervical stenosis.

Vascular compromise also seems to play an important role in CM and is responsible for deterioration in the later clinical course. Several experimental investigations substantiate the importance of histopathological changes in intramedullary vessels due to tractive and shear forces rather than anterior spinal artery compression.[3,4] Hypermobility that provokes further load to the compressed spinal canal is one of the main biomechanical reasons for progressing CM.[5]

Clinical symptoms

Typical symptoms of CM are well known. The common clinical features of the disease are the presence of spastic paraparesis or tetraparesis accompanied by gait disturbances, coordination abnormalities as well as clumsiness with fine motor skills.[1] Nuchal, shoulder, arm and/or radicular pain, although present in large number of patients with CM, are not reliable in terms of clinical diagnosis. The deterioration can proceed either in a stepwise fashion or gradually; however, in most cases, acute CM is an acute aggravation.

The differential diagnosis includes lesions of peripheral nerves, soft disc herniation, polyneuropathy, myopathy, systemic spinal diseases, (autoimmune) inflammation, deformities, spinal tumours and vascular lesions.

Evaluation and diagnoistic tools

A neuroradiological evaluation is mandatory for neurosurgical management. The basic diagnostic tool to demonstrate osteophytic spurs or other gross pathologies is the plain X-ray. Although computed tomography (CT) provides adequate information regarding a narrow canal and the bony structure, magnetic resonance tomography (MRI) has already become the major diagnostic tool in CM.[6-8] Soft tissue, disc herniation and compression of the spinal cord can be evaluated well by MRI (Fig. 1). On the other hand, assessment of bone is limted. T2-weighted

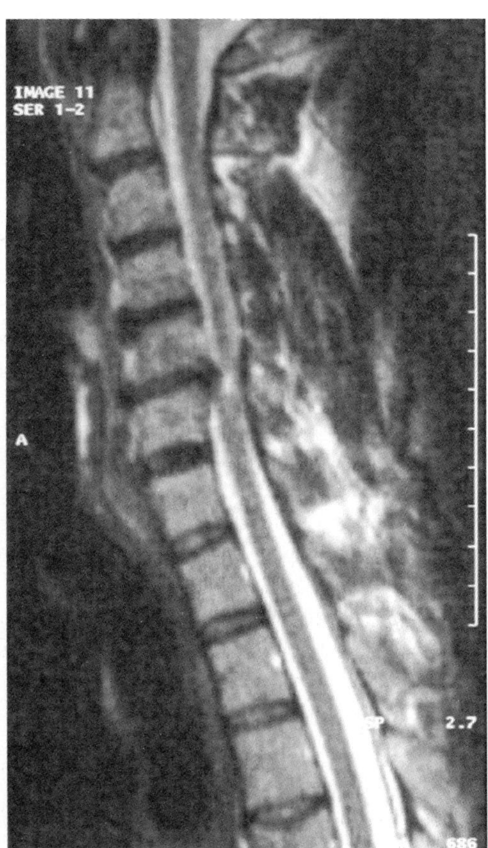

Fig. 1. MRI of disc herniation at C5–C6 level with spinal cord compression and discrete sign of intramedullary hyperintensity. The patient presented with acute onset of cervical myelopathy.

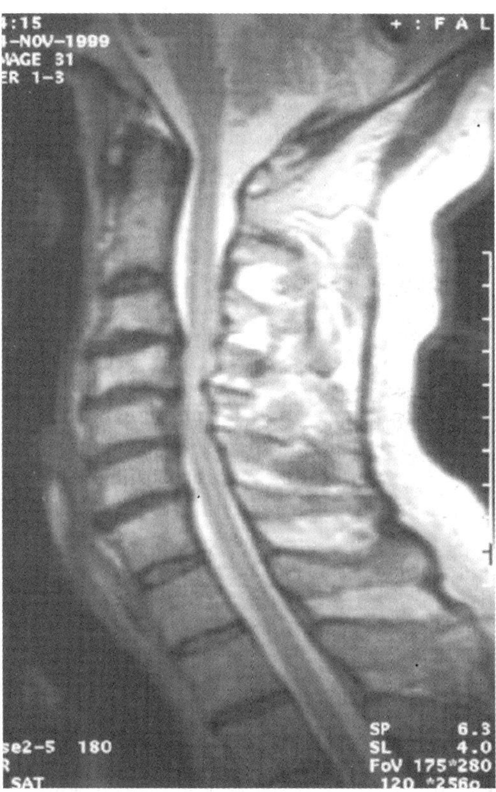

Fig. 2. MRI of multilevel osteochondrotic changes of the middle cervical spine. Anterior and posterior compression of the spinal cord due to osteophytes with intramedullary hyperintensity. Preoperatively, the patient presented with deterioration over years with subacute symptoms.

images can rule out intramedullary structural changes but the typical hyerintensity tend to exaggerate the magnitude of spinal cord compression (Fig. 2). Plain X-rays, CT and MRI also have their value for postoperative demonstration of surgical decompression.

Additionally, the electrophysiological evaluation is a helpful tool for preoperative assessment but does not influence the indication for operation. In fact, electrophysiology helps in distinguishing CM from other differential diagnoses. Usually somato-sensory evoked potentials are used for intraoperative monitoring.[9,10] Magnetic stimulation will be more relevant in the future, particularly for patients with severe CM.[11]

Treatment

Conservative

Only older literature[12] exists about the long-term non-operative treatment of CM. As mentioned above, the clinical course can be variable. This chronic disease may follow a stepwise fashion or gradually progress with slight and short intervals of remission. In case of severe CM conservative treatment with long-ranging immobilization is not acceptable for the patient and operative decompression is advised.

Operative (microsurgical decompression)

Earlier, operative treatment of CM was confined mostly to laminectomy.[13–17] Nowadays, the anterior approaches as compared to the posterior procedures are widely used for operative decompression of distinct cervical stenosis as well as tumour and trauma.[5,18–24] The posterior approach is still used in case of foraminotomies to extirpate soft disc herniation or mainly in Japan for open-door laminoplasties.[25,26]

Based on the pathophysiological concept of ventral compression due to osteophytic spurs and/or disc herniation the anterior approaches

have became widely accepted. Basically, these microsurgical procedures are conducted with a microscope and microinstruments (Fig. 3).[5,22–24]

The patient is placed supine on the table for the operation. The standard approach along the medial border of the sternocleidomastoid muscle to the anterior spine is employed using intraoperative fluoroscopy to define the correct level. Further procedure depends on the extent of compression. CM due to a soft disc herniation is treated by removing the intervertebral disc as well as the sequestered disc herniation and the posterior longitudinal ligament. After that an ablation of the dorsal osteophytes with micropunches and microdrill is mandatory. Depending on the surgeon's preference, a ventral fusion is mostly performed. The need is widely accepted and commonly titan or carbon cages, surgical cement or iliac crest grafts are used (Fig. 4). The goal is to spread apart the intervertebral space with expansion of the neuroforamina and radicular decompression. It is not the method of fusion but the extent and consistency of microsurgical decompression that is crucial to success, which necessitates a microscope.

In case of long-segment ventral osteophytes a uni- or multisegment resection of the medial vertebral bodies and the adjacent discs can be carried out. As mentioned above the operative success depends on the radical nature of microsurgical epidural decompression. In the standard approach, an appropriate bone graft is harvested from the iliac crest, brought into right position, and fixed with screws and ventral plate (Fig. 5).

Postoperatively, the adequacy of decompression is verified by CT. Follow-up treatment comprise rapid mobilization with consequent physical therapy.

Complications

Complications of the techniques described are extremely rare provided that the microsurgical principles are observed. Our own series of the

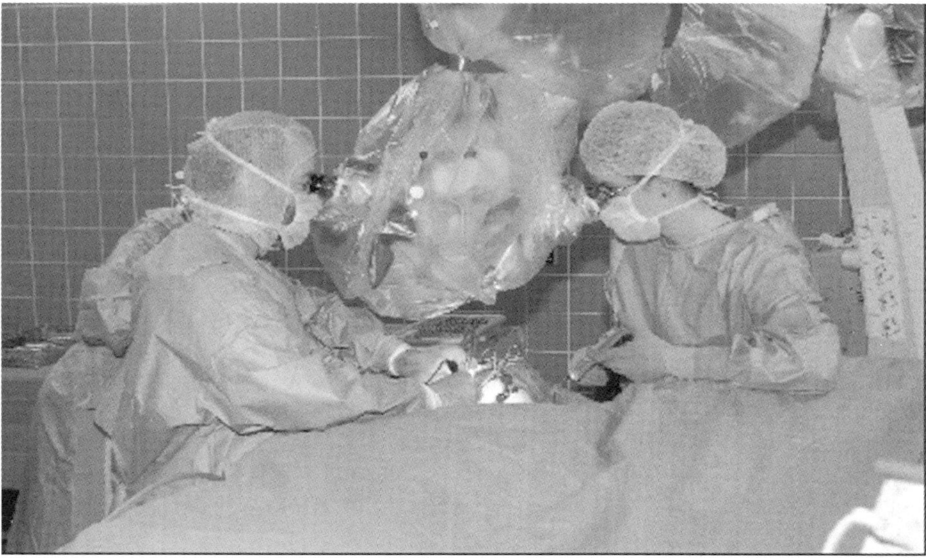

Fig. 3. Application of the microscope during a microsurgical cervical spine procedure and the constant availability of the C-arm.

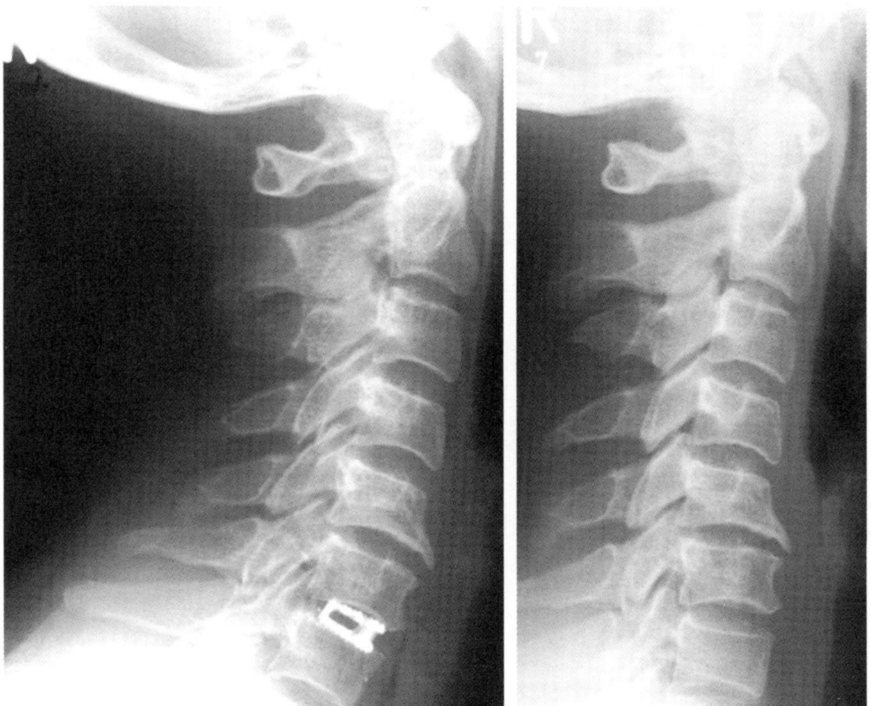

Fig. 4. Postoperative X-ray (left) of the cervical spine after microsurgical anterior discectomy, fusion with titan cage and ablation of osteophytes. Restitution of the physiological cervical lordosis. Preoperative X-ray is shown on the right.

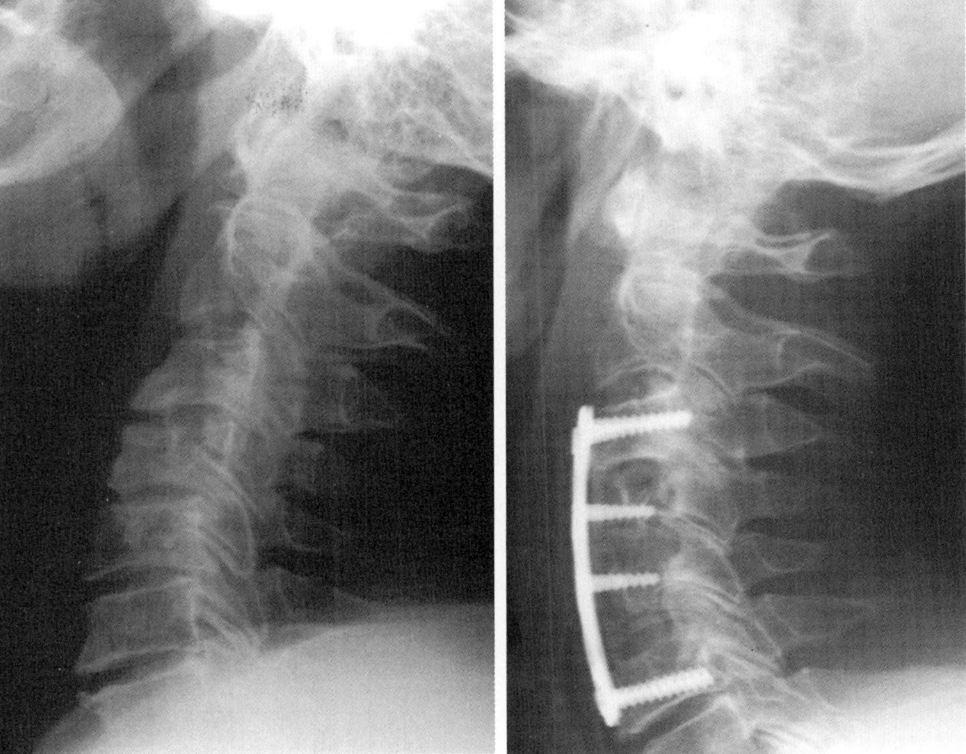

Fig. 5. Preoperative (left) and postoperative (right) X-ray of the cervical spine: corprectomy C4–C5 with iliac crest graft interponat and anterior fusion with plate due to multilevel osteochondrosis and spinal stenosis.

past 10 years consist of more than 1000 patients with a mortality rate of 0.21% (1 multimorbid, bedridden patient with progressive high-grade myelopathy died postoperatively from a pulmonary embolism). Other relevant complications such as wound healing disorders, transient neurological deterioration, or loosening of the screws are rare (<3%). Clinical improvement depends on the preoperative extent and duration of CM. More than 75% of patients show a significant clinical and electrophysiological decrease of preoperative symptoms.[5] Subjective recovery is about 90%, which is mostly due to relief from pain. However, about 10% of the operated, particularly those who have complex osteodegenerative changes, suffer a recurrent deterioration in the long-term follow-up. Our experiences are congruent with the results of comprehensive studies in the literature.

Conclusion

CM is a severe disease pattern, which consists of an acute or a chronic deterioration. The clinical symptoms and the diagnostic evaluation are well defined. The operative decompression should be utilized early in the clinical course and in a consequent microsurgical manner, if needed with instrumentation. The operative outcome depends on the extent and duration of preoperative symptoms, the correct strategic procedure, and the intensity of microsurgical decompression.

References

1. Clark CR. Cervical spondylotic myelopathy: History and physical findings. *Spine* 1988;**13**:847–9.
2. Bohlman HH, Emery SE. The pathophysiology of cervical spondylosis and myelopathy. *Spine* 1988;**13**:843–6.
3. Cusick JF. Pathophysiology and treatment of cervical spondylotic myelopathy. *Clin Neurosurg* 1991;**37**:661–81.
4. Mair WG, Druckman R. The pathology of spinal cord lesions and their relation to the clinical features in protrusion of cervical intervertebral discs: A report of four cases. *Brain* 1953;**76**:70–91.
5. Seifert V. Anterior decompressive microsurgery and osteosynthesis for the treatment of multi-segmental cervical spondylosis. Pathophysiological considerations, surgical indication, results and complications: A survey. *Acta Neurochir (Wien)* 1995;**135**:105–21.
6. Badami JP, Norman D, Barbaro NM, *et al.* Metrizamide CT myelography in cervical myelopathy and radiculopathy: Correlation with conventional myelography and surgical findings. *AJR Am J Roentgenol* 1985;**144**:675–80.
7. Karnaze MG, Gado MH, Sartor KJ, *et al.* Comparison of MR and CT myelography in imaging the cervical and thoracic spine. *AJR Am J Roentgenol* 1988;**150**:397–403.
8. Mehalic TF, Pezzuti RT, Applebaum BI. Magnetic resonance imaging and cervical spondylotic myelopathy. *Neurosurgery* 1990;**26**:217–26, discussion 226–7.
9. Hattori S, Saiki K, Kawai S. Diagnosis of the level and severity of cord lesion in cervical spondylotic myelopathy. Spinal evoked potentials. *Spine* 1979;**4**:478–85.
10. Yiannikas C, Shahani BT, Young RR. Short-latency somatosensory-evoked potentials from radial, median, ulnar, and peroneal nerve stimulation in the assessment of cervical spondylosis. Comparison with conventional electromyography. *Arch Neurol* 1986;**43**:1264–71.
11. Lo YL, Chan LL, Lim W, *et al.* Systematic correlation of transcranial magnetic stimulation and magnetic resonance imaging in cervical spondylotic myelopathy. *Spine* 2004;**29**:1137–45.
12. Arnasson O, Carlsson CA, Pellettieri L. Surgical and conservative treatment of cervical spondylotic radiculopathy and myelopathy. *Acta Neurochir (Wien)* 1987;**84**:48–53.
13. Casotto A, Buoncristiani P. Posterior approach in cervical spondylotic myeloradiculopathy. *Acta Neurochir (Wien)* 1981;**57**:275–85.
14. Fager CA. Posterior surgical tactics for the neurological syndromes of cervical disc and spondylotic lesions. *Clin Neurosurg* 1978;**25**:218–44.
15. Hirabayashi K, Watanabe K, Wakano K, *et al.* Expansive open-door laminoplasty for cervical spinal stenotic myelopathy. *Spine* 1983;**8**:693–9.
16. Jeffreys RV. The surgical treatment of cervical myelopathy due to spondylosis and disc degeneration. *J Neurol Neurosurg Psychiatry* 1986;**49**:353–61.
17. Kimura I, Oh-Hama M, Shingu H, Cervical myelopathy treated by canal-expansive laminaplasty. Computed tomographic and myelographic findings. *J Bone Joint Surg Am* 1984;**66**:914-20.
18. Camins MB, Rosenblum BR. Osseous lesions of the cervical spine. *Clin Neurosurg* 1991;**37**:722–39.
19. Caspar W, Barbier DD, Klara PM, Anterior cervical fusion and Caspar plate stabilization for cervical trauma. *Neurosurgery* 1989;**25**:491–502.
20. Dickman CA, Sonntag VK. Cruciate paralysis after a traumatic upper cervical spine injury. *Spine* 1992;**17**:1268.
21. Goffin J, Plets C, Van den Bergh R. Anterior cervical fusion and osteosynthetic stabilization according to Caspar: A prospective study of 41 patients with fractures and/or dislocations of the cervical spine. *Neurosurgery* 1989;**25**:865–71.
22. Seifert V. Anterior approaches in multisegmental cervical spondylosis. In: Schmidek HH (ed). *Operative techniques.* Philadelphia: Saunders & Co.; 2006:1849–64.
23. Seifert V, Stolke D. Multisegmental cervical spondylosis: Treatment by spondylectomy, microsurgical decompression, and osteosynthesis. *Neurosurgery* 1991;**29**:498–503.
24. Seifert V, Zimmermann M, Stolke D, *et al.* Spondylectomy, microsurgical decompression and osteosynthesis in the treatment of complex disorders of the cervical spine. *Acta Neurochir (Wien)* 1993;**124**:104–13.
25. Epstein N. Posterior approaches in the management of cervical spondylosis and ossification of the posterior longitudinal ligament. *Surg Neurol* 2002;**58**:194–207, discussion 207–8.
26. Koshu K, Tominaga T, Yoshimoto T. Spinous process-splitting laminoplasty with an extended foraminotomy for cervical myelopathy. *Neurosurgery* 1995;**37**:430–4, discussion 434–5.

13

Brachial plexus traction injuries in adults: The role of neurotization in the management

DHANANJAYA I. BHAT, BHAGAVATULA INDIRA DEVI

Brachial plexus injury in adults is a common clinical problem. It is a devastating type of injury, especially if the dominant upper limb is involved. Road traffic accidents, particularly those involving motorcycles, are a common cause of brachial plexus injuries.[1] In an epidemiological review in 1997, Midha[2] found that road accidents account for more than half of such injuries. The individuals are usually young males and many are the only earning member of the family. This places both a psychological and financial burden on the family, and is a burden on society as well.

We briefly describe the anatomy and pathophysiology of brachial plexus injury in adults. We will go on to enumerate the surgical options, focusing mainly on traction injuries, and describe our experience in their management.

Anatomy

The brachial plexus is formed from the ventral rami of C5 to T1 spinal nerves, with varying contribution from C4 and T2. The C5 and C6 roots merge to form the upper trunk. The C7 continues as the middle trunk, and the C8 and T1 roots combine to form the lower trunk within the posterior triangle of the neck. Each trunk has an anterior and a posterior division beneath the clavicle, and further branching results in the lateral, posterior and medial cords, which are named relative to their relationship with the axillary artery below the clavicle. The nerve supply to the rhomboids and serratus anterior comes from the proximal parts of the ventral roots of C5 and C5, C6, C7, respectively. The ventral roots of C8 and T1 have white rami communications with the cervical sympathetic chain. Thus, injury to these roots causes Horner syndrome.[3]

Pathophysiology

Brachial plexus injuries occur in about 1.2% of polytrauma victims, with motor vehicle accidents being the commonest cause.[2] Of the patients with brachial plexus lesions, 59%–70% have associated injuries, which may include polytrauma, head/spine injuries, clavicle fracture, shoulder joint injuries, vascular injuries and chest injuries.[1,4] Brachial plexus injuries may be either of the open or closed type and may be either supraclavicular, retroclavicular or infraclavicular. Up to 15% of cases have more than a single lesion along the neural element. Supraclavicular lesions are more common than infraclavicular lesions in stretch injuries. Retroclavicular lesions are very infrequent. Closed injuries are generally traction injuries in which the head and shoulder are forcibly pushed away from one another, resulting in severe stretch of soft tissues, including nerves and less frequently, vessels. These traction forces can result in mild conduction blockage, causing temporary paralysis (neuropraxia) or a more severe degree of injury in the form of axonotmesis or neuronotmesis. The structural damage to the nerve can result in either pre-ganglionic or post-ganglionic injuries. In pre-ganglionic injuries, the roots are avulsed from the spinal cord or ruptured in their intradural course proximal to the dorsal root ganglion or at the level of the ganglion in the intervertebral foramen. There is no Wallerian degeneration of the sensory axons in the peripheral nerve because the axons remain in continuity with the cell body of the ganglion; likewise there is no neuroma formation. Post-ganglionic injuries occur distal to the dorsal root ganglion and are physiologically similar to other peripheral nerve injuries with Wallerian degeneration of both sensory and motor fibres. They may be associated with a scar, neuroma formation or structural discontinuity of the nerve.[5,6]

The C5, C6 and C7 roots are attached to the transverse processes through transverse radicular ligaments, which protect them to a certain extent from being avulsed directly from the spinal cord. They are more prone to rupture distal to the spinal cord following stretch injuries, when varying lengths of proximal stump are left attached to the spinal cord. The absence of these radicular ligaments and the right-angled relation of the C8 and T1 roots with the cord make them more susceptible to avulsion injuries.[7] The upper and middle trunks are more commonly involved than the lower trunk. The posterior and lateral cords take the brunt of damage in infraclavicular lesions. The medial cord almost always escapes.[6]

Infraclavicular lesions occur following violent hyperextension of the shoulder and are frequently associated with fracture of the shaft of the humerus or injury to the shoulder joint. They are associated with a higher incidence of vascular injuries.[8] The majority of plexus injuries in the adult are closed avulsion or traction injuries and they involve predominantly the upper trunk (Erb palsy) in up to 70%, lower trunk (Klumpke palsy) in up to 20% and the whole of the plexus in 10% of cases.[9] However, in tertiary centres, pan-brachial plexus (C5 to T1 roots) injuries seem to be more common (39%–57%), followed by C5, C6 and C5–C7 root injuries (15%–20% each). Isolated C8–T1 root injuries are rare (8%). This difference may be due to a referral bias, with many upper plexus injuries improving spontaneously and thus not being referred to a centre.[1,9,10]

Clinical features

During the acute stage of the problem, the management of associated vascular, bony, chest, head and spine injuries takes priority. Later on, once the patient is stable, during follow-up, or when the patient has presented for several days or months following the injury, individual testing of the muscles with concomitant application of anatomical knowledge aids in localizing the level of the lesion. Special attention needs to be paid to the following.[6,8–10]

- Tinel sign indicates a post-ganglionic lesion and may provide some evidence of axonal regeneration. However, the presence of this sign does not guarantee a good clinical recovery. The absence of Tinel sign distal to the injury along the nerve after an appropriate time interval suggests no regeneration or total disruption of the nerve.
- The presence of perception of deep pain and sympathetic function in a flail anaesthetic limb indicates that the nerve fibres are probably not completely cut. The smaller unmyelinated fibres subserving the above functions are more

resilient to traction forces than the large myelinated fibres carrying motor and superficial sensory signals. Therefore, it is essential to look for changes in sweating, skin temperature and colour.

- Burning paraesthesias which may be associated with lightning shooting pain along the upper limb are highly suggestive of a proximal injury with root avulsion.
- Horner syndrome is suggestive of C8–T1 root avulsions from the cord or injury to the roots close to the cord.
- Along with Horner syndrome, look for wasting of paraspinal muscles and rhomboid and serratus anterior muscle wasting. The presence of any one of these indicates pre-ganglionic injuries or injuries close to the intervertebral foramen. These findings preclude direct nerve repair or anastomosis between the proximal and distal stumps of the injured nerve. Neurotization, or nerve transfer, is then the only treatment option.

Investigations

X-ray

X-rays of the cervical spine and chest may give an indication of the severity of the injury. Severe, pre-ganglionic injuries may be associated with transverse process fractures, haemidiaphramatic palsy (phrenic nerve injury), fracture of the first rib or clavicle, or chest injuries. Look for rib fractures on the same side as the plexus injury because their presence may indicate associated intercostal nerve (ICN) injury, which precludes this nerve from being a potential donor nerve for repair of the injured plexus elements.[11]

CT myelogram

In a normal individual, the anterior and posterior roots can be visualized as linear filling defects in the contrast-filled subarachnoid spaces. In cases of brachial plexus injury, the computed tomography (CT) myelogram may demonstrate a cerebrospinal fluid pouch (pseudo-meningocele), suggesting a significant degree of traction and breach in the sleeve that is causing extradural leak of cerebrospinal fluid. This suggests an associated nerve root avulsion from the spinal cord. In these conditions the anterior and posterior roots cannot be visualized. However, sometimes there is a pseudomeningocele without an avulsion of the root.[11]

MRI

The nerve root appears as a low signal intensity in the fat of the neural foramina on T1-weighted images. This is not seen when there is a root avulsion. Magnetic resonance imaging (MRI) can also demonstrate the brachial plexus in the neck, the presence of a large neuroma and the presence of a pseudomeningocele (Fig. 1).[11]

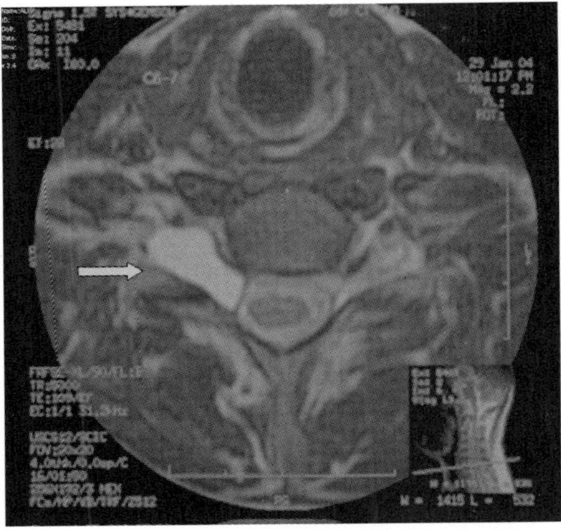

Fig. 1. MRI demonstrating a pseudomeningocele at C6–C7 level on the right side (arrow)

Neurophysiological studies

Nerve conduction studies (NCS) and electro-myography (EMG) are useful in localizing the injury, identifying the degree of injury, prognosticating and assessing recovery. They are not useful earlier than 7–10 days post-injury as the distal part of the nerve does not degenerate immediately and continues to conduct for several days. Motor responses can be elicited for 3–4 days after the injury and electrical activity may persist for 6–7 days. The nature of the lesion takes up to 6 weeks to manifest. Hence, when NCS and EMG are performed after 6 weeks, they can be good predictors of the prognosis. They are also useful in the postoperative period to detect regeneration before it becomes clinically evident.[6,12]

Treatment

In acute injuries, the treatment of vascular damage and other life-threatening conditions takes priority. If the presence of a haematoma accompanied by progressive neurological deficits due to plexus compression is detected, it must be explored immediately. Acute open injuries with clean-cut lacerations must be explored within 72 hours and direct repair or repair with an interposed graft can be done. In the case of infected ragged edges, the stumps can be tagged and re-explored later, when the cut ends can be sutured with grafts.[6]

The management of closed traction injuries is very challenging (Fig. 2). The standard initial treatment is to wait watchfully, so as to allow spontaneous recovery of the injured neural elements and prevent unnecessary premature resection of recovering nerves. Waiting also allows the lesion to become better demarcated. However, as the number of days of denervation increases, the muscles tend to undergo atrophy and fibrosis, and are replaced by fat. This makes the delayed repair of nerves effectively sub-optimal. Thus, a balance has to be maintained between waiting and taking action. Some believe in

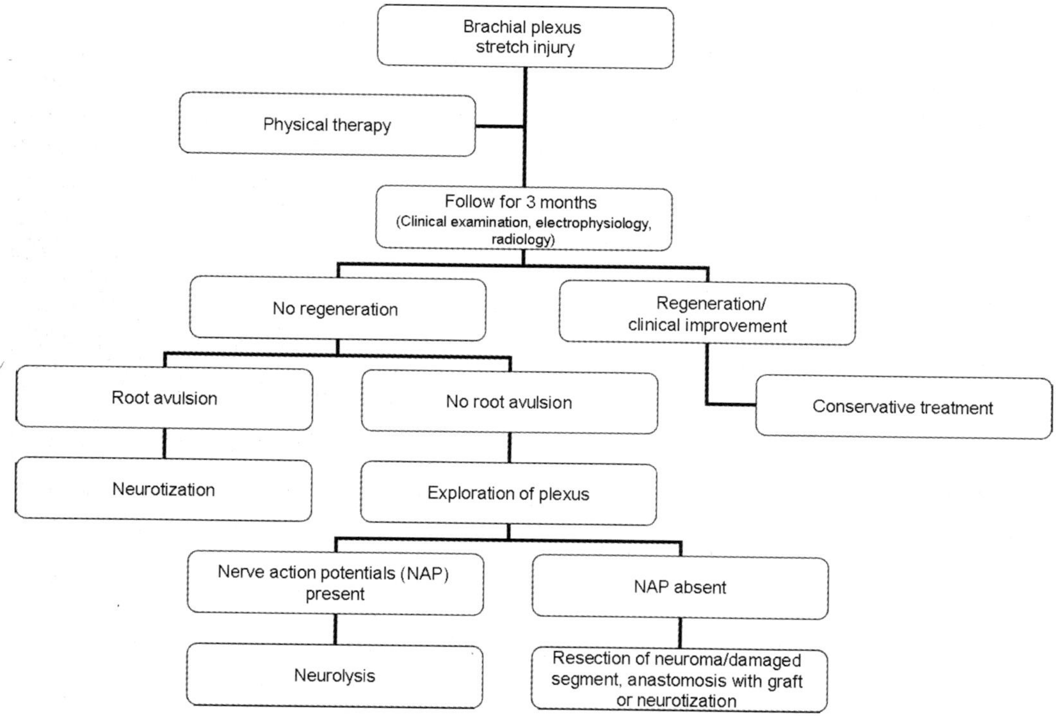

Fig. 2. Management algorithm for traction injuries of brachial plexus

performing early surgeries, i.e. within 6 weeks of the injury,[13] while others have obtained good results even after a time interval of up to 7–9 months.[14,15] In their series of 204 patients, Terzis *et al.*[16] found that a duration of denervation of less than 6 months was important for re-innervation of the biceps. On an average, most surgeons agree upon a time interval of 3–6 months.[1,6,17]

During this period of observation, physical therapy is important. The goal is to maintain the normal range of movement of all the joints, maintain the bulk of the muscles, improve strength, prevent wasting and shortening of tendons, and manage pain. All this is to optimize recovery once muscle re-innervation takes place. Regular clinical and electrophysiological tests are performed at intervals.

During follow-up, if there are signs of recovery, conservative treatment with physical and occupational therapy is continued. Between 40% and 66% of patients with only upper trunk complete injury have varying degrees of recovery, up to 30% improving significantly. However, patients with pan-brachial plexus injuries with a flail anaesthetic limb have a poor chance of recovering spontaneously (only around 4% have some recovery).[10,18] Incomplete loss of function usually improves with time.

If there are no signs of recovery or there is suboptimal recovery, then surgical intervention may be contemplated. Surgical repair can be considered earlier if the injury is severe and complete, with avulsion of roots, as judged by the clinical examination and electrophysiology.

Surgical options

During the exploration of the brachial plexus, motor and sensory nerve action potentials (NAPs) are recorded across the injured segments. In case there are regenerative motor NAPs, an external and internal neurolysis of the injured segment is performed, i.e. the scar tissue surrounding the nerve is incised and removed, thus freeing the nerve (external neurolysis). Sometimes, due to excess scarring, longitudinal incisions have to be made within the nerve in order to separate the fascicles and free from fibrosis (internal neurolysis). Recovery following this procedure is encouraging, especially for the C5 and C6 roots and for upper trunk injuries. Midha *et al.* have reported an 84% improvement following neurolysis.[10,17]

When a neuroma in continuity is encountered, NAPs are recorded across it. If there are regenerative NAPs, then neurolysis is sufficient. The absence of NAPs indicates lack of functioning neural elements within the lesion. The neuroma is then resected and serial transverse sectioning of the proximal stump is done till a viable fascicular pattern is obtained. Following this, the gap is bridged with an autograft (in most cases it is the sural nerve). Again, the results of grafting are good and recovery varies from slightly less than 50%–82%.[10,19] If the sensory NAPs are normal, it indicates that the sensory fibres are intact and there is probably a pre-ganglionic injury. This is further confirmed by the absence of somatosensory evoked potentials in the contralateral sensory cortex. The presence of pre-ganglionic injury precludes repair of the nerve roots directly or with a graft. Neurotization is then the only option.[10,17,20]

Neurotization is a procedure in which a functioning nerve is used as a donor. It is cut proximal to its target muscle and the proximal stump is sutured to the denervated (injured) distal nerve stump of the plexus, with or without an intervening graft. Neurotization was first attempted by Letievant in 1873 and later by Tuttle in 1913.[17] In 1973, Kotani *et al.* neurotized the musculocutaneous nerve with the ICN for the first time.[21] At present, neurotization is the standard treatment for pre-ganglionic injuries. The commonly used donor nerves are the ICNs, phrenic nerve, accessory nerve, branches of the cervical plexus and components of the brachial plexus, like the ulnar nerve, medial pectoral nerve and contralateral C7 nerve. Usually, the recipient nerve is the musculocutaneous nerve.

The other recipient nerves include the axillary and suprascapular nerves. In performing such a procedure, the original function of the donor nerve is sacrificed for a more beneficial function in the upper limb.[10,17]

Whatever may be the surgical intervention, the results are better for the C5 and C6 distributions (especially elbow flexion). The results for the distal musculature, especially the C8 and T1 distribution (i.e. wrist and fingers), are uniformly poor.[10]

For pre-ganglionic injuries, direct implantation of the distal ruptured roots into the spinal cord is an exciting option. A few case studies relating to this procedure have been published and these showed some recovery of proximal muscle function. However, the results are not good enough to justify its becoming a standard surgical procedure.[22,23]

Reconstructive surgeries are used when neural repair has failed. These procedures include tendon and muscle transfers (pedicle and free muscle) in order to bring about elbow flexion and wrist and finger movements. However, in pan-brachial plexus injuries, most of the muscles of the limb are paralysed, so the possibility of such transfer is limited. Functional improvements in distal limb movements are poor even with these procedures.[10,24]

Goals of surgery

In upper brachial plexus injury, the primary goal of surgery would be to restore elbow flexion, followed by stabilization of the shoulder and/or restoring abduction. Elbow flexion can be achieved by neurotizing the musculocutaneous nerve with the intercostal nerve, medial pectoral nerve, ulnar nerve or spinal accessory nerve. The shoulder can be stabilized by neurotization of the suprascapular nerve with the spinal accessory nerve or by arthrodesis of the joint. Shoulder abduction and stabilization can also be obtained by intercostal-axillary nerve anastomosis.[10,24]

In pan-brachial plexus injury with an anaes-thetic flail upper limb, the top priority is to restore elbow flexion. This will allow the patient to use his limb like a strut, as a paperweight, as a platform on which objects may be balanced, as a hook for hanging objects, or to turn simple levers.[10] Many surgeons perform shoulder stabilization for optimal use of elbow flexion. However, others feel that it may not be necessary as restoration of the power of the biceps itself stabilizes the shoulder.[24] We, too, feel that it is unnecessary to neurotize the supracapsular nerve for shoulder stabilization.

Reconstructive procedures are used as salvage procedures. The goals of reconstruction are to restore some degree of elbow flexion and shoulder stability. These secondary procedures have the advantage of not being time-dependent, as results are seen immediately after surgery.[10,24]

Surgical procedure

Surgery is performed under general anaesthesia. The patient is placed supine and strapped to the bed, with the shoulder of the affected limb abducted and externally rotated. The ipsilateral hip is flexed, internally rotated and adducted with the knee flexed, exposing the calf so as to be able to harvest the sural nerve. A sand bag is placed beneath the ipsilateral shoulder and hip. The musculocutaneous nerve is exposed in the arm, in the groove between the biceps and brachialis muscle, and is traced till its attachment to the biceps muscle. Generally, the third ICN is exposed in the midaxillary line along the lower border of the rib up to the midclavicular line (Fig. 3). The nerve is cut and the proximal stump mobilized. One then measures the approximate length of the graft required to connect the ICN with the musculocutaneous nerve without any tension even during maximum abduction. An appropriate length of the sural nerve is harvested by making multiple transverse incisions over the calf, from above the lateral malleolus (Fig. 4). One can obtain a sural nerve graft of up to 30 cm in length. The graft is then tunnelled subcutaneously

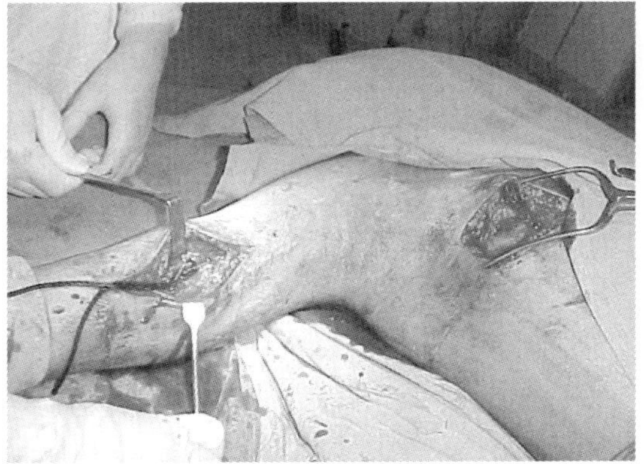

Fig. 3. Exposure of the musculocutaneous N and the intercostal nerve

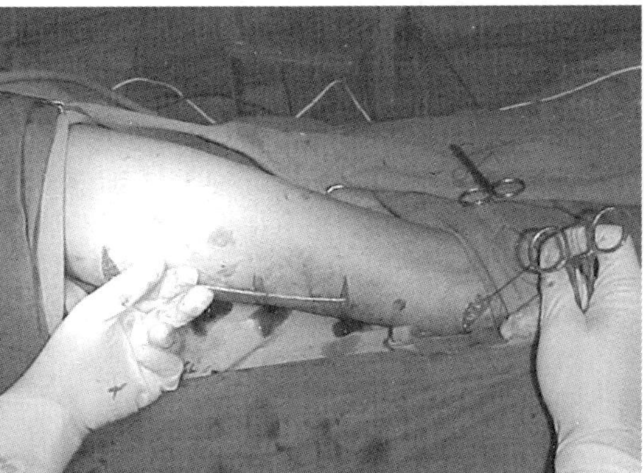

Fig. 4. Sural nerve graft harvested from calf

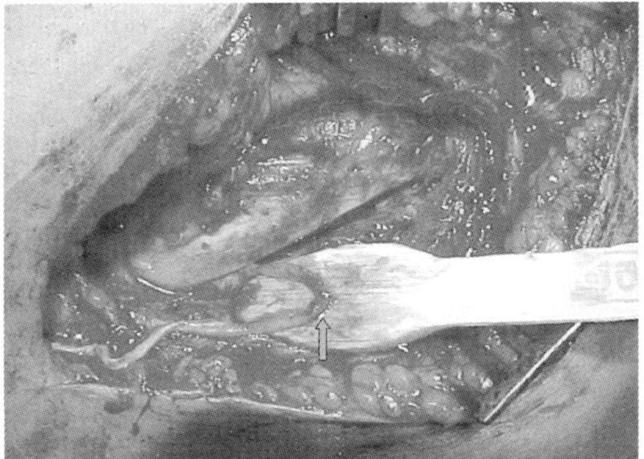

Fig. 5. ICN sutured to the sural nerve (arrow) in the intercostal space

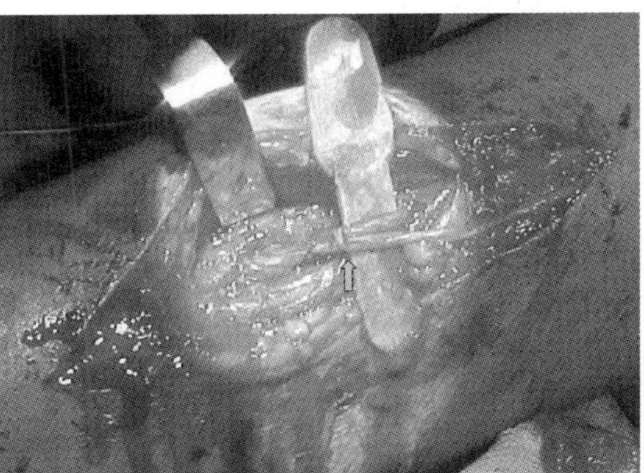

Fig. 6. Musculocutaneous nerve sutured to the sural nerve (arrow) in the arm

across the axilla. One end is anastomosed with the cut end of the intercostal nerve, using 8-0 mersilk epineural stitches (Fig. 5). Similarly, the other end of the graft is sutured to the cut distal end of the musculocutaneous nerve, as close as possible to its entry into the biceps muscle in order to achieve optimal results (Fig. 6). When the ICN is too thin compared to the musculocutaneous nerve, a lower ICN is also used for neurotization of the musculocutaneous nerve.

Postoperatively the limb is supported with an arm sling for about three weeks. Physiotherapy is resumed as soon as possible, usually within a few days of surgery. Good physiotherapy is very essential for augmenting the success of regeneration. The patient is advised to inhale deeply when trying to flex his elbows as during the initial stage of regeneration, there is a synkinetic movement between inspiration and elbow flexion, with inspiration facilitating flexion. Slowly, however, the patient learns to dissociate the two and is eventually able to perform elbow flexion independent of inspiration, due to plasticity at the cortical and probably the spinal cord level too.

Plexus injury pain

Following brachial plexus injury, patients may experience severe, disabling pain in the upper limb. The pain is commonly associated with avulsion injuries and is seen in up to 80% of cases of complete brachial plexus palsy. It has been postulated that the pain arises because spinal cord differentiation causes the dorsal horn neurons to fire spontaneously due to lack of peripheral sensory input following root avulsion.[25] This pain may resolve spontaneously in many cases.[10] Wynn Parry, who reported on 404 patients with pain following brachial plexus injury, found that more than 50% of them had some relief in three years.[26]

Interestingly, many studies have shown that there is significant relief from pain in up to 80% of patients 2–10 years after surgery. There may be relief from pain as early as the first postoperative day to several months after surgery. Pain has been found to decrease not only after direct surgeries on the plexus (such as neurolysis or excision of neuromas and grafting), but also after neurotization procedures (such as intercostal to musculocutaneous nerve anastomosis). Many patients correlate relief from pain with recovery of motor functions. It has also been observed that if there is no recovery after surgery, then the pain persists.[8,27–28] Amitryptilline and gabapentin can be tried to relieve the patient's pain, but may not be very useful. In refractory cases, central destructive procedures, like dorsal root entry zone lesioning, performed by an expert can be useful.[10]

NIMHANS experience

We analysed 51 patients who were surgically treated for brachial plexus injuries from 1997 to 2003. The mean age was 28.7 years and 43 of the patients were male. Motor vehicle accidents accounted for 85% of the injuries. Twenty-three (45%) patients had associated systemic injuries. Forty-six (90%) had closed traction injuries, and the remaining five had open injuries. Pan-brachial plexus injury with a flail limb was seen in 22 patients (43%). In 18 cases, the C5 and C6 roots were involved, with 8 of them having involvement of C7 root also. Upper trunk injury was seen in 9 patients. In one case the C8 and T1 roots were involved, and in another the

infraclavicular posterior cord was involved. Clinical and nerve conduction studies showed a pre-ganglionic type of injury in 42 patients and post-ganglionic injury in the rest. Neurotization was performed for all these patients, without supraclavicular exploration. A total of 55 nerves were neurotized (33 musculocutaneous, 18 axillary and 2 radial and 2 ulnar nerves). In most cases, the intercostal nerve was used as a donor nerve. In two cases, neurotization was performed using the medial pectoral nerve and split median nerve as the donor.

In our experience, there were no major postoperative complications. In two cases, small pleural tears occurred during dissection of the ICN. These did not require intercostal drainage and recovery was uneventful.

Early signs of recovery may appear 6–8 months after surgery. However, the average time is 12–13 months, while in some cases, 18 months elapse before signs of recovery are noted.[29] Our average follow-up period for 36 patients was of 22 months' duration. In the case of musculocutaneous nerve neurotization, there was a functionally useful recovery in 54.1% of patients, while in the case of axillary nerve neurotization, the percentage was 60%. None of the patients with ulnar or radial nerve repair improved, except for one patient with radial nerve injury who regained some elbow extension. The critical time interval within which surgical improvements could be expected was five-and-a-half months. Four of the five patients who had presented with preoperative pain had some relief from pain.[30]

At present, there are no randomized controlled studies showing the superiority of one procedure over the other. In general, the success rate for musculocutaneous and axillary nerve neurotization with different donor nerves varies greatly and is between 30% and 90%.[8,29,31,32,33] Samardzic *et al.*[29] reported overall and useful recovery rates of 50% and 57%, respectively, following ICN to musculocutaneous nerve neurotization and 63% and 33% overall and useful recovery rates following ICN to axillary nerve neurotization. Narakas *et al.*[14] Dubuisson *et al.*[1] and Kawai *et al.*[31] reported recovery rates of 50%–64% following neurotization. This compares well with our results, except for the quality of recovery of the axillary nerve, which was significantly higher in our patients.

Conclusions

Brachial plexus injury is a disabling condition, with a complex pathophysiology and clinical features. There is still no consensus regarding the management of these injuries. Recovery may be spontaneous in the case of mild injuries, but severe ones often require surgical intervention. The results of surgery together with good physiotherapy are encouraging but far from satisfactory, especially for pan-brachial plexus and lower plexus injuries. Neurotization is a simple and elegant procedure and should always be considered before undertaking any reconstructive procedure, especially for pre-ganglionic upper brachial plexus injuries.

References

1. Dubuisson AS, Kline DG. Brachial plexus injury: An survey of 100 consecutive cases from a single service. *Neurosurgery* 2002;**51**:673–83.
2. Midha R. Epidemiology of brachial plexus injuries in a multitrauma population. *Neurosurgery* 1997;**40**:1182–8.
3. Drake LR, Vogl W, Mithcell AW (eds). *Gray's anatomy for students.* Philadelphia: Elsevier; 2005:656–65.
4. Narakas AO. The treatment of brachial plexus injuries. *Int Orthop* 1985;**9**:29–36.
5. Fry CF. Action potential and nervous conduction. *Surgery* 2005;**23**:425–9.
6. Mannan K, Carlstedt T. Injuries to the brachial plexus. *Surgery* 2006;**24**:409–14.
7. Sunderland S. Meningeal neural relations in the intervertebral foramen. *J Neurosurg* 1974;**40**:756–63.
8. Rolfe Birch. Injuries to the brachial plexus; controversies and possibilities. In: Mayberg MR, Winn HR (eds). *Peripheral nerve issues: Controversies and evolving treatments, Neurosurgery Clinics of North America.* Philadelphia:WB Saunders; 2001;**12**:285–94.
9. Mehta S, Tan S, Power DM. Instructional course lecture: Assessment and early management of traumatic brachial plexus injury. *The Internet Journal of Hand Surgery* 2007, Volume 1, Number 1.
10. Midha R. Stretch injuries to brachial plexus. In: DH Kim, Midha R, Murovic JA, Spinner RJ (eds). *Nerve injuries: Operative results for major nerve injuries, entrapments and tumors.* 2nd ed. Philadelphia: Elsevier; 2008:325–62.
11. Rankine JJ. Adult traumatic brachial plexus injury. *Clin Radiol* 2004;**59**:767–74.
12. Chaudhry V, Cornblath DR. Wallerian degeneration in human nerves: Serial electrophysiological studies. *Muscle Nerve* 1992;**15**:687–93.
13. Yamada S, Lonser RR, Iacono RP, *et al.* Bypass coaptation procedures for cervical nerve root avulsion. *Neurosurgery* 1996;**38**:1145–52.
14. Narakas AO, Hentz VR. Neurotization in brachial plexus injuries. Indication and results. *Clin Orthop Relat Res* 1988;**237**:43–56.
15. Samii M, Carvalho GA, Nikkhah G, *et al.* Surgical reconstruction of the musculocutaneous nerve in traumatic brachial plexus injuries. *J Neurosurg* 1997;**87**:881–6.
16. Terzis JK, Vekris MD, Soucacos PN. Outcomes of brachial plexus reconstruction in 204 patients with devastating paralysis. *Plast Reconstr Surg* 1999;**104**:1221–40.
17. Kandenwein JA, Kretschmer T, Engelhardt M, *et al.* Surgical interventions for traumatic lesions of the brachial plexus: A retrospective study of 134 cases. *J Neurosurg* 2005;**103**:614–21.
18. Wynn Parry C. The management of traction lesions of the brachial plexus and peripheral nerve injuries to the upper limb: A study in teamwork. *Injury* 1980;**11**:265–85.
19. Songcharoen P. Brachial plexus injury in Thailand: A report of 520 cases. *Microsurgery* 1995;**16**:35–9.
20. Sulaiman WAR, Kline DG. Nerve surgery: A review and insights about its future. *Clin Neurosurg* 2006;**53**:38–47.
21. Kotani PT, Matsuda H, Suzuki T. Trial surgical procedure of nerve transfer to avulsion injuries of the plexus brachialis, in Orthopaedic Surgery and Traumatology. International Congress Series No. 291. *Amsterdam Excerpta Medica* 1973:348–50.
22. Bertelli JA, Ghizoni MF. Brachial plexus avulsion injury repairs with nerve transfers and nerve grafts

directly implanted into the spinal cord yield partial recovery of shoulder and elbow movements. *Neurosurgery* 2003;**52**:1385–90.

23. Carlstedt T, Praveen A, Hallin R, *et al.* Spinal nerve root repair and reimplantation of avulsed ventral roots into the spinal cord after brachial plexus injury. *J Neurosurg* 2000;**93** (Suppl 2):237–47.

24. Bentolila V, Nizard R, Bizot P, *et al.* Complete traumatic brachial plexus palsy: Treatment and outcome after repair. *J Bone and Joint Surg* 1999;**81**:20–8.

25. Bertelli JA, Ghizoni MF. Pain after avulsion injuries and complete palsy of the brachial plexus: The possible role of nonavulsed roots in pain generation. *Neurosurgery* 2008;**62**:1104–14.

26. Wynn Parry CB. Brachial plexus injuries. *Br J Hosp Med* 1984;**32**:130–9.

27. Berman JS, Taggart M, Anand P. Pain relief from preganglionic injury to the brachial plexus by late intercostal transfer. *J Bone Joint Surg Br* 1996;**78**:759–60.

28. Berman JS, Birch R, Anand P. Pain following human brachial plexus injury with spinal cord avulsion and the effect of surgery. *Pain* 1998;**75**:199–207.

29. Samardzic M, Rasulic L, Grujicic D, *et al.* Results of nerve transfers to the musculocutaneous and axillary nerves. *Neurosurgery* 2000;**46**:93–103.

30. Moiyadi AV, Indira Devi B, *et al.* Brachial plexus injuries: Outcome following neurotization with intercostal nerve. *J Neurosurg* 2007;**107**:308–13.

31. Kawai H, Kawabata H, Masada K, *et al.* Nerve repairs for traumatic brachial plexus palsy with root avulsion. *Clin Orthop Relat Res* 1988;**237**:75–86.

32. Nagano A. Treatment of brachial plexus injury. *J Orthop Sci* 1998;**3**:71–80.

33. Malessy MJ, Thomeer RT. Evaluation of intercostal to musculocutaneous nerve transfer in reconstructive brachial plexus surgery. *J Neurosurg* 1998;**88**:266–71.

14

Grade 1 degenerative spondylolisthesis in patients >60 years of age: Routine fusion is necessary

RAMAKRISHNA EASWARAN, S. SUNDARRAJAN

Degenerative spondylolisthesis was first described in the medical literature by MacNab in 1950, as spondylolisthesis with intact neural arch.[1] Although Cloward perfected the technique of posterior lumbar interbody fusion using an iliac autograft in the 1960s, only a few surgeons could master this exacting technique.[2] The recognition of spinal stenosis as an essential concomitant of degenerative spondylolisthesis led to treatment with decompression alone.[3] The Hamlet-like question, 'to fuse or not to fuse' has been a recurring theme in meetings on the spine, with orthopaedic surgeons and neurosurgeons on opposite sides of the divide. The light shed on this dilemma pales in comparison with the heat generated by arguments that have been emotionally driven rather than factually so. The spinal implant industry has added a plethora of devices that further confound the issue. In today's parlance 'fusion' has become synonymous with 'instrumented fusion'.

In this chapter we have reviewed fusion surgery for degenerative spondylolisthesis. Also given is an account of our surgical approach to the problem of degenerative spondylolisthesis, especially in the elderly.

Background

Epidemiology

Degenerative spondylolisthesis (DSO) is found most commonly at the L4–L5 level, with decreasing frequency at L3–L4, L2–L3, L5–S1 and L1–L2 levels. Women of 40–60 years of age exhibit slippage in a 2:1 to 10:1 ratio when compared with men.[4] The male patients are typically older, i.e. in their sixth or eighth decades. The factors associated with an increased incidence of DSO are listed in Table 1.[5–11]

Clinical features

DSO may be incidentally detected on radiographic survey of patients with no spinal symptoms. Some patients have only brief and rare episodes of non-disabling back or leg pain related to an acute strain; they respond quickly to conservative treatment. Natural history studies show a very low rate of clinical progression in these patients.[12] Such patients do not need surgery, but clinical and radiographic follow up

Table 1. Factors predisposing to DSO

Women[5]

Oophorectomized women—3 times greater incidence[6]

Osteoporosis—leading to elongation of the pars[7]

Sagittal orientation of facets (sagittal facet angle >45° increases risk 25-fold)[8]

Specific factors for L4–L5 level DSO

   —Narrow L4 inferior articular process[9]

   —Sacralization of L5[9]

   —Horizontalization of the lamina and the facets[10]

Specific factors for L5–S1 level DSO[11]

   —Slender L5 transverse process

   —Greater inclination of sacral table

   —Less deep location of the L5 vertebra in the pelvis

is advisable. Back pain may become less severe over time, as the degeneration progresses to the Kirkaldy–Willis phase 3 of restabilization.[12]

The typical patient with DSO presents with lower back pain, sciatica and claudicatory leg pain in various permutations.[13] The symptoms do not improve on forward bending, as in the case of spinal stenosis. The patients tend to support their trunk with their arms.[14] The symptoms respond poorly to conservative methods. The symptomatic patients have a real risk of further clinical and radiological progression and are hence candidates for surgery.[12]

Investigations

It is not enough to obtain a supine lateral radiograph of the lumbar spine, as 15% of vertebral slips reduce on lying down.[14] Good radiographs can pick up olisthesis missed by supine MRI (Fig. 1).[15] Standing flexion and extension radiographs are indicated for assessing the dynamic change in the grade of olisthesis in the sagittal plane (Fig. 2). Lateral flexion X-rays are useful in showing translatory slips in the coronal plane.[14] DSO is generally Meyerding grade I or II (low grade). Progression to a higher grade does not occur in the absence of previous decompression surgery. CT shows spondylolysis better than oblique X-rays (Fig. 1D). Elongation of the pars and sclerosis arising from healed pars defect are also seen. MRI gives a wealth of information about the neural structures, disc, end plates and facet joints. The distended facet sign has recently been described to be associated with position-dependent spinal stenosis in dynamic DSO.[16] Axial loaded MRI and dynamic MRI can be done in a few centres only.[17] All patients undergoing surgery are, in addition, evaluated with non-contrast spiral CT with multiplanar reconstruction. Intrathecal contrast CT myelography is used for those in whom MRI cannot be performed (usually because of the presence of a metal artefact in the postoperative patient). Nerve conduction studies are

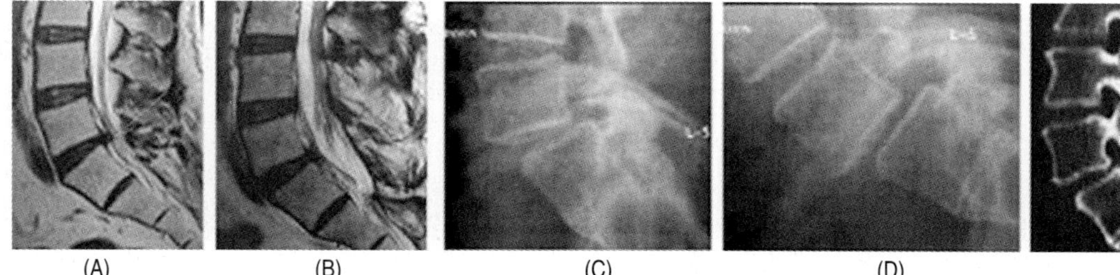

(A)   (B)   (C)   (D)   (E)

Fig. 1. Adult occult isthmic spondylolisthesis. (A) A 57-year-old man with L4–L5 disc prolapse and canal stenosis. He underwent L3–L4–L5 laminectomy and L4–L5 discectomy elsewhere, but had worsening dynamic and static back pain and sciatica. (B) MRI 2 years later showed adequate canal restoration, but did not show spondylolisthesis. (C) Standing radiograph in extension showed grade 1 L4–L5 slip. (D) On flexion it increases to grade 2. (E) CT shows the defect in the L4 isthmus missed by MRI and radiographs.

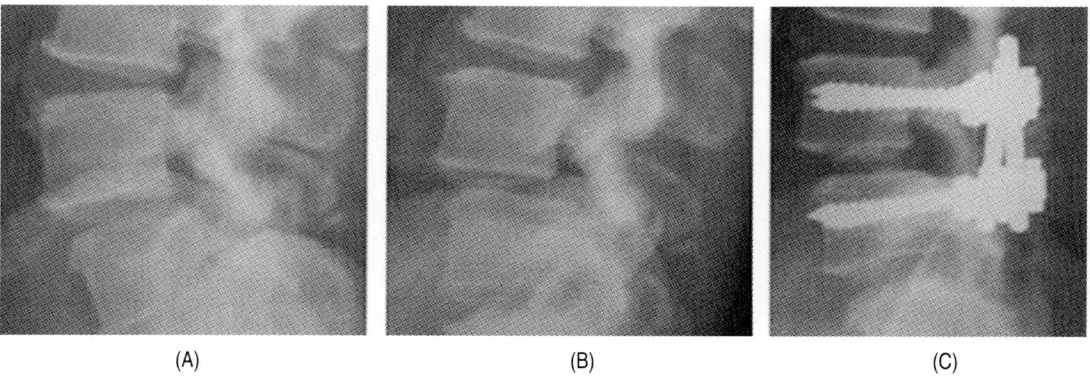

Fig. 2. Role of dynamic X-rays. (A) Lateral radiograph in extension shows hardly any spondylolisthesis. (B) Radiograph in flexion shows grade 1 L4–L5 DSO. (C) Symptoms resolved with decompression and *in situ* instrumented posterior interbody fusion (PLIF).

performed mainly to pick up co-existing peripheral neuropathy. Provocative and contrast discography or facet blocks are not commonly used in the setting of DSO. They might help in deciding if fusion surgery needs to be extended beyond the level of the olisthesis.[18]

Surgery

There is now categorical evidence from prospective trials showing that any operation is preferable to non-operative management in DSO.[19] The twin aims of surgery are to relieve pain and to prevent progressive worsening or recurrence of symptoms. Decompression of the nerve roots is traditionally the most important treatment for DSO. The details of decompression surgery and its merits can be found in Chapter 15 of this volume. Over the years, decompression surgery has become less invasive and more focused.

The aim of fusion is to obtain a stable spine and a pain-free patient. Fusion addresses the instability caused by the disease and aggravated by the decompression procedure. A variety of fusion procedures are available. These include intertransverse fusion, posterolateral fusion (PLF), posterior interbody fusion (PLIF), transforaminal interbody fusion (TLIF), anterior interbody fusion (ALIF) and circumferential (270° or 360°) fusion. Autografts, allografts (locally banked cadaveric bone or commercially available femoral rings) and xenografts (bovine bone) are used in various combinations. The autograft may be obtained from the lumbar spine during decompression or separately from the iliac crest. Morbidity at the iliac crest donor site is considerable. Persistent iliac pain was reported by a third of the patients 2 years after surgery in a recent prospective study.[20] This has prompted a switch to the use of local bone or cages. Cages for interbody fusion are made of titanium, carbon fibre, ceramic or polyethyletherketone. They come in various shapes, such as threaded cylinders, spiked cuboids, tapered cuboids or the expandable variety. ALIF relies more on cages, as the neural structures do not come in the way of implanting large cages. With instrumentation becoming almost universal, it may not be necessary to get blocks of bone; morsellated chips obtained during decompression fuse just as well (Fig. 3). Good results have been reported with chip grafts in both PLIF and PLF.[21,22]

There is no consensus on the use of instrumentation in lumbar fusion. The reasons for performing instrumented fusion are summarized in Table 2. The fusion rate is higher with the use of instrumentation, but this does not automatically mean a better clinical outcome.[23]

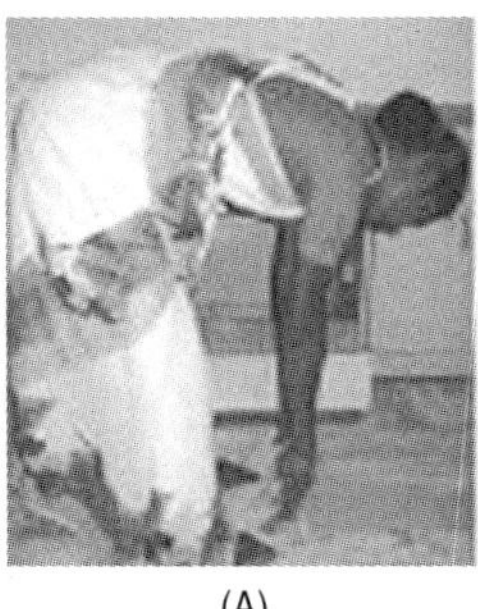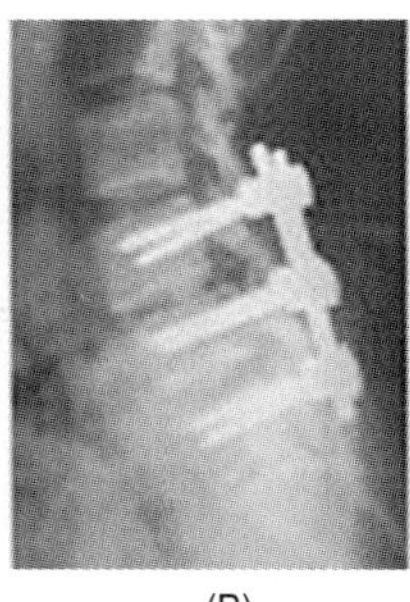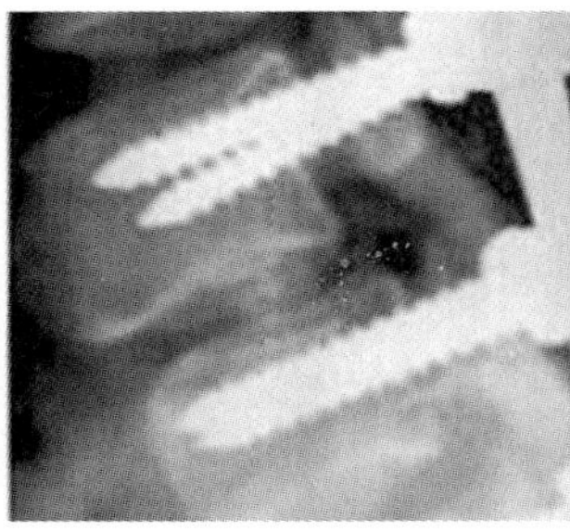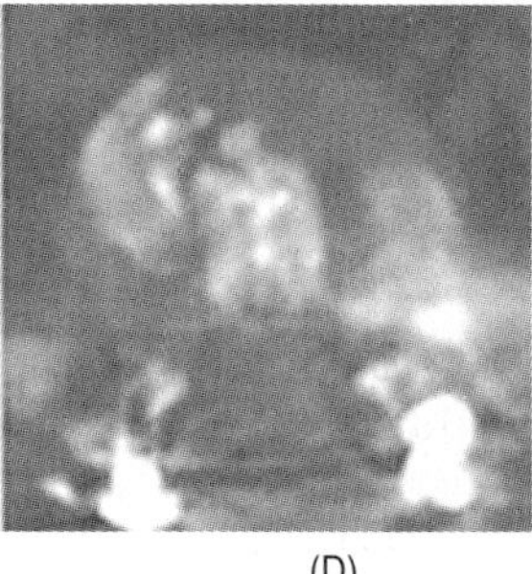

(A)   (B)   (C)   (D)

Fig. 3. Results 6 weeks after 2-segment instrumented PLIF for DSO. (A) Range of lumbar flexion. (B) Lateral radiograph. (C) Note onset of fusion of the chip PLIF grafts in L3–L4 space. (D) Consolidation of graft in CT.

Table 2. Reasons for using instrumentation in lumbar fusion

Immediate stabilization

Quicker ambulation and return to work

Correction of spondylolisthesis

Correction of kyphosis or scoliosis

Maximize chances of fusion

Use in situations in which fusion chances are lower (osteoporosis, smokers)

Minimize the chances of recurrence of spondylolisthesis or stenosis

Better clinical outcome

Fusion does not necessarily decrease the range of movement of the whole lumbar spine (Fig. 3). The previously used posterior instrumentation using sublaminar wires and Luque rods or a Hartshill rectangle has now become supplanted by transpedicular screws.[24] Because they provide three column support, pedicle screws are the stablest of devices.[25] The vertebral slip can be corrected by distraction-lordosing or by using reduction screws. It is acceptable to obtain *in situ* fusion as long as the nerve root space is well decompressed, as the degree of slip is usually low in DSO. Recent advances include percutaneous placement of pedicle screws and use of neuro-navigation for proper placement of the screw.[26,27] Recombinant human bone morphogenic protein has been used to increase the chances of fusion and it might even obviate the need for a bone graft, but its cost is prohibitive.[28]

Critical appraisal of surgery for degenerative spondylolisthesis

There is a large body of literature supporting decompression alone for managing DSO.[4,29] There is an equally large one favouring fusion surgery.[1,23,30,31] It must be noted that decompression is an indispensable step in any fusion procedure. Therefore, the debate is not on 'decompression *versus* fusion', but on 'non-fusion *versus* fusion' procedures. Though some surgeons perform fusion after decompression in all patients with DSO, others are more selective in that fusions are restricted to those patients with dynamic instability rather than mere static olisthesis.[4,32] We can conceptualize the debate by examining the arguments used by the non-fusion and fusion camps. The arguments in favour of performing non-fusion surgery (decompression alone) and those against performing fusion surgery (decompression + fusion +/– instrumentation) have been covered in Chapter 15 of this volume. The truth behind such arguments is critically examined here.

The pros for performing fusion are summarized below:

Arguments for performing fusion surgery (decompression + fusion +/– instrumentation)

- The source of symptoms is not only the fixed nerve compression, but dynamic instability also contributes greatly. A successful fusion relieves symptoms better than decompression alone and prevents further progression of olisthesis.
- Recent advances have helped in making fusion surgery safe, simple and patient-friendly. The more experienced the surgeon, the lower the complication rate.
- Though adjacent level degeneration does occur after fusion, it is overestimated and may not be clinically relevant.
- Sufficient biomechanical, clinical and radiological evidence exists in the literature favouring fusion surgery.
- The use of instrumentation has increased the fusion rates.
- The increased cost of instrumentation is offset by a quicker return to occupation.

Arguments against performing non-fusion surgery (decompression alone)

- Decompression involves removal of the ligaments, disc and facet joints in part or in whole, and weakening of muscle. Decompression thus results in biomechanical weakening of the spine already damaged by degenerative disease. All these factors lead to further spinal instability and clinical deterioration.
- In spite of a temporary relief from root pain after decompression, patients can continue to have disabling back pain and subsequent recurrence of root pain.
- When fusion is not being perfomed, the surgeon hesitates to do the required degree of decompression for fear of inducing further instability. Inadequate lateral canal decompression is a common cause of failed back surgery syndrome.
- Should the patient ultimately need a fusion, it means having to perform two operations, which leads to a greater cost and longer convalescence.
- Not fusing an unstable or potentially unstable

spine could be grounds for litigation.

Let us examine some of these issues in detail.

Is nerve root compression the sole cause of pain?

There are several contributors to pain in the back and leg, apart from static compression on the nerve root by the intervertebral disc or a narrow canal. In a study comparing MRI and discography, the loss of disc height was significantly associated with symptoms.[33] Interbody fusion with a graft or cage aims to restore the disc height and hence eliminates one more source of pain. Residual back pain correlated better with the Modic end plate signal changes than with the residual protrusion of the disc in a 2-year follow-up study of microdiscectomy and sequestrectomy.[34] The sinuvertebral nerve (recurrent nerve of Luschka) innervates the annulus, posterior longitudinal ligament, dura and the facet joint capsule. Pain in the back and leg can arise from its nociceptive nerve endings, even without any root compression.[35] The pain in the back and leg has been shown to be alleviated by preoperative percutaneous transpedicular external fixation.[36] It is therefore simplistic to assume that mere decompression will relieve the pain fully.

Progression of spondylolisthesis after decompression

Standing flexion–extension radiographs revealed spondylolisthesis not shown by MRI in 7% of 90 patients undergoing single-level discectomy in a recent study.[15] This indicates new instability after discectomy in a previously stable motion segment. One can easily imagine the effects of discectomy in a level that is already olisthetic. This is indeed brought out by one study of decompression for spinal stenosis, in which progressive postoperative spondylolisthesis

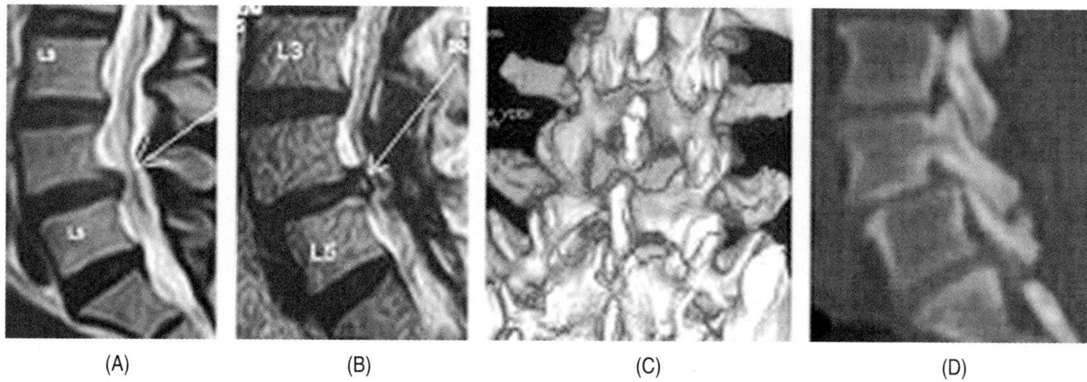

(A)   (B)   (C)   (D)

Fig. 4. Progression of spondylolisthesis after laminotomy for DSO. (A) MRI of 61-year-old woman with L4–L5 disc prolapse and grade 1 DSO. (B) Sagittal T2 MRI 1 year after bilateral laminotomy/discectomy (done elsewhere)—the patient had unrelieved back and leg pain. (C) CT reconstruction to show the small laminar fenestrations and intact facets. (D) Parasagittal CT reconstruction clearly shows intact pars and grade 1 DSO. Symptoms were relieved by instrumented PLIF.

occurred in 31% of patients with normal pre-operative alignment and in 73% of patients with preoperative subluxation.[37] Subluxation was seen in 66% of patients undergoing decompression for DSO in an early series.[14] Even in patients who had normal sagittal balance, there was a 15% incidence of spondylolisthesis in the post-operative follow up of patients undergoing removal of three or more facets.[38]

Epstein has been championing decompression alone in stenosis/DSO.[4] That such enthusiasts are converting to primary fusion is evident from the increase in fusion rates from 3.7%, in her initial 191 cases, to 17% in the subsequent 129 cases. In another recent series by the same author, 5 of 45 patients undergoing laminectomy alone for synovial cysts/stenosis developed postoperative olisthy.[39] Of 35 patients with cysts/stenosis and preoperative grade 1 DSO, olisthy increased after surgery to grade 2 in 11 patients in 2 years.[39] In biomechanical studies, the integrity of the disc has been proved to be even more important than the ligaments in providing stability.[40] In Epstein's series, of the 8 patients undergoing re-operation for instability, 5 had had a discectomy done in the first procedure, and this indicates the biomechanical contribution of the disc to stability.[4] In a 10-year follow up of 145 non-surgically managed patients with DSO, progressive spondylolisthesis was observed in 49 patients (34%). Those who had claudication initially had a greater incidence of clinical worsening over time as opposed to those presenting with only backache.[12] We contend that the more conservative methods of performing decompression have been necessitated by the dissatisfaction of surgeons and patients with a full-fledged laminofacet-ectomy–discectomy. The major reason for the dissatisfaction is the instability after such a procedure. That even minimal decompression procedures are not free from the risk of inducing further instability is illustrated by a case from our series (Fig. 4).

Correlation between radiological and clinical progression of spondylolisthesis

It is true that post-decompression increase in olisthesis might not be always symptomatic, as is the case in patients being clinically well despite a poor looking radiograph. In an 18-month follow-up study, asymptomatic olisthesis was seen to occur in 83% of 23 patients with DSO.[41] From a study of natural history, it can be guessed that a longer follow up would have revealed a greater number of symptomatic patients worsening.[12] This was indeed the case in an 11-year follow-up study of 50 patients undergoing decompression alone for lumbar canal stenosis.[32] Women with a preoperative slip and those whose slip increased after surgery had a documented clinical progression of symptoms and needed reoperation.[32] As lumbar spondylosis is a progressive disease, it is tempting for the decompressionist to lay the blame for worsening of the condition on ageing changes. A study of 119 patients revealed that the laminectomized levels showed greater changes in spondylolisthesis, disc space angle, and disc space height than in un-operated levels; the outcome correlated with radiographic changes.[42] This study proves that progression of spondylolisthesis is not caused by ageing but by the effect of decompression surgery.[42] Another factor that mars the result is bone re-growth after decompression, which was observed to a symptomatic degree in 40% of 40 patients in one series; bone re-growth was less in those undergoing primary fusion.[43]

Is lumbar instability a mere radiological finding or a clinically relevant issue?

The range of normal variation in lumbar movement is large, as shown by radiographic studies on asymptomatic volunteers.[44] Normal lumbar vertebral levels should have <3 mm of dynamic anteroposterior (AP) translation (<8% of vertebral body width). Although 42% of the normal subjects had at least one level with a static olisthesis of >3 mm in either flexion or extension, only 5% had a dynamic AP translation of >3 mm.[45] Based on biomechanical studies, a sagittal plane translation of >4.5 mm (>15% of vertebral body) or a sagittal plane rotation of >5° has been suggested to indicate lumbar in-stability.[46] It is necessary to define instability not merely by radiographic criteria but also by clinical criteria. The checklist formulated by White and Panjabi gives 2 points each to loss of function or surgical destruction of the anterior and posterior elements, 2 points each to the sagittal plane translation and rotation, 3 points to cauda equina damage, and 1 point to antici-pation of dangerous loading; if the total comes to 5 or more, the spine is held to be unstable.[46] Unilateral medial facetectomy increased the range of motion in flexion, and unilateral total facetectomy rendered the spine unstable in a biomechanical study.[47] Even fenestration and discectomy have been proved to cause instability in biomechanical studies.[48] From the foregoing account, it is obvious that lumbar instability is an established, clinically relevant concept and that decompression operations contribute to this instability.

Is there evidence that fusion produces better results?

The papers extolling decompression alone were mostly written in the 1970s and 1980s. At that time there was no clear definition of the outcome measures. The clinical results were evaluated by the operating surgeon in nebulous terms, such as good, fair or bad. From the 1990s, standardized outcome measures, self-evaluated by the patient or by an independent observer, came into vogue. Examples are the Prolo (functional and economic) Scale, Low Back Outcome Score, Denis Pain and Work Scale, Oswestry Disability Index, Short Form-36 (SF-36), Roland–Morris Disability Questionnaire and Japanese Orthopedic Associa-tion Score.[49]

Decompression surgery has been compared with primary fusion using proper outcome measures in a few prospective controlled trials. A prospective study published in 1991 showed an excellent or a good outcome at 4 years in 96% of those undergoing fusion, whereas only 44% of the decompression group experienced a similar result.[1] The fusion patients fared better in every clinical and radiological outcome measure studied. Age and sex did not influence the outcome of fusion. A systematic review in 2007 of 13 randomized trials and comparative observational studies showed that a satisfactory clinical outcome was significantly more likely with fusion than with decompression alone (p<0.05).[50] However, it must be admitted that these reviewers have commented on the low methodological quality of the studies in general.

The next lower level of evidence favouring fusion comes from retrospective series. A meta-analysis of such studies up to 1993 indicated success rates of 69%, 86% and 90% for decompression, non-instrumented fusion and instrumented fusion, respectively.[51] It should not be forgotten that procedures, such as PLF and PLIF, have a long history and have given good results in the hands of expert surgeons. An example is Yamamoto's series of 67 patients with DSO who had PLIF, with nearly two-thirds of them without pedicle screw augmentation. The ultimate fusion rate was 94% (including delayed fusion and collapsed fusion), and 89% were reported to be in the excellent or good category.[52] This is to be compared with the 64%–80% good results observed in most series for initial decompression alone.[4]

Long-term follow-up results of fusion are also available. In a minimum 5-year follow-up study of instrumented posterolateral fusion for DSO, 83% of patients were satisfied with the result. There was no pseudarthrosis, stenosis or progression of spondylolisthesis at the operated level.[53] In a study that specifically measured patient-relevant outcomes, 93% fusion was achieved and 93% of patients were satisfied with the result of instrumented fusion for DSO.[54] It is remarkable that in a study with an average of 17 years of follow-up, out of 24 patients undergoing circumferential fusion for isthmic spondylolisthesis, none reported backache.[55] In an 11-year follow-up study, patients with DSO had a lower incidence of re-operation after fusion surgery than after decompression alone (17% *vs.* 28%; p=0.002).[56]

On the basis of the above findings, it can be concluded that there is excellent proof favouring primary fusion in DSO.

Is fusion surgery more prone to complications, especially in the elderly?

The fear of higher complications in the elderly stems from the report of Deyo showing an 18% complication rate in those over the age of 75 years.[57] It must be remembered that this report studied all types of lumbar surgery and not specifically fusions. Major complications of fusions were rare (2%) in another study.[53] The transmuscular approach to pedicle screw fixation described later in this chapter results in less blood loss, shorter operating time and reduced hospital stay. Percutaneous options are now available for placing pedicle screws.[27] Unilateral pedicle screw instrumented fusion has proven to be as effective as a bilateral procedure in a randomized trial.[58] TLIF with instrumentation has been advocated as a less invasive procedure.[59] Laparoscopic or minimally invasive ALIF (mini-ALIF) approaches also reduce the blood loss and give comparably good results.[60] Using allografts or cages instead of autografts helps shorten operating time, reduces blood loss and avoids donor site morbidity. In a recent Japanese study no differences were seen in the outcome of lumbar fusion across ages, with elderly people being no more vulnerable to complications than the younger ones.[61] In our opinion, a patient who is medically fit for a decompression procedure should be able to withstand the additional 1½–2 hours required for instrumented fusion. Use of instrumentation allows early ambulation and this reduces the complications caused by recumbency. There is, of course, a learning curve for instrumented fusion or ALIF, but is this not so for any other operation, such as endoscopic spine surgery or disc replacement?

Is fusion better than pseudarthrosis?

There was once an opinion that patients developing pseudarthrosis might also have good clinical results. In an early prospective study, the results were excellent or good in the 9 patients developing pseudarthrosis of the 25 patients undergoing arthrodesis for DSO.[1] However, a recent long-term prospective study conclusively shows benefits of a solid fusion over pseudarthrosis with respect to back and lower limb symptomatology.[30] In 47 patients with DSO followed up for 5–14 years, the clinical outcome was excellent to good in 86% of patients with a solid arthrodesis, but in only 56% of patients with a pseudarthrosis.[30] It must also be noted that with the addition of instrumentation to fusion, the probability of achieving a solid fusion is greater (p<0.05).[50] Successful arthrodesis occurred in 82% of the instrumented cases versus 45% of the non-instrumented cases of DSO (p=0.0015), as reported in a paper that won the 1997 Volvo Award for clinical studies.[23] Using pedicle screw instrumentation, 'insert–rotate' type of interbody spacers and bone graft, the pain and outcome measures were significantly improved in a set of 36 patients with DSO, with a mean age of 65 years, and a follow up for a mean of 2 years. The outcome was rated as good or excellent by 91% of patients. Mean preoperative slip reduced from 20.2% to 1.7% (92% correction; p<0.001). Mean focal lordosis increased from 13° to 16° (26% increase). There were no device-related procedural complications.[62] These well-designed studies show that fusion is a desirable clinical goal in DSO.

Does spondylolisthesis progress after fusion?

DSO is a 'wear and tear' problem and the stimulus for continued degeneration is the stress on the motion segment produced by physiological loads. Fusion should ideally abolish motion at the segment and halt further degeneration in that segment. This is indeed the case with circumferential fusion.[63] This aim is also well achieved with successful interbody fusion.[62] Further progression of spondylolisthesis is sometimes seen with uninstrumented postero-lateral fusion, as there is no anterior column stabilization by this procedure.[55] In a study of 44 patients followed for a minimum of 2 years, the rate of progression of the spondylolisthesis was least with instrumented fusion, intermediate with non-instrumented fusion and highest with decompression alone.[64]

Adjacent level degeneration

Solid fusion with or without instrumentation eliminates motion in the operated segment. This throws additional stress on the neighbouring motion segments causing an accelerated degeneration. The rate of adjacent level disease was 18 out of 125 instrumented fusion levels in a follow up of 3–4 years.[65] Next-segment disease included spondylolisthesis (39%), spinal canal stenosis due to disc herniation and/or facet hypertrophy (33%), stress fracture of the adjacent vertebral body (28%), and scoliosis (17%). Postmenopausal women and smokers had increased risk.[65] Though these figures raise concern, it must be remembered that the radiological degeneration at an adjacent level may have no bearing on the clinical outcome. In a study of 45 patients followed up for 5 years, there was no evidence that postoperative narrowing of the adjacent disc affects the clinical outcome of L4–L5 instrumented posterior lumbar interbody fusion.[66] With longer follow-up, some patients will need surgery at the adjacent level. The rate of symptomatic degeneration at an adjacent segment warranting either decompression or arthrodesis was predicted to be 16.5% at 5 years and 36.1% at 10 years.[67]

Cost and complications of instrumentation

There is no denying the cost of implants such as titanium pedicle screws and cages. Titanium has imaging advantages but is more expensive.

Stainless steel implants have higher torsional resistance and are cheaper. They are particularly useful for long segment instrumentation.[68] Intraoperative complications of pedicle screws were observed in 1.2% of 648 screws placed; they included screw misplacement, nerve root injury, dural tear and pedicle fracture.[69] Postoperative complications were seen in 1.5% of patients and they included screw back-out, slipping of rod, screw breakage and the need for device removal to treat infection.[69] Screw failure is more common when interbody fusion has not been achieved.[70] A higher re-operation rate was noted in patients undergoing instrumented fusion compared with those with uninstrumented fusion.[71] The risk of instrumentation-related complications is a small price to pay for the advantages of instrumentation. Dickman obtained 96% fusion rates with pedicle screws in 104 cases followed up for a mean of 20 months.[72] Screw breakage may not be symptomatic and patients may achieve solid fusion before, or in spite of, device failure.[72]

Which type of fusion?

Posterolateral fusion is easier and safer to perform than PLIF, which requires root retraction.[73] However, the fusion rates are higher with interbody fusion, as the graft is placed under compression and there is a wider area of bone contact.[2] PLIF also allows restoration of disc height. The PLF mass sometimes becomes exuberant and gives rise to secondary neural compression. This is not the case with PLIF.[70,74] Circumferential (270° or 360°) fusion gives the most stable fusion.[55,63] A systematic review in 2006 could not find any substantial difference between the various fusion techniques for isthmic, low-grade adult spondylolisthesis, but it was in favour of instrumented fusion.[75] In a long-term study of functional outcome, patients with DSO (compared with those with adult isthmic spondylolisthesis) had better outcome when the PLF was supported by instrumentation.[71]

Results of anterior fusion

The transperitoneal approach has now become supplanted by an open mini extraperitoneal anterior or anterolateral approach. Fusion rates of 79%–100% have been reported in the literature. In a series of 46 patients, 81% were pain-free and 88% returned to their jobs after fusion surgery. The complications arising from this approach were iliac vein injury and ileus. The complications related to fusion were non-union, collapsed union and cage migration.[76] The best indication for the anterior approach is previous posterior surgery. The results with ALIF have been demonstrated in 33 patients with failed back surgery syndrome (including 13 with spondylolisthesis), in whom the back pain, leg pain, and functional status improved significantly to 76%, 80% and 67%, respectively.[77] The rate of adjacent level disease was lower (by nearly half) with ALIF compared with PLIF.[78] The least angular motion was noted with ALIF and the greatest with unilateral PLF in a finite element analysis.[79] Recently, an anterior tension band plating technique has also been described to prevent settling of the graft or cage.[80] In cases in which a pedicle screw support is needed, it has been done percutaneously after the ALIF procedure.[27]

Special situations

1. Osteoporosis and DSO

Postmenopausal and age-associated osteoporosis is common in patients with DSO. Though osteoporosis does not delay bone healing, the quality of autologous donor bone is likely to be poor and the fusion mass is likely to have less strength. Hence, instrumented fusion has been recommended for osteoporotic patients.[81] Care must be taken to prevent iatrogenic fracture during surgery.[82] Pedicle screws cannot be used in spines with bone mineral density (BMD) of

<0.3–0.4 g/sq cm. Screw loosening is common.[83] It can be avoided by using the maximal feasible diameter of the screw, converging the screws, adding cross-connectors, and by not tapping the drill channel or by doing under tapping.[84] As the use of large diameter screws can increase the risk of pedicle fracture, it has been suggested that the screw should not exceed 70% of the outer pedicle diameter if the BMD is 0.7 g/sq cm.[82] The screw path can be augmented with polymethylmethacrylate bone cement.[85] Less rigid titanium implants are available for osteoporotic bone. Pre- and post-operative medical therapy for osteoporosis and extended use of orthosis are essential.

2. Degenerative scoliosis and DSO

This is a clear indication for instrumented fusion as deformity correction is essential. In a review of studies on spinal instability and stenosis with scoliosis, it was found that non-fusion surgery produced inferior results compared with instrumented fusion.[86]

3. Adult isthmic spondylolysis

Isthmic spondylolysis is a common pathology in adolescents and young adults, a substantial proportion of whom have minimal or no symptoms in young age. Symptoms develop as they grow older and as degenerative stenosis and worsening of spondylolisthesis occur.[87] It is sometimes difficult to detect the spondylolysis unless oblique radiograph or CT is done; it can be missed in patients imaged with MR alone[15] (Fig. 1). Adult onset isthmic spondylolisthesis has also been reported.[88] Patients with isthmic spondylolisthesis can progress to a higher grade over time or after decompression without fusion. The results of fusion are gratifying in this subgroup of patients, but the type of fusion which achieves the best result is not clearly documented in the literature.[89] Instrumentation is recommended to correct the slip.

Our approach

Value of team approach

In our centre, the neurosurgeon and an orthopaedic surgeon form a team. This has enabled us to bring together our unique training, attitudes and skills in managing spondylolisthesis. Thus we are able to safely offer instrumented fusion for patients who have been denied surgery or offered only decompressive surgery elsewhere.

Preoperative evaluation

The extent of disablement in daily activities resulting from pain is the most important factor in deciding on surgery. Minor neurological deficits do not dictate surgery. Medical evaluation and management are vital to avoid complications, especially in the older patient. We get flexion–extension lateral views in the standing posture, especially when the MRI does not show spondylolisthesis (Figs 1, 2). Preoperative helical CT pediculometry (measurement of the pedicle width, length of the screw path and inclination to the sagittal plane) is done in every case being taken up for surgery. Although the standard axial plane inclination of the pedicle in the lower lumbar level is held to be 15°, we have encountered cases where it is up to 25°–35° at L5 and S1 (Fig. 5A). Midline sagittal reconstruction helps to accurately measure the degree of spondylolisthesis. Parasagittal reconstructions are the best to depict subtle defects in the pars interarticularis (Fig. 1).

Disadvantages of the conventional midline approach

Having had a difficult time in placing pedicle screws through the midline approach, we

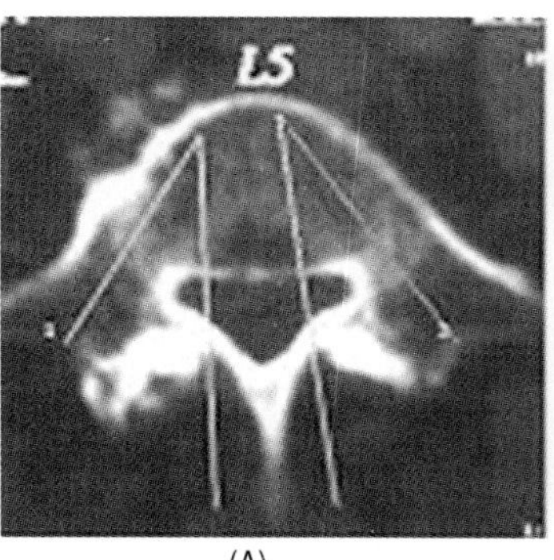
(A)

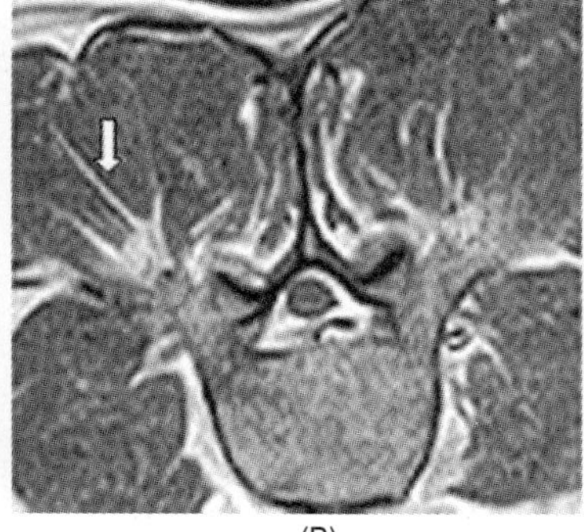
(B)

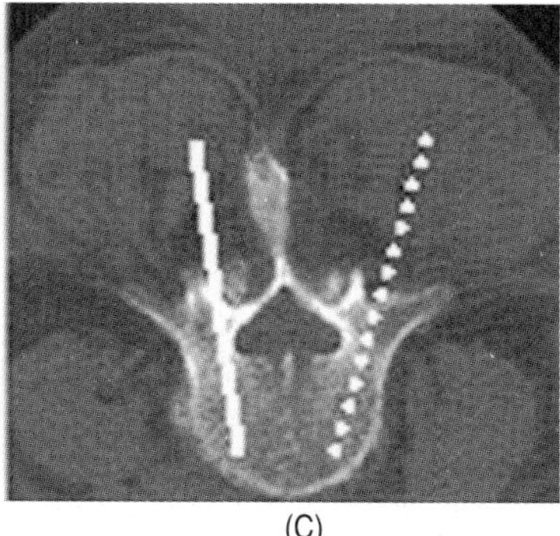
(C)

Fig. 5. Transmuscular approach. (A) Wide pedicle angulation at L5 measured by CT pediculometry: 29° (left) and 34° (right). (B) Axial MRI showing the plane in the multifidus muscle used for the transmuscular approach (arrowhead). (C) Direction of pedicle screw in conventional midline approach (solid line) and improved direction with paraspinous transmuscular approach (dashed line).

switched to the bilateral paraspinous transmuscular approach, akin to the approach originally described by Wiltse for PLF.[90] The disadvantages we encountered with the midline approach are listed in Table 3.

Operative technique of bilateral paraspinous transmuscular open approach to pedicle screw placement

The patient is placed in the prone jack-knife position over radiolucent bolsters to effect as much postural reduction of the slip as possible. The pedicles are marked on the skin with AP and lateral image intensifier screening, and the incision is made 3 cm above and below the highest and lowest pedicle to be instrumented. This midline skin incision is shorter than the conventional one for the midline approach. The lumbar fascia is exposed to 3 cm on either side of the midline. Paired fascial incisions are made 2–3 cm from midline, depending on the bulk of the muscle. Longitudinal monopolar diathermy dissection is done through and through the fibres of erector spinae (superficial) muscle. Above the L3 level, the plane inside the deeper placed multifidus muscle is well developed and is used for reaching the lateral border of facet, which can be palpated through the muscle. Below L3 level

Table 3. Disadvantages of the midline approach to open lumbar pedicle screw placement

---

Erector spinae muscle damage

   —Prolonged retraction

   —Ischaemic damage

   —Physical trauma

Bulk of muscle

   —Prevents lateral starting of screw track
      convergence of screws difficult
      medial pedicle breach, risk to nerve root
      poorer purchase, especially in osteoporotic bone
      needs cross-connector to prevent toggling

   —Interferes with instruments

   —Anatomical landmarks obscured, especially when
      facets are hypertrophic

Longer incision, skin necrosis from retraction

Longer duration of surgery

Blood loss, need for drain

Longer recovery time, pain

---

the intramultifidus plane can sometimes be entered (Fig. 5B). If not, the deep muscle is also split longitudinally. The microlumbar hook retractor and magnification help in performing this exposure. Dissection of the deep muscle and soft tissue is done directly only over the pedicle entry point. This entry point is identified from the conventional anatomical landmarks, and it lies a few millimetres lateral to the point that would be entered from the midline approach. The transmuscular approach starts more laterally, passes more centrally in the pedicle and ends up with better triangulation than with the midline approach (Fig. 5C). The muscle does not get in the way of the drills and taps. After finishing the work on one pedicle, the hook retractor is moved to the next level on the same side and then the same procedure is repeated on the opposite side.

Once all the pedicle screws are placed, midline exposure is done just at the areas required for decompression. This often is unilateral or bilateral laminofacetectomy at one level. Microdiscectomy and packing of the chips of bone obtained from the decompression into the disc space for interbody fusion are integral steps of this surgery. We then return to the transmuscular approach for reduction and secure placement of the vertical connecting rods. Closure of the paraspinous muscle and fascia on either side and in the midline can be completed rapidly. Drains and blood transfusions are only rarely needed. The advantages of the bilateral paraspinous transmuscular approach are listed in Table 4.

Postoperatively, the patient is ambulated as early as possible, generally by day 2 or 3 and discharged by day 4 or 5. Back exercises are taught and activity gradually increased in the second week after the sutures are removed. Most patients resume low levels of activity in the 3rd to 4th week. Corsets are not used routinely. Follow up standing radiographs in flexion and extension are taken at 3 months and at 1 year.

Over the past 7 years, we have performed 79 instrumented lumbar fusions for adult spondylolisthesis and 36 for DSO (43 for isthmic spondylolisthesis). The last 30 cases of instrumented lumbar fusions (over the past 2½ years) have been done through the bilateral paraspinous transmuscular approach. The age of 27 patients in the DSO group was 60 years or more. We have been impressed by the ease and patient-friendliness of this approach (Fig. 3). From this short experience, we are of the impression that primary instrumented fusion at the time of

Table 4. Advantages of the bilateral paraspinous transmuscular approach for open lumbar pedicle screw placement

Reduced muscle damage
—No prolonged retraction
—No ischaemia
—No physical injury
No bulk of muscle
—To prevent lateral starting of screw track and convergence and so least possibility of breaching medial pedicle wall
—To interfere with instruments
—To obscure anatomical landmarks
No cross-connector assembly needed in single level fusion due to converging track
Better intraoperative AP imaging-no interference from air within the exposure
Shorter incision, no skin necrosis
Shorter time of surgery
Minimal blood loss, no need for drain
Shorter recovery time, less pain, less need for analgesic
Offers many advantages of percutaneous pedicle screw placement at no additional cost

decompression gives the best results in grade 1 DSO, even in the elderly. It gives the best relief from symptoms and the complication rate is at an acceptable level. Furthermore, we have not observed device failure or progression of symptoms post-procedure.

Conclusion

Decompression alone can relieve symptoms in some patients with degenerative low-grade spondylolisthesis. The question is, should we do only what is just adequate or should we offer the best current choice? Gone are the days when an age of 60 years was considered as 'old age'. In an increasingly health conscious society, a large percentage of 'senior citizens' lead a physically active life. We must do everything possible to make them resume their activities as fully, as quickly and as surely as possible. Based on personal experience and a critical analysis of the evidence in the literature, instrumented PLIF–PLF appears to be the best current choice for DSO. Mere chronological age is not the sole criterion to decide on fusion, but the general health and level of activity of the patient are important considerations.

References

1. Herkowitz HN, Kurz LT. Degenerative lumbar spondylolisthesis with spinal stenosis. A prospective study comparing decompression with decompression and intertransverse process arthrodesis. *J Bone Joint Surg Am* 1991;**73**:802–8.

2. Ramani PS. Introduction, Chap 1. In: Ramani PS (ed). *Posterior lumbar interbody fusion.* Bombay: Associated Personnel Services Publ; 1989.

3. Epstein NE, Epstein JA, Carras R, *et al.* Degenerative spondylolisthesis with an intact neural arch: A review of 60 cases with an analysis of clinical findings and the development of surgical management. *Neurosurgery* 1983;**13**:555–61.

4. Epstein N. Surgical management of lumbar stenosis: Decompression and indications for fusion. *Neurosurg Focus* 1997;**3**:Article 1.

5. Love TW, Fagan AB, Fraser RD. Degenerative spondylolisthesis. Developmental or acquired? *J Bone Joint Surg Br* 1999;**81**:670–4.

6. Imada K, Matsui H, Tsuji H. Oophorectomy predisposes to degenerative spondylolisthesis. *J Bone Joint Surg Br* 1995;**77**:126–30.

7. Tabrizi P, Bouchard JA. Osteoporotic spondylolisthesis: A case report. *Spine* 2001;**26**: 1482–85.

8. Boden SD, Riew KD, Yamaguchi K, *et al.* Orientation of the lumbar facet joints: Association with degenerative disc disease. *J Bone Joint Surg Am* 1996;**78**:403–11.

9. Sato K, Wakamatsu E, Yoshizumi A, *et al.* The configuration of the laminas and facet joints in degenerative spondylolisthesis. A clinicoradiologic study. *Spine* 1989;**14**:1265–71.

10. Nagaosa Y, Kikuchi S, Hasue M, *et al.* Pathoanatomic mechanisms of degenerative spondylo-listhesis: A radiographic study. *Spine* 1998;**23**:1447–51.

11. Hosoe H, Ohmori K. Degenerative lumbosacral spondylolisthesis: Possible factors which predispose the fifth lumbar vertebra to slip. *J Bone Joint Surg Br* 2008;**90**:356–9.

12. Matsunaga S, Ijiri K, Hayashi K. Nonsurgically managed patients with degenerative spondylolisthesis: A 10–18-year follow-up study. *J Neurosurg* 2000;**93** (2 Suppl):194–8.

13. Möller H, Sundin A, Hedlund R. Symptoms, signs and functional disability in adult spondylolisthesis. *Spine* 2000;**25**:683–9.

14. Linville DA. Spinal stenosis, degenerative spondylolisthesis and scoliosis. Chap 41 Vol. II. In: Canale TS (ed). *Campbell's operative orthopaedics.* St Louis: Mosby; 2003:2061–80.

15. Kizilkilic O, Yalcin O, Sen O, *et al.* The role of standing flexion–extension radiographs for spondylolisthesis following single level disk surgery. *Neurol Res* 2007;**29**:540–3.

16. Ben-Galim P, Reitman CA. The distended facet sign: An indicator of position-dependent spinal stenosis and degenerative spondylolisthesis. *Spine J* 2007;**7**: 245–8.

17. Jayakumar P, Nnadi C, Saifuddin A, *et al.* Dynamic degenerative lumbar spondylolisthesis: Diagnosis with axial loaded magnetic resonance imaging. *Spine* 2006;**31**:E298–E301.

18. Antti-Poika I, Soini J, Tallroth K, *et al.* Clinical relevance of discography combined with CT scanning. A study of 100 patients. *J Bone Joint Surg Br* 1990;**72**: 480–5.

19. Weinstein JN, Lurie JD, Tosteson TD, *et al.* Surgical versus nonsurgical treatment for lumbar degenerative spondylolisthesis. *N Engl J Med* 2007;**356**:2257–70.

20. Sasso RC, LeHuec JC, Shaffrey C. Iliac crest bone graft donor site pain after anterior lumbar interbody fusion: A prospective patient satisfaction outcome assessment. *J Spinal Disord Tech* 2005;**18** (Suppl): S77–S81.

21. Simmons JW. Posterior lumbar interbody fusion with posterior elements as chip grafts. *Clin Orthop Relat Res* 1985;**193**:85–9.

22. Kho VK, Chen WC. Posterolateral fusion using laminectomy bone chips in the treatment of lumbar spondylolisthesis. *Int Orthop* 2008;**32**:115–19.

23. Fischgrund JS, Mackay M, Herkowitz HN, *et al.* 1997 Volvo Award winner in clinical studies. Degenerative lumbar spondylolisthesis with spinal stenosis: A prospective, randomized study comparing decompressive laminectomy and arthrodesis with and without spinal instrumentation. *Spine* 1997;**22**:2807–12.

24. Ogilvie JW, Bradford DS. Sublaminar fixation in lumbosacral fusions. *Clin Orthop Relat Res* 1991;**269:** 157–61.

25. Goel VK, Ebraheim NA, Biyani A, *et al.* Role of mechanical factors in the evaluation of pedicle screw type spinal fixation devices. *Neurol India* 2005;**53:** 399–407.

26. Ringel F, Stoffel M, Stüer C, *et al.* Minimally invasive transmuscular pedicle screw fixation of the thoracic and lumbar spine. *Neurosurgery* 2006;**59** (4 Suppl 2): ONS361–ONS366.

27. Foley KT, Gupta SK, Justis JR, *et al.* Percutaneous pedicle screw fixation of the lumbar spine. *Neurosurg Focus* 2001;**10:**E10.

28. Katayama Y, Matsuyama Y, Yoshihara H, *et al.* Clinical and radiographic outcomes of postero-lateral lumbar spine fusion in humans using recombinant human bone morphogenetic protein-2: An average five-year follow-up study. *Int Orthop* 2008. [Epub ahead of print].

29. Kristof RA, Aliashkevich AF, Schuster M, *et al.* Degenerative lumbar spondylolisthesis-induced radicular compression: Nonfusion-related decompression in selected patients without hypermobility on flexion–extension radiographs. *J Neurosurg* 2002;**97** (3 Suppl):281–6.

30. Kornblum MB, Fischgrund JS, Herkowitz HN, *et al.* Degenerative lumbar spondylolisthesis with spinal stenosis: A prospective long-term study comparing fusion and pseudarthrosis. *Spine* 2004;**29:**726–33.

31. Ghogawala Z, Benzel EC, Amin-Hanjani S, *et al.* Prospective outcomes evaluation after decompression with or without instrumented fusion for lumbar stenosis and degenerative Grade I spondylolisthesis. *J Neurosurg (Spine)* 2004;**3:**267–72.

32. McCullen GM, Bernini PM, Bernstein SH, *et al.* Clinical and roentgenographic results of decompression for lumbar spinal stenosis. *J Spinal Disord* 1994;**7:**380–7.

33. Buirski G, Silberstein M. The symptomatic lumbar disc in patients with low-back pain. Magnetic resonance imaging appearances in both a symptomatic and control population. *Spine* 1993;**18:** 1808–11.

34. Barth M, Diepers M, Weiss C, *et al.* Two-year outcome after lumbar microdiscectomy versus microscopic sequestrectomy—part 2: Radiographic evaluation and correlation with clinical outcome. *Spine* 2008;**33:**273–9.

35. Gilchrist RV, Isaac Z, Bhat AL. Innervation of the anterior spinal canal: An update. *Pain Physician* 2002;**5:**167–71.

36. van der Schaaf DB, van Limbeek J, *et al.* Temporary external transpedicular fixation of the lumbosacral spine. *Spine* 1999;**24:**481–4.

37. Fox MW, Onofrio BM, Onofrio BM, *et al.* Clinical outcomes and radiological instability following decompressive lumbar laminectomy for degenerative spinal stenosis: A comparison of patients undergoing concomitant arthrodesis versus decompression alone. *J Neurosurg* 1996;**85:**793–802.

38. Shenkin HA, Hash CJ. Spondylolisthesis after multiple bilateral laminectomies and facetectomies for lumbar spondylosis. Follow-up review. *J Neurosurg* 1979;**50:**45–7.

39. Epstein N. Lumbar laminectomy for the resection of synovial cysts and coexisting lumbar spinal stenosis or degenerative spondylolisthesis: An outcome study. *Spine* 2004;**29:**1049–55.

40. Crawford NR, Cagli S, Sonntag VK, *et al.* Biomechanics of grade I degenerative lumbar spondylolisthesis—Part 1: *In vitro* model. *J Neurosurg* 2001;**94** (1 Suppl):45–50.

41. Herron LD, Trippi AC. L4–5 degenerative spondylolisthesis. The results of treatment by decompressive laminectomy without fusion. *Spine* 1989;**14:**534–8.

42. Tuite GF, Doran SE, Stern JD, *et al.* Outcome after laminectomy for lumbar spinal stenosis—Part II: Radiographic changes and clinical correlations. *J Neurosurg* 1994;**81:**707–15.

43. Postacchini F, Cinotti G. Bone regrowth after surgical decompression for lumbar spinal stenosis. *J Bone Joint Surg Br* 1992;**74:**862–9.

44. Hayes MA, Howard TC, Gruel CR, *et al.* Roentgenographic evaluation of lumbar spine flexion–extension in asymptomatic individuals. *Spine* 1989;**14:**327–31.

45. Boden SD, Wiesel SW. Lumbosacral segmental motion in normal individuals. Have we been measuring instability properly? *Spine* 1990;**15:** 571–6.

46. White AA 3rd, Panjabi MM. *Clinical biomechanics of the spine* (2nd edn). Philadelphia: Lippincot; 1990.

47. Abumi K, Panjabi MM, Kramer KM, *et al.* Biomechanical evaluation of lumbar spinal stability after graded facetectomies. *Spine* 1990;**15:**1142–7.

48. Lu WW, Luk KD, Ruan DK, *et al.* Stability of the whole lumbar spine after multilevel fenestration and discectomy. *Spine* 1999;**24:**1277–82.

49. Fujiwara A, Kobayashi N, Saiki K, *et al.* Association

of the Japanese Orthopaedic Association Score with the Oswestry Disability Index, Roland–Morris Disability Questionnaire and short-form 36. *Spine* 2003;**28**:1601–7.

50. Ryan MC, Gruszczynski AT, Braunsfurth HA, *et al.* The surgical management of degenerative lumbar spondylolisthesis: A systematic review. *Spine* 2007;**32**:1791–98.

51. Mardjetko SM, Connolly PJ, Shott S. Degenerative lumbar spondylolisthesis. A meta-analysis of the literature 1970–1993. *Spine* 1994;**19** (Suppl 20): 2256S–2265S.

52. Yamamoto T, Ohta N, Minobe Y, *et al.* Posterior lumbar interbody fusion for degenerative spondylolisthesis. Chap 16. In: Ramani PS (ed). *Posterior lumbar interbody fusion.* Bombay: Associated Personnel Services Publ; 1989:177–86.

53. Booth K, Bridwell KH, Eisenberg BA, *et al.* Minimum 5-year results of degenerative spondylolisthesis treated with decompression and instrumented posterior fusion. *Spine* 1999;**24**:1721.

54. Nork SE, Hu S, Workman KL, *et al.* Patient outcomes after decompression and instrumented posterior spinal fusion for degenerative spondylolisthesis. *Spine* 1999;**24**:561–69.

55. Remes V, Lamberg T, Tervahartiala P, *et al.* Long-term outcome after posterolateral, anterior and circumferential fusion for high-grade isthmic spondylolisthesis in children and adolescents: Magnetic resonance imaging findings after average of 17-year follow-up. *Spine* 2006;**31**:2491–9.

56. Martin BI, Mirza SK, Comstock BA, *et al.* Reoperation rates following lumbar spine surgery and the influence of spinal fusion procedures. *Spine* 2007;**32**:382–7.

57. Deyo RA, Cherkin DC, Loeser JD, *et al.* Morbidity and mortality in association with operations on the lumbar spine. The influence of age, diagnosis, and procedure. *J Bone Joint Surg Am* 1992;**74**:536–43.

58. Fernandez-Fairen M, Sala P, Ramirez H, *et al.* A prospective randomized study of unilateral versus bilateral instrumented posterolateral lumbar fusion in degenerative spondylolisthesis. *Spine* 2007;**32**: 395–401.

59. Houten JK, Post NH, Dryer JW, *et al.* Clinical and radiographically/neuroimaging documented outcome in transforaminal lumbar interbody fusion. *Neurosurg Focus* 2006;**20**:E8.

60. Chung SK, Lee SH, Lim SR, *et al.* Comparative study of laparoscopic L5–S1 fusion versus open mini-ALIF, with a minimum 2-year follow-up. *Eur Spine J* 2003;**12**:613–7.

61. Okuda S, Oda T, Miyauchi A, *et al.* Surgical outcomes of posterior lumbar interbody fusion in elderly patients. *J Bone Joint Surg [Am]* 2006;**88**: 2714–20.

62. Sears W. Posterior lumbar interbody fusion for degenerative spondylolisthesis: Restoration of sagittal balance using insert-and-rotate interbody spacers. *Spine J* 2005;**5**:170–9.

63. Heary RF, Bono CM. Circumferential fusion for spondylolisthesis in the lumbar spine. *Neurosurg Focus* 2002;**13**:Article 3.

64. Bridwell KH, Sedgewick TA, O'Brien MF, *et al.* The role of fusion and instrumentation in the treatment of degenerative spondylolisthesis with spinal stenosis. *J Spinal Disord* 1993;**6**:461–72.

65. Etebar S, Cahill DW. Risk factors for adjacent-segment failure following lumbar fixation with rigid instrumentation for degenerative instability. *J Neurosurg* 1999;**90** (2 Suppl):163–9.

66. Miyakoshi N, Abe E, Shimada Y, *et al.* Outcome of one-level posterior lumbar interbody fusion for spondylolisthesis and postoperative intervertebral disc degeneration adjacent to the fusion. *Spine* 2000; **25**:1837–42.

67. Ghiselli G, Wang JC, Bhatia NN, *et al.* Adjacent segment degeneration in the lumbar spine. *J Bone Joint Surg Am* 2004;**86-A**:1497–503.

68. Korovessis P, Baikousis A, Deligianni D, *et al.* Effectiveness of transfixation and length of instrumentation on titanium and stainless steel transpedicular spine implants. *J Spinal Disord* 2001; **14**:109–17.

69. Faraj AA, Webb JK. Early complications of spinal pedicle screw. *Eur Spine J* 1997;**6**:324–6.

70. La Rosa G, Cacciola F, Conti A, *et al.* Posterior fusion compared with posterior interbody fusion in segmental spinal fixation for adult spondylolisthesis. *Neurosurg Focus* 2001;**10**:Article 9.

71. Bjarke Christensen F, Stender Hansen E, Laursen M, *et al.* Long-term functional outcome of pedicle screw instrumentation as a support for posterolateral spinal fusion: Randomized clinical study with a 5-year follow-up. *Spine* 2002;**27**:1269–77.

72. Dickman CA, Fessler RG, MacMillan M, *et al.* Transpedicular screw-rod fixation of the lumbar spine: Operative technique and outcome in 104 cases. *J Neurosurg* 1992;**77**:860–70.

73. Madan S, Boeree NR. Outcome of posterior lumbar interbody fusion versus posterolateral fusion for

spondylolytic spondylolisthesis. *Spine* 2002;**27:** 1536–42.

74. Coric D, Branch CL. Posterior lumbar interbody fusion in the treatment of symptomatic spinal stenosis. *Neurosurg Focus* 1997;**3:**Article 5.

75. Jacobs WC, Vreeling A, De Kleuver M. Fusion for low-grade adult isthmic spondylolisthesis: A systematic review of the literature. *Eur Spine J* 2006; **15:**391–402.

76. Rauzzino MJ, Shaffrey CI, Nockels RP, *et al.* Anterior lumbar fusion with titanium threaded and mesh interbody cages. *Neurosurg Focus* 1999;**7:** Article 7.

77. Duggal N, Mendiondo I, Pares HR, *et al.* Anterior lumbar interbody fusion for treatment of failed back surgery syndrome: An outcome analysis. *Neurosurgery* 2004;**54:**636–43.

78. Min JH, Jang JS, Lee SH. Comparison of anterior- and posterior-approach instrumented lumbar interbody fusion for spondylolisthesis. *J Neurosurg Spine* 2007;**7:**21–6.

79. Bono CM, Khandha A, Vadapalli S, *et al.* Residual sagittal motion after lumbar fusion: A finite element analysis with implications on radiographic flexion–extension criteria. *Spine* 2007;**32:**417–22.

80. Aryan HE, Lu DC, Acosta FL Jr, *et al.* Stand-alone anterior lumbar discectomy and fusion with plate: Initial experience. *Surg Neurol* 2007;**68:**7–13.

81. Hu SS. Internal fixation in the osteoporotic spine. *Spine* 1997;**22** (24 Suppl):43S–48S.

82. Hirano T, Hasegawa K, Washio T, *et al.* Fracture risk during pedicle screw insertion in osteoporotic spine. *J Spinal Disord* 1998;**11:**493–7.

83. Soshi S, Shiba R, Kondo H, *et al.* An experimental study on transpedicular screw fixation in relation to osteoporosis of the lumbar spine. *Spine* 1991;**16:** 1335–41.

84. Carmouche JJ, Molinari RW, Gerlinger T, *et al.* Effects of pilot hole preparation technique on pedicle screw fixation in different regions of the osteoporotic thoracic and lumbar spine. *J Neurosurg Spine* 2005;**3:**364–70.

85. Frankel BM, Jones T, Wang C. Segmental poly-methylmethacrylate-augmented pedicle screw fixation in patients with bone softening caused by osteoporosis and metastatic tumor involvement: A clinical evaluation. *Neurosurgery* 2007;**61:**531–7.

86. Fraser JF, Huang RC, Girardi FP, *et al.* Pathogenesis, presentation, and treatment of lumbar spinal stenosis associated with coronal or sagittal spinal deformities. *Neurosurg Focus* 2003;**14:**Article 6.

87. Floman Y. Progression of lumbosacral isthmic spondylolisthesis in adults. *Spine* 2000;**25:**342–47.

88. Virta LJ. The development of isthmic lumbar spondylolisthesis in an adult. A case report. *J Bone Joint Surg Am* 1994;**76:**1397–98.

89. Kwon BK, Albert TJ. Adult low-grade acquired spondylolytic spondylolisthesis: Evaluation and management. *Spine* 2005;**30** (6S Supplement): S35–S41.

90. Vialle R, Wicart P, Drain O, *et al.* The Wiltse paraspinal approach to the lumbar spine revisited: An anatomic study. *Clin Orthop Relat Res* 2006;**445:** 175–80.

15

Grade 1 degenerative lumbar spondylolisthesis in patients >60 years of age: Routine fusion is not necessary

VEDANTAM RAJSHEKHAR

Degenerative spondylolisthesis of the lumbar spine in individuals >60 years of age is a common cause of lumbar canal stenosis (LCS), which leads to back and leg pain. The most favourable management strategy for this condition is debatable. Patients with listhesis of grade 2 or higher may benefit significantly from fusion (with or without instrumentation) surgery. But in patients with grade 1 listhesis, especially in elderly patients, there is no class 1 evidence to suggest that decompression and fusion provides better outcomes than decompression alone.

In this chapter, I will provide evidence from the literature on why decompression alone might be a better strategy in elderly patients (>60 years of age) with a stable grade 1 degenerative spondylolisthesis causing canal stenosis.

Definition of grade 1 listhesis

Grade 1 listhesis is defined as a slip of 3–14 mm in the sagittal plane between the lumbar vertebral bodies, without causing dynamic instability (i.e. <3 mm movement on dynamic lateral X-rays of the lumbar spine).[1] This review relates specifically to elderly patients >60 years of age.

Aim of treatment

The major aim of surgery for LCS is to provide relief from neurological deficits in the lower limbs, and alleviate the symptoms of neurogenic bladder dysfunction and neurogenic claudication. Surgery should not be offered solely to address back pain. Matsunaga *et al.*, in a remarkable study, followed up 145 patients with degenerative spondylolisthesis for 10–18 years.[2] Of the 110 patients who presented with back pain, with or without leg pain, 85 (77%) showed improvement after a 10-year follow up. The 35 who showed no improvement were heavy manual labourers. Patients with neurogenic claudication and bladder dysfunction deteriorated without surgical intervention.

Matsunaga and co-workers concluded that patients with back pain alone should not undergo surgery, as the disc height decreases over time, resulting in spontaneous relief of the back pain.[2] The average age of their patients was 58.6 years. Hence, it can be argued that their recommendation for conservative therapy in patients with back pain alone is probably more justified in patients >60 years of age.

Minimally invasive decompression surgery

Decompression surgery for LCS, in the presence of spondylolisthesis, has evolved over the years from complete laminectomy and bilateral facetectomies to more radical techniques for decompression, but which minimize injury to the ligamentous and bony structures.[3–7] Decompression surgery for spondylolisthesis should aim to spare the facets as much as possible because they are an important stabilizing structure; loss in their integrity increases the mobility of the vertebral bodies in the sagittal plane.

Thus, the essence of surgery is to decompress the neural elements, both the thecal sac and the nerve roots (i.e. central and lateral canals, and root canals), without worsening the instability of the spine. This can be achieved by carefully studying the images of the spine of the patient. The offending elements responsible for causing the compression are most frequently the inferior third or half of the lamina of the cephalad vertebra and thickened ligamentum flavum. Medially placed hypertrophied facets (facet tropism) can add to the neural compression. A strategy of excising only the compressing bony and ligamentous structures without entering the facet joints should be planned.

Coronal hemilaminectomy is one such strategy, whereby the lower third or half of the cephalad lamina is removed with minimal removal of the spine and the interspinous ligament.[3] The thickened ligamentum flavum is removed extensively, both in the midline and laterally from under the facets, until the dural tube and roots are seen to be free of any compression. This, in effect, increases the interapophysiolaminar space (IALS). Should decompression of the lateral canals be required, the inferior facets of the superior vertebra may be undercut, without entering the joint space of the facet. The surgery, which takes from 45 to 60 min, is performed under an operating microscope to reduce muscle retraction and avoid injury to the dural tube.

Other methods include the port-hole technique, hemilaminotomy and hemilaminectomy with bilateral decompression, using the microscope and high-speed drills, all of which spare the supraspinous ligaments and the facets, and achieve good decompression of the spinal and lateral canals.[5–7] These techniques are theoretically less destabilizing than the traditional laminectomies and facetectomies practised earlier and hence are eminently suitable when using decompression alone in patients with grade 1 spondylolisthesis.

Evidence supporting the use of decompression alone

Epstein studied 320 patients with an average age of 66 years who had degenerative spondylolisthesis and who underwent a laminectomy.[8] During an average follow up of at least 10 years, 80% of patients showed good to excellent outcomes, 9.3% needed primary fusions, 3% required secondary fusions and <1% required tertiary fusions. Thus, with over 85% of patients not requiring any fusion, it can be concluded that laminectomy is an effective surgical procedure. Likewise, Young *et al.* found that only 2 of 50 patients with grade 1 spondylolisthesis who were managed with laminectomy alone required subsequent fusion.[4]

Herron and Trippi found that 20 of 24 patients with degenerative spondylolisthesis had a good outcome following laminectomy without fusion and 3 had a fair outcome, in spite of a slight increase of 1 mm in slippage after surgery.[9] Sanderson and Wood reported that in 19 patients above the age of 65 years (average age 72.2 years) who underwent a laminectomy (with medial facetectomy if required) for spondylolisthesis, the outcome was good to excellent in 84%.[10] They concluded that if the dynamic lateral radiographs did not reveal any instability in patients with degenerative L4–L5 listhesis, then decompression alone with preservation of the facets and the pars interarticularis provided good results. Johnsson *et al.* reported that most patients who had undergone decompression alone remained asymptomatic despite postoperative progression of preoperative slippage.[11] It must be noted that the patients reported in these series were suffering from listhesis that was more than grade 1. Hence, it is reasonable to argue that for patients with grade 1 listhesis, the outcome of decompression without fusion is likely to be better than that reported for patients with higher grades of listhesis.

Katz *et al.* reported the results of a study in a cohort of 93 patients with grade 1 degenerative spondylolisthesis.[12] Fifty-two patients underwent laminectomy without arthrodesis, 26 had non-instrumented arthrodesis, and 27 had instrumented arthrodesis. On average, the patients who did not undergo arthrodesis were 8 years older than those who did and had significantly more levels decompressed. Linear regression models showed no significant association between treatment groups and either improvement in back pain or in walking capacity at 6 and 24 months in spite of the decompression group being older and having more levels of compression.

A port-hole technique was proposed by Kleeman *et al.*[6] for the treatment of lumbar canal stenosis in elderly patients. This technique is similar to coronal hemilaminectomy but spares the interspinous ligament and the spinous process. Kleeman and co-workers[6] used this technique to treat 15 patients with grade 1 non-lytic listhesis. Over a 4-year follow up, 80% of patients showed a good outcome. They recommend the use of this technique in elderly patients with grade 1 listhesis to avoid using fusion.

Matsudaira *et al.*, in a comparative observational study performed in 2005 on patients with grade 1 degenerative spondylolisthesis, reported that the decompression group with laminoplasty in fact had a better outcome than those who had additional instrumented fusion.[13] This suggests that if the decompression does not destabilize the spine further then fusion is not necessary.

Advantages of decompression alone

Decompression surgery is quicker than decompression and fusion surgery and is therefore better tolerated by older patients. Blood loss is less than when fusion is done and the lack of an implant minimizes the likelihood of infection. The cost of surgery is also less, as there is no cost of implant and hospitalization is shorter when compared with fusion surgery (Table 1). In addition, there is no donor site morbidity. Fusion surgery can always be performed should the patient require it in the future. However, it should be noted that fusion surgery has been shown to be associated with higher postoperative mortality and morbidity, apart from its higher cost (Table 2).[14]

Deyo *et al.* reported on the outcome of lumbar fusion surgery in a large cohort of elderly Medicare patients (average age of 72 years).[14]

Table 1. Advantages of decompression alone

- Shorter surgery
- Lower mortality
- Lower morbidity (blood transfusion; pulmonary complications; urinary tract infection, etc.)
- Lower infection rates
- Shorter hospitalization
- No donor site morbidity
- Less expensive
- Lower reoperation rates
- Similar outcomes as fusion
- Option of fusion available, if necessary

Table 2. Disadvantages of fusion

- Higher mortality and morbidity
- More expensive
- Higher reoperation rates
- Adjacent segment disease
- Fusion does not correlate with clinical outcome
- Clinical outcomes similar to decompression alone
- Pseudarthrosis

Patients undergoing fusion had a complication rate that was 1.9 times greater than those who had surgery without fusion. The blood transfusion rate was 5.8 times higher, nursing home placement rate 2.2 times more, and hospital charges 1.5 times higher (all p<0.0005) in those who underwent fusion. The mortality at 6 weeks post-surgery was double in patients undergoing fusion (p=0.025). Reoperation rates at 4 years were no lower for patients who had fusion surgery and the results were similar in most diagnostic subgroups. Deyo *et al.* concluded that 'indications for fusion among older patients require better definition, preferably based on outcomes from prospective controlled studies'.[14]

The rate of major postoperative complications is 3.7% in patients undergoing fusion and decompression versus 2.2% in those undergoing decompression alone.[15] Deyo *et al.* reported a higher incidence of nerve root injury in those undergoing fusion compared with those undergoing decompression alone.[14] In 1997, Katz *et al.* reported that the average cost of a laminectomy in the USA was US$ 14,700 whereas it was US$ 30,200 for laminectomy and fusion.[12]

Fusion also increases the probability of precipitating a secondary degenerative slippage above the fusion site. Lee reported this in 2 of 18 patients who had undergone fusion surgery and were followed up for 8.5 years.[16] Evaluation of recurrent symptoms in patients who have undergone fusion is also a problem, as it is unclear whether the recurrent symptoms are caused by a failure of fusion or recurrent stenosis, although the latter is a more likely cause.

Finally, not all fusion procedures lead to a favourable long-term outcome. In many patients, the slippage progresses because of pseudo-arthrosis, and a secondary fusion procedure is needed. It has been reported that reoperation rates are much higher in patients undergoing fusion than those undergoing decompression alone.[14] Katz *et al.* reported that repeat surgery rates were 2%, 15% and 7% for the no fusion, uninstrumented fusion and instrumented fusion groups, respectively.[12]

Evidence supporting the need for fusion

A poor outcome following decompression alone is seen when the decompression involves extensive facetectomy, in which more than one-third of the facet is removed or when the pars interarticularis is violated. Johnsson *et al.* reported poor results following extended laminectomies and complete bilateral facetectomies in 61 patients with spondylolisthesis.[17]

A meta-analysis of the literature performed in 1993 showed that decompression alone gave a good outcome in 69% of patients compared with 90% of those treated with decompression and fusion.[18] However, randomized studies were not used in the meta-analysis.[19,20] In non-randomized studies there is a risk of selection bias with sicker patients being subjected to decompression alone and relatively healthier patients undergoing the more demanding fusion procedure. This is the case with the study by Ghogawala *et al.* who compared the outcomes in patients with grade 1 spondylolisthesis undergoing either fusion (14 patients) or decompression alone (20 patients).[1] They concluded that those undergoing fusion had better outcomes on the Short-Form 36 scores and Oswestry Disability Index. As the results were reported after only a 1-year follow-up, it is possible that a longer follow-up might have shown a different outcome.

On reviewing the literature, it is evident that there are major lacunae in the reports of studies in patients with grade 1 degenerative spondylolisthesis. Apart from there being a lack of randomization, only a few of the reported studies comparing decompression and fusion focused on patients above 60 years of age. They invariably report the results in patients with all grades of listhesis. Finally, the surgical procedures are not standardized and the decompression is more extensive than recommended by this author. There is also a possibility that a discoidectomy might have been performed in some of the patients.

Martin *et al.*, on reviewing the debate of

decompression versus fusion for degenerative spondylolisthesis, concluded that there was moderate evidence that fusion provided a better outcome than decompression.[21] Although instrumented fusion resulted in better fusion rates, the clinical outcomes were similar in the instrumented and uninstrumented fusion groups.[21] It is interesting to note that if the main aim of fusion is to achieve a better clinical outcome, then the better fusion rates attained with instrumentation did not achieve this result. Martin *et al.* also conceded that the available studies, both randomized and non-randomized, suffered from major methodological flaws and concluded that properly conducted randomized controlled trials were needed to settle the issue.[21]

Conclusion

The author strongly recommends that discretion be exercised in the use of fusion for older patients (>60 years of age) with grade 1 degenerative spondylolisthesis. Decompression alone is sufficient in the vast majority of such patients. In those with hypermobility, as determined by dynamic X-rays and lateral decubitus X-rays of the lumbar spine, fusion may be needed. However, these patients account for 5%–10% of this group and hence the other >90% of patients should not be exposed to the risks and cost of fusion surgery. Randomized controlled studies with a long-term follow-up are clearly needed to resolve this issue.[21] Even if fusion is found to be superior in providing benefit in the short term, the cost–benefit ratio and the risk of complications should be carefully weighed before selecting the optimal surgical procedure.

References

1. Ghogawala Z, Benzel EC, Amin-Hanjani S, *et al.* Prospective outcomes evaluation after decompression with or without instrumented fusion for lumbar stenosis and degenerative grade I spondylolisthesis. *J Neurosurg (Spine 1)* 2004;**3**:267–72.

2. Matsunaga S, Ijiri K, Hiyashi K. Nonsurgically managed patients with degenerative spondylolisthesis: A 10- to 18-year follow-up study. *J Neurosurg (Spine 2)* 2000;**93**:194–8.

3. Epstein NE, Epstein JA, Carras R, *et al.* Degenerative spondylolisthesis with an intact neural arch: A review of 60 cases with an analysis of clinical findings and the development of surgical management. *Neurosurgery* 1983;**13**:555–61.

4. Young S, Veerapen R, O'Laoire SA. Relief of lumbar canal stenosis using multilevel subarticular fenestrations as an alternative to wide laminectomy: A preliminary report. *Neurosurgery* 1988;**23**:628–33.

5. Cavusoglu H, Kaya RA, Turkmenoglu ON, *et al.* Midterm outcome after unilateral approach for bilateral decompression of lumbar spinal stenosis: A 5-year prospective study. *Eur Spine J* 2007;**16**: 2133–42.

6. Kleeman TJ, Hiscoe AC, Berg EE. Patient outcome after minimally destabilizing lumbar stenosis decompression: The 'port-hole' technique. *Spine* 2000;**25**: 865–70.

7. Costa F, Sassi M, Cardia A, *et al.* Degenerative lumbar spinal stenosis: Analysis of results in a series of 374 patients treated with unilateral laminotomy for bilateral microdecompression. *J Neurosurg (Spine)* 2007;**7**:579–86.

8. Epstein NA. Surgical management of lumbar stenosis: Decompression and indications for fusion. *Neurosurg Focus* 1997;**3**:Article 1.

9. Herron LD, Trippi AC. L4–5 degenerative spondylolisthesis. The results of treatment by decompressive laminectomy without fusion. *Spine* 1989;**14**:534–8.

10. Sanderson PL, Wood PL. Surgery for lumbar spinal stenosis in old people. *J Bone Joint Surg Br* 1993;**75**: 393–7.

11. Johnsson KE, Redlund-Johnell I, Uden A, *et al.* Preoperative and postoperative instability in lumbar spinal stenosis. *Spine* 1989;**14**:591–3.

12. Katz JN, Lipson SJ, Lew RA, *et al.* Lumbar laminectomy alone or with instrumented or non-instrumented arthrodesis in degenerative lumbar spinal stenosis. Patient selection, costs and surgical outcome. *Spine* 1997;**22**:1123–31.

13. Matsudaira K, Yamakazi T, Seichi A, *et al.* Spinal stenosis in grade I degenerative lumbar spondylolisthesis: A comparative study of outcomes following laminoplasty and laminectomy with instrumented spinal fusion. *J Orthop Sci* 2005;**10**: 270–76.

14. Deyo RA, Ciol MA, Cherkin DC, *et al.* Lumbar spine fusion. A cohort study of complications, re-

operations and resource use in the Medicare population. *Spine* 1993;**18:**1463–70.

15. Weir B, de Leo R. Lumbar stenosis: Analysis of factors affecting outcome in 81 surgical cases. *Can J Neurol Sci* 1981;**8:**295–8.

16. Lee CK. Accelerated degeneration of the segment adjacent to a lumbar fusion. *Spine* 1988;**13:**375–7.

17. Johnsson KE, Willner S, Johnsson K. Postoperative instability after decompression for lumbar spinal stenosis. *Spine* 1986;**11:**107–10.

18. Mardjetko SM, Connolly PJ, Shott S. Degenerative lumbar spondylolisthesis. A meta-analysis of the literature, 1970–1993. *Spine* 1994;**19:**S2256–S2265.

19. Bridwell KH, Sedgewick TA, O'Brien MF, *et al.* The role of fusion and instrumentation in the treatment of degenerative spondylolisthesis with spinal stenosis. *J Spinal Disord* 1993;**6:**461–72.

20. Kuntz KM, Snider RK, Weinstein JN, *et al.* Cost-effectiveness of fusion with and without instrumentation for patients with degenerative spondylolisthesis and spinal stenosis. *Spine* 2000;**25:**1132–9.

21. Martin CR, Gruszczynski AT, Braunsfurth HA, *et al.* The surgical management of degenerative lumbar spondylolisthesis: A systematic review. *Spine* 2007;**32:**1791–8.

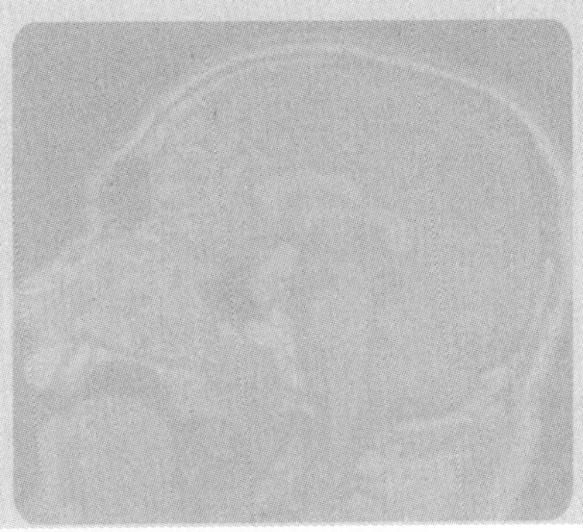

Epilepsy

16

Epilepsy and autonomic dysfunction

P. SATISHCHANDRA, C. PRADHAN, T.N. SATHYAPRABHA

Epilepsy is a common neurological disorder. Prevalence studies conducted in 2001 estimated that approximately 5.5 million people in India (5.33/1000 population) were affected.[1] Global trends show a similar prevalence.[1]

Up to 70% of new-onset epilepsy cases are satisfactorily controlled with a single drug; 15% are managed successfully with polypharmacy, i.e. taking 2–3 different drugs, and approximately 15% who are refractory to the above are forced to seek newer or experimental therapies. Of these approximately 5% opt for epilepsy surgery. Almost 10% of all epilepsy patients remain refractory to all forms of treatment.[2]

Activation of the autonomic nervous system has been well documented in patients receiving electroconvulsive therapy (ECT) and in those with spontaneous symptomatic seizures during ictus.[3,4] Autonomic dysfunction has been noted to extend well into the interictal period and could be the only sign during this phase of clinical calm. Several studies have shown that the hallmark of clinical seizure onset is a decreased variability in the heart rate and decreased sympathetic tone resulting from autonomic activation.[5,6,7] Autonomic dysfunction is more prominent in refractory epilepsy and could be caused by uncontrolled electrical stimulation and/or chronic functional changes in the related neuroanatomical regions of the brain.

Sudden unexplained death in epilepsy (SUDEP) remains an important cause of mortality in refractory epilepsy.[5] Although the exact mechanisms of SUDEP are presently unclear, autonomic dysfunction is said to play a significant role.

Neurophysiology of autonomic activation in epilepsy

Autonomic symptoms in epilepsy are believed to result from the involvement of autonomic centres in the brain due to seizure foci, seizure propagation, or as a behavioural manifestation of the episode itself. A pattern of autonomic involvement during seizures, which coincided with the progress of the seizure wave front across the temporal lobe, was described by Van Buren as early as 1958.[4] In 1999, Novak *et al.*, using time frequency analysis, described combined parasympathetic and sympathetic activation, rapid parasympathetic withdrawal approximately 30 sec before seizure onset, and sympathetic activation peaking at the time of seizure onset in complex partial seizures of temporal lobe origin.[6] This pattern indicates propagation of the electrical activity through spatially separated autonomic centres. Similar observations were reported in patients who had seizures induced by ECT.[7] Pre-ictal elevation of cardiac parasympathetic activity can be used as a predictor for secondary generalization of seizures.

Most authors agree that overactivity of the parasympathetic system is a preferential outcome in left hemisphere involvement and sympathetic activation in the right hemisphere.[8,9,10] Studies on the central autonomic areas have shown that stimulating the left insular cortex causes parasympathetic symptoms and stimulating the right insular cortex causes sympathetic symptoms.[8,10]

Temporal lobe epilepsy (TLE) is notorious both for its refractoriness and for the autonomic symptoms that are an inevitable consequence of the disease. These symptoms appear because the entorhinal–cortex–hippocampus complex is believed to be the site of origin of seizure activity in the majority of these patients. Neuronal discharges in the mesial temporal structures, viz. the amygdala and hippocampus, are synchronized with the cardiac and respiratory cycles. Seizure foci in the temporal lobe propagate easily to the autonomic centres in the brain. Local stimulation of the amygdala is insufficient to alter the heart rate, for which propagation through the entire limbic system is necessary. The longer time lag seen between seizure spikes and induced cardiac changes in frontal lobe foci compared with seizures in temporal lobe foci could be because of the greater distance of the frontal lobe from the limbic system.[9,11]

Ictal autonomic changes

Ictal autonomic changes can produce cardiovascular, respiratory, gastrointestinal, cutaneous, pupillary, urinary and genital symptoms.[12] These autonomic changes can elicit visceral, emotional and sexual symptoms. Ictal activation of the central autonomic network frequently leads to hallucinations, and less often to the illusion of visceral or corporeal sensations. Sympathetic responses predominate during most seizures. The responses include tachycardia, T-wave flattening and increased blood pressure. Ictal bradycardia followed by tachycardia, persistent

bradycardia and asystole are particular features in patients with frontal lobe seizures and in those with pre-existing parasympathetic autonomic dysfunction. Conduction and rhythm abnormalities have also been documented during ictus; they include the following: atrial fibrillation, sinus arrhythmia, atrial and ventricular premature depolarization, bundle-branch block, *torsade de pointes*, ST-segment and T-wave abnormalities, and QT prolongation.[9,13]

Other ictal autonomic changes may include flushing, erythema, cyanosis, blanching, piloerection, mydriasis and miosis with hippus. Apnoea, hypoventilation, hyperventilation, ascending abdominal sensations, dyspepsia, pain, hunger, increased borborygmi, nausea, vomiting, belching, incontinence, frequency of micturition, urge to defaecate, faecal incontinence, and bladder incontinence and/or urgency are also common manifestations. Erotic feelings, sexual arousal, erectile dysfunction, genital sensations and orgasm are rare ictal phenomena.[9,14]

Interictal autonomic changes

Long-standing and chronic epilepsy is invariably associated with abnormal autonomic function. Reduced heart rate variability has been documented in patients with both refractory as well as long-standing, well-controlled epilepsy.[11] Ictal autonomic dysfunction has been associated with the pathogenesis of SUDEP.[15] Diehl and colleagues demonstrated an interictal increase in the sympathetic modulation of cerebral blood flow velocities in epilepsy patients.[16]

We have demonstrated significant interictal autonomic dysfunction in patients with refractory epilepsy. Of the 73 patients with refractory epilepsy on rational polytherapy, 56.2% had definite or severe involvement of two or more cardiac autonomic tests. It is hoped that this study will stimulate further research on SUDEP and other causes of death in patients with long-standing, chronic epilepsy.[17] The long-term modulation of central autonomic centres in patients with refractory epilepsy seems to be due to functional changes or epileptiform discharges. Models of neuronal plasticity and learning also suggest that seizure discharges in autonomic centres, as in any other area of the brain, probably initiate a vicious cycle, which explains the severity of autonomic dysfunction in long-standing and uncontrolled seizures. Indeed, the hallmark of refractory epilepsy is the interictal spikes seen in an electroencephalograph (EEG) which might suggest subclinical electrical seizures.[9] Neuroimaging studies have demonstrated a variety of organic lesions in patients with refractory epilepsy, but these do not seem to be associated with increased autonomic dysfunction, which suggests that it may be possible to reverse autonomic dysfunction in some of these groups of epilepsy patients.[18]

Antiepileptic drugs and autonomic dysfunction

Autonomic dysfunction in epilepsy was previously partly attributed to the use and withdrawal of anticonvulsants, especially carbamazepine.[19] Administration of this drug has been shown to decrease heart rate variability and causes parasympathetic hypofunction.[19] Studies by our group and by Berilgen *et al.* have shown no significant association between autonomic dysfunction and the use of anticonvulsants.[17,20] Berilgen *et al.* have also suggested that autonomic changes are amenable to antiepileptic medication.[20] A wide range of autonomic disturbances, including arrhythmia, hypotension and respiratory depression, are known to be associated with AEDs.[9] Hypotension is seen with valproic acid, phenytoin, benzodiazepines and barbiturates; the latter two drugs can also cause respiratory depression. Carbamazepine and oxcarbamazepine have anticholinerigc side-effects, and can cause arrhythmias, respiratory depression and conduction defects. Phenytoin is known to cause arrhythmias. Gastrointestinal disturbances have been noted with ethosuximide, felbamate and valproic acid.[9]

SUDEP

The mortality rate in patients with epilepsy is 2–3 times greater than that in the general population; SUDEP may account for 8%–17% of these deaths.[21] Risk factors include a younger age at onset, a duration of illness >10 years, male sex, symptomatic epilepsy, generalized tonic–clonic seizures, increased seizure frequency, subtherapeutic antiepileptic drug (AED) levels, change in the AED, polypharmacy with AEDs, and surgical intervention for seizures.[22] Most cases of SUDEP occur during the third and fifth decades.[22] In addition to the underlying cerebral pathology in SUDEP, the pathological findings at autopsy in patients with symptomatic epilepsy include cerebral oedema, signs of hypoxia in the hippocampal area, and sclerosis of the amygdalae. In addition, mild to moderately severe pulmonary oedema with protein-rich fluid and alveolar haemorrhage may also be seen. Non-fatal cardiac pathological findings include fibrosis of the conductive system.[9]

Various pathophysiological events may contribute to SUDEP. Respiratory events, including airway obstruction, central apnoea, bradyarrhythmias and neurogenic pulmonary oedema, are probable terminal events. Catecholamine surges that occur during repeated seizures can also result in fibrosis of the cardiac conduction system and arrhythmias, during both the ictal and interictal periods. This can lead to cardiac arrest and acute cardiac failure, and may contribute significantly to SUDEP.[23]

Sudden death in epilepsy occurs more commonly during rapid eye movement (REM) sleep. This was thought to be paradoxical as REM is known to be seizure protective.[24] Lather *et al.* described pre-terminal seizures occurring in 30%–80% of SUDEP cases. Another possible mechanism for SUDEP is the 'lock stem phenomenon', which is synchronization of cardiac sympathetic and vagal cardiac neural discharges with epileptogenic discharge.[25] Use of carbamazepine is associated with impaired cardiac regulation and with increased risk of

SUDEP. Decreased heart rate variability is known to increase the vulnerability of the cardio-regulatory centres, leading to an increase in ventricular automaticity, which in turn predisposes to arrhythmias. This is particularly crucial, as autonomic cardiac arrhythmias may contribute significantly to the phenomenon of SUDEP.[9]

Modulation of autonomic dysfunction in epilepsy

Yoga and other stress-alleviating biofeedback mechanisms decrease autonomic arousal, and have been shown to reduce seizures both in terms of frequency and EEG parameters.[26,27] As the relationship between stress and epilepsy is well documented, stress-alleviating methods can reduce seizure frequency.[27] A prospective study demonstrated a clear benefit of yoga in reducing parasympathetic dysfunction and seizure frequency.[28]

The exact mechanisms, although unknown, might be brain plasticity and the neurochemical changes arising from the practice of yoga.[28] Yogic breathing increases sensory–motor rhythm, which is a 12–15 Hz rhythm found frequently in waking states and which may be beneficial in preventing SUDEP.[29] Yoga might also play an important role in interrupting the vicious cycle of stress and epilepsy. With evidence indicating that SUDEP is secondary to para-sympathetic dysfunction, modulation of central parasympathetic output through yoga may be preventative.[28]

Vagal nerve stimulation

Left vagal nerve stimulation (VNS) is another effective therapeutic intervention for medically refractory partial-onset seizures as it eliminates the possibility of drug interactions or life-threatening adverse effects of AEDs. Studies have shown a long-term decrease in mean seizure frequency of 40%–50%, and a short-term decrease in mean seizure frequency of 20%–30% in patients who are >12 years of age.[30]

Studies using several animal models have shown that VNS inhibits seizures; high-intensity, high-frequency stimulation of the C fibres is known to produce desynchronization of the cortical EEG.[31] VNS increases seizure threshold by causing widespread release of gamma-amino-butyric acid (GABA) and glycine in the brain. Low-frequency stimulation causes synchronization; although it also increases free and total GABA levels in the cerebrospinal fluid, it usually does not prevent the occurrence of seizures.[32]

Investigators have also suggested that the anticonvulsant effects of VNS may be caused by indirect modulation of the reticular activating system, central autonomic network, limbic system, diffuse noradrenergic projection system and locus coeruleus.[33] VNS causes measurable changes in cerebral blood flow in the cerebellum, thalamus and cortex, and may activate inhibitory structures in the brain. VNS also alters vagal parasympathetic efferent activities, but these are independent of its anti-seizure effects. Adverse effects are reported in 5% of patients with high-frequency stimulation. They include hoarseness, throat pain, coughing, dyspnoea, paraesthesiae, and muscular pain, all of which decrease with time.[30]

Conclusion

Activation of the autonomic nervous system is a well known ictal phenomenon in patients with epilepsy. This activation is known to extend well into the interictal phase. Numerous studies have shown decreased heart rate variability and decreased sympathetic tone caused by autonomic activation.[4–7] Autonomic dysfunction is more prominent in patients with refractory epilepsy and it could be caused by uncontrolled electrical stimulation and chronic functional changes in the related neuroanatomical regions of the brain. SUDEP remains an important cause of mortality in refractory epilepsy. Several mechanisms for

SUDEP have been proposed. Of these, autonomic dysfunction, leading to central apnoea, arrhythmias and cardiac failure play a crucial role. Non-pharmacological methods, used in addition to drug therapy, may be useful in the management of epilepsy-related autonomic dysfunction. These methods include vagal nerve stimulation, yoga, meditation and behavioural modification.

References

1. Sridharan R, Murthy BN. Prevalence and pattern of epilepsy in India. *Epilepsia* 1999;**40**:631–6.
2. Radhakrishnan K. *Medically refractory epilepsy*. In: Radhakrishnan K (ed). Trivandrum, India: Sree Chitra Tirunal Institute for Medical Sciences and Technology; 1999:1–40.
3. Brown ML, Huston PE, Hines HM, *et al*. Cardiovascular changes associated with electroconvulsive shock in monkeys; cerebral blood flow, blood pressure and cardiac rate measurements before, during and after electroconvulsive shock. *Arch Neurol Psychiatry* 1953;**69**:609–14.
4. Van Buren JM. Some autonomic concomitants of ictal automatism: A study of temporal lobe attacks. *Brain* 1958;**81**:505–28.
5. Nashef L, Walker F, Allen P. Apnoea and bradycardia during epileptic seizures: Relation to sudden death in epilepsy. *J Neurol Neurosurg Psychiatry* 1996;**60**:297–300.
6. Novak V, Reeves AL, Novak P, *et al*. Time frequency mapping of RR interval during complex partial seizures of temporal lobe origin. *J Auton Nerv Syst* 1999;**77**:195–202.
7. Lai I, Yang C, Kuo T, *et al*. Immediate impact of electroconvulsive therapy on cardiac autonomic function in schizophrenia: A preliminary study. *Schiz Res* 2008;**100**:353–5.
8. Oppenheimer SM, Kedem G, Martin WM. Left-insular cortex lesions perturb cardiac autonomic tone in humans. *Clin Auton Res* 1996;**6**:131–40.
9. Nouri S, Balish M. Epilepsy and the autonomic nervous system. In: Bromfield EB, Talavera F, Cavazos JE, *et al*. (eds). *eMedicine*. WebMD. http://www.emedicine.com/neuro/TOPIC658.htm [accessed on 6 October 2008].
10. Zhang ZH, Rashba S, Oppenheimer SM. Insular cortex lesions alter baroreceptor sensitivity in the urethane-anesthetized rat. *Brain Res* 1998;**813**:73–81.
11. Ansakorpi H, Korpelainen JT, Huikuri HV, *et al*. Heart rate dynamics in refractory and well controlled temporal lobe epilepsy. *J Neurol Neurosurg Psychiatry* 2002;**76**:26–30.
12. Baumgartner C, Lurger S, Leutmezer F. Autonomic symptoms during epileptic seizures. *Epileptic Disord* 2001;**3**:103–16.
13. Reynolds EH. Do anticonvulsants alter the natural course of epilepsy? Treatment should be started as early as possible. *BMJ* 1995;**310**:176–7.
14. Devinsky O. Effects of seizures on autonomic and cardiovascular function. *Epilepsy Curr* 2004;**4**:43–8.
15. Hirsch C, Martin D. Unexpected death in young epileptics. *Neurology* 1971;**21**:682–90.
16. Diehl B, Diehl RR, Stodieck SR, *et al*. Spontaneous oscillations in cerebral blood flow velocities in middle cerebral arteries in control subjects and patients with epilepsy. *Stroke* 1997;**28**:2457–9.
17. Sathyaprabha TN, Satishchandra P, Netravathi K, *et al*. Cardiac autonomic dysfunctions in chronic refractory epilepsy. *Epilepsy Res* 2006;**72**:49–56.
18. Wieshmann U. Clinical application of neuroimaging in epilepsy. *J Neurol Neurosurg Psychiatry* 2003;**74**:466–70.
19. Hennessy MJ, Tighe MG, Binnie CD, *et al*. Sudden withdrawal of carbamazepine increases cardiac sympathetic activity in sleep. *Neurology* 2001;**57**:1650–4.
20. Berilgen MS, Sari T, Bulut S, *et al*. Effects of epilepsy on autonomic nervous system and respiratory function tests. *Epilepsy Behav* 2004;**5**:513–16.
21. Walczak TS, Leppik IE, D'Amelio M, *et al*. Incidence and risk factors in sudden unexpected death in epilepsy: A prospective cohort study. *Neurology* 2001;**56**:519–25.
22. Ficker DM, So EL, Shen WK. Population-based study of the incidence of sudden unexplained death in epilepsy. *Neurology* 1998;**51**:1270–4.
23. Terrence CF Jr, Wisotzkey HM, Perper JA. Unexpected unexplained death in epileptic patients. *Neurology* 1975;**25**:594–8.
24. Ferri R, Curzi-Dascalova L, Arzimanoglou A, *et al*. Heart rate variability during sleep in children with partial epilepsy. *J Sleep Res* 2002;**11**:153–60.
25. Lathers CM, Schraeder PL, Weiner FL. Synchronization of cardiac autonomic neural discharge with epileptogenic activity: Lockstep phenomenon. *Electroencephalogr Clin Neurophysiol* 1987;**67**:247–59.

26. Kaplan BJ. Biofeedback in epileptics: Equivocal relationship of reinforced EEG frequency to seizure reduction. *Epilepsia* 1975;**16**:477–85.

27. Panjwani U, Selvamurthy W, Singh SH, *et al.* Effect of *sahaja yoga* practice on seizure control and EEG changes in patients of epilepsy. *Indian J Med Res* 1996;**103**:165–72.

28. Sathyaprabha TN, Satishchandra P, Pradhan C, *et al.* Modulation of cardiac autonomic balance with adjuvant yoga therapy in patients with refractory epilepsy. *Epilepsy Behav* 2008;**12**:245–52.

29. Murthy PJNV, Janakiramaiah N, Gangadhar BN, *et al.* P300 amplitude and antidepressant response to *sudarshan kriya yoga* (SKY). *J Affect Disord* 1998;**50**: 45–8.

30. Schachter SC, Saper CB. Vagus nerve stimulation. *Epilepsia* 1998;**39**:677–86.

31. Rielo D, Benbadis SR. Vagal nerve stimulation. In: Murro AM, Talavera F, Cavazos JE, *et al.* (eds). eMedicine. WebMD. http://www.emedicine.com/ neuro/TOPIC559.htm [accessed on 6 October 2008].

32. Henry TR. Therapeutic mechanisms of vagus nerve stimulation. *Neurology* 2002;**24** (Suppl 4):S31–S37.

33. George MS, Nahas Z, Bohning DE, *et al.* Vagal nerve stimulation and deep brain stimulation. In: Stein DJ, Kupfer DJ, Schatzberb AF (eds). *American Psychiatric Publishing Textbook of mood disorders.* Virginia: American Psychiatric Publishing Inc. 2005:337–49.

17

Myoclonic epilepsy

S. PRABHAKAR, MANISH MODI

Myoclonic epilepsies are a collection of syndromes, in which myoclonic seizures are a prominent feature. 'Myoclonus' is derived from the Greek words for muscle and turmoil.[1] Myoclonic seizures are defined as brief, sudden, involuntary muscle contractions that vary in their distribution and manifestations.[2]

Classification of myoclonus

Myoclonus can be clinically described under the following subheadings[1]

- In terms of bodily involvement, a myoclonic seizure can be focal (i.e. confined to one region), regional (i.e. affecting two or more contiguous regions) or generalized (i.e. affecting the whole body).
- In terms of frequency, a myoclonic seizure can consist of a single jerk or repetitive jerks. Repetitive myoclonic jerks can further be rhythmic or arrhythmic.
- In terms of amplitude, the seizure can be small (i.e. no joint movement) or massive (i.e. movement of the extremities, trunk or head).
- In terms of side of involvement, the seizure can occur unilaterally or bilaterally, and further, symmetrically or asymmetrically.
- Electrophysiologically, myoclonus can be epileptic or non-epileptic. In general, epileptic myoclonus has an electroencephalograph (EEG) correlate of spike, multispikes, spike–wave or multispike wave complexes.[3] However, the pathophysiology is not that simple. In many diseases involving the cortex, such as Creutzfeldt–Jacob disease, Alzheimer's disease, post-hypoxic brain damage and metabolic encephalopathies, myoclonus is a prominent feature. However, there is no EEG discharge associated with the jerk. Perhaps there is some subcortical pathology to explain the myoclonus in these disorders. The other explanation is that the epileptiform cortical discharges are so spatially restricted that they do not reach the scalp.
- The Commission of Paediatric Epilepsy of the International League against Epilepsy has defined four types of myoclonus, i.e. cortical, thalamo-cortical, reticular reflex and negative myoclonus.[4] Negative myoclonus has been defined as muscular inhibitions that induce brief, brisk movements resembling myoclonic seizures. Negative myoclonus may originate in the cerebral cortex, cerebellum, brain stem or spinal cord.[5]

Classification of myoclonic epilepsies

Myoclonic epilepsy syndromes can be epileptic or non-epileptic and can also be divided into inherited and acquired forms (Fig. 1).[1,6] The recent availability of genetic studies has greatly enhanced

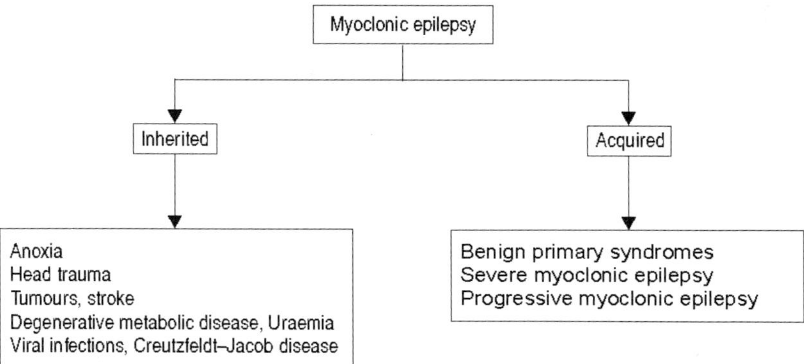

Fig. 1. Flow chart showing types and causes of myoclonic epilepsies

our understanding of many inherited myoclonic epilepsy syndromes. The vast majority of myoclonic epilepsy syndromes are idiopathic or cryptogenic and genetic factors are important, as indicated by the frequency of epilepsy in family members. There is evidence that functional impairment of the ion channel may represent the pathophysiological substrate for at least some of the non-progressive myoclonic epilepsies, while a gene defect that causes accumulation of abnormal material in various organs, including the brain, is responsible for progressive myoclonic epilepsies.[6]

Acquired myoclonic seizures may develop as a consequence of anoxia, head trauma, stroke, tumours, metabolic encephalopathies such as uraemia, viral infections and degenerative disorders of the central nervous system. In aggregate, acquired myoclonic seizures are much more common than the inherited syndromes, but have attracted much less interest in the neurological literature.[3] The inherited myoclonic epilepsies can be classified on the basis of age of onset from the practical point of view (Table 1).

Myoclonic epilepsy in the newborn

Early myoclonic encephalopathy

Fragmentary, erratic and severe myoclonus begins neonatally or during the first month of life and is followed by partial seizures and tonic spasms. Myoclonus involves the muscles of the face and extremities, and the seizures may be occasional to almost continuous. Among the multiple prenatal causes are inborn errors of metabolism, such as methyl malonic acidaemia and non-ketotic hyperglycaemia. The EEG shows

Table 1. Classification of myoclonic epilepsies by age of onset

Neonatal period
- Early myoclonic encephalopathy

Infancy and early childhood
- Benign myoclonic epilepsy of infancy (5 months to 5 years)
- Severe myoclonic epilepsy of infants or Dravet syndrome (2 months to 1 year)
- Myoclonic-astatic epilepsy (7 months to 6 years, usually after 2 years)

Late childhood and adolescence
- Myoclonic absence epilepsy (1–12 years)
- Juvenile myoclonic epilepsy (6–22 years)
- Photosensitive myoclonic epilepsy

Variable age
- Epilepsies with prominent distal myoclonus or Angelman syndrome (3 months to 20 years)
- Autosomal dominant cortical reflex myoclonus and epilepsy (12–59 years)
- Familial adult myoclonic epilepsy (19–73 years)

Progressive myoclonic epilepsies

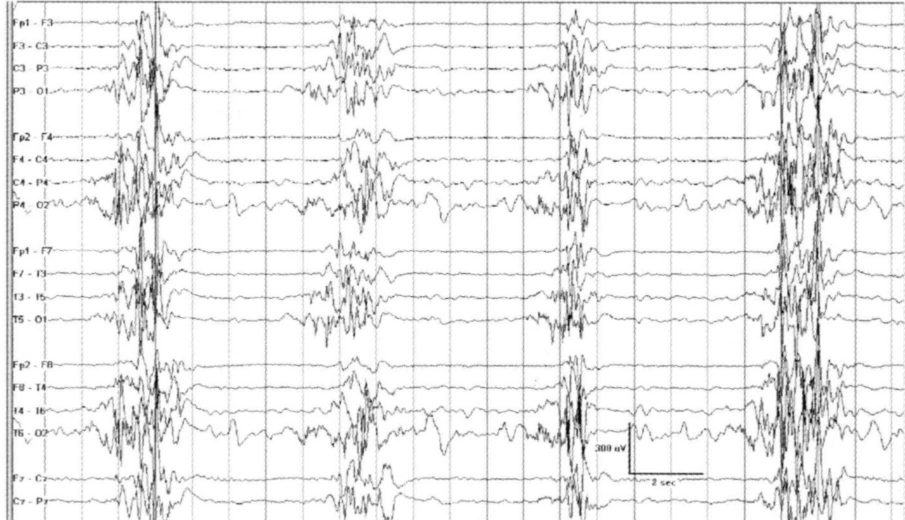

Fig. 2. EEG showing burst suppression pattern in a case of early myoclonic epilepsy

bursts of spikes, sharp waves and slow waves, separated by periods of electrical silence (suppression bursts) (Fig. 2).[7]

Myoclonic epilepsy in infancy and early childhood

Benign myoclonic epilepsy of infancy

The age of onset of seizures ranges from 5 months to 5 years in otherwise normal children. The myoclonic jerks are initially mild and gradually increase in frequency to multiple daily events. There is nodding of the head or upward rolling of the eyes, accompanied by brisk abduction of the upper limbs. The jerks may be asymmetrical and vary in intensity. Myoclonic jerks may be triggered by tapping or acoustic stimuli in some patients. The EEG may show normal background activity. Spike and wave discharges are seen concomitant with myoclonic jerks. In general, the outcome is favourable for these patients and treatment is withdrawn in the case of most patients older than 6 years of age at follow-up.[8]

Myoclonic astatic epilepsy (MAE)

This epilepsy appears between the age of 7 months and 6 years, the peak incidence being between 2 and 6 years. Brief, massive, axial and symmetric jerks, involving the neck, shoulders, arms and legs, often result in nodding of the head, abduction of the arms and flexion of the legs at the knees. Each jerk is followed by an abrupt loss of muscle tone that causes the patient to drop to the floor and may lead to injuries. The episodes usually last less than 2–3 sec. The EEG shows bursts of spike/polyspike and wave complex at 2–4 Hz. Myoclonic astatic epilepsy is self-limited and the seizures abate within 3 years in 50%–90% of patients.[6,9]

Severe myoclonic epilepsy of infancy (SMEI) (Dravet syndrome)

Severe myoclonic epilepsy of infancy is characterized by multiple types of seizures, including myoclonus, intractability despite treatment and an unfavourable evolution. Initially, in the case of an otherwise normal child, febrile seizures lasting several minutes to hours begin between the age of 2 months and 1 year. Afebrile seizures occur a few months later. In the second and third years of life, myoclonic and atypical absences appear. Myoclonic seizures appear at the age of 1–5 years as massive, generalized myoclonic jerks, involving the axial muscles and causing the patient to fall to the ground. The EEG shows normal background activity for the first few years, but this becomes slower over time. Generalized or asymmetric spike/polyspike waves appear later in the course of the disease. SEMI is highly refractory to medication and the patient shows only mild improvement with valproate and benzodiazepines.[6,10]

Myoclonic epilepsies of late childhood and adolescence

Myoclonic (or clonic) absence epilepsy

The age of onset of this type of epilepsy ranges from 1–12 years, the peak being reached at around 7 years. There is a preponderance of male patients (70%). More than two-thirds of patients have additional generalized tonic–clonic seizures. Almost 50% of patients suffer from cognitive impairment, which gradually becomes severe. Myoclonic absences are resistant to drug therapy.[6]

Juvenile myoclonic epilepsy

The age of onset ranges from 6 to 22 years, the percentage of females affected (61%) being higher than that of males. Myoclonic jerks usually appear between the age of 12 and 16 years and generalized tonic–clonic seizures peak at about 16 years. The myoclonic jerks are sudden and spontaneous, affecting mainly the arms and shoulders symmetrically. They rarely involve the lower extremities or the entire body. Most jerks occur within 20–30 min of waking up in the morning. Sleep deprivation is the most effective trigger. Infrequent generalized tonic–clonic

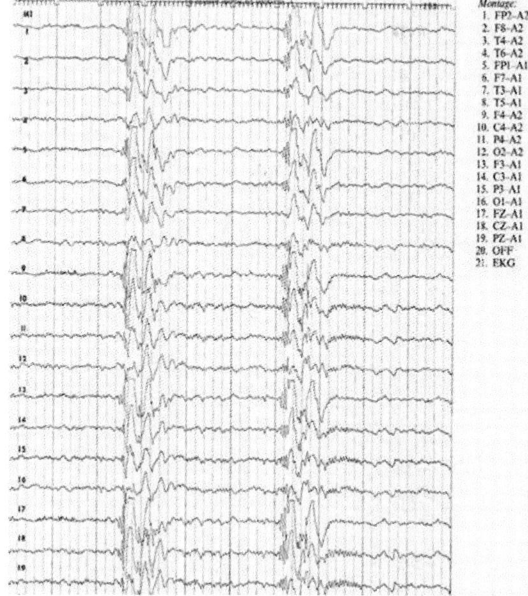

Fig. 3. EEG showing generalized polyspike and wave pattern in a case of juvenile myoclonic epilepsy

seizures occur in approximately 85% of patients. These seizures are usually precipitated by sleep deprivation, stress or alcohol. Short absence attacks sometimes occur independently of jerks. The EEG shows normal background activity. Approximately 30%–40% of patients have a photoparoxysmal response and characteristic spike and wave, as well as generalized polyspike and wave, complexes (Fig. 3). The ictal EEG consists of generalized symmetric discharge of high frequency (10–16 per sec), followed by several slow waves.[11] Monotherapy with sodium valproate controls the jerks and other attacks in approximately 85% of patients. In resistant cases, low doses of clobazam or clonazepam can be effective. Other drugs like lamotrigine, topiramate and levertiracetam have been used as an alternative or add-on in cases that are difficult to treat.[6,11]

Photosensitive myoclonic epilepsy

Visually induced generalized myoclonic jerks are usually symmetric and affect mainly the upper extremities. Usually, they produce nodding of the head and slight abduction of the arm. Myoclonic attacks may be provoked by watching television or playing video games. In the case of mentally retarded patients especially, myoclonic attacks are induced when they wave a hand between their eyes and a source of light, flutter their eyelids before a source of light or stare at patterned surfaces. In the EEG, the jerks are seen to be associated with the photoparoxysmal response. The EEG consists of a bilateral polyspike or polyspike and wave discharge. This form of myoclonic epilepsy is resistant to drug therapy.[12]

Myoclonic epilepsies with variable age of onset

Epilepsies with prominent distal myoclonus: Angelman syndrome

These patients present with moderate-to-severe mental retardation, lack of development of language functions, microbrachycephaly, inappropriate laughter, ataxic gait, tremors, epilepsy and jerky movements. Rapid distal jerking of fluctuating amplitude causes a coarse tremor, combined with dystonic limb posturing. On EEG, bilateral jerks of myoclonic absences show rhythmic repetition at 2.5 Hz and are time locked with a cortical spike.[13]

Table 2. Types of progressive myoclonic epilepsies and their definite diagnosis

---

Unverricht–Lundborg disease
    CSTB gene mutation

Lafora disease
    Lafora bodies in skin biopsy or EPM2A mutation

Myoclonic epilepsy with ragged red fibres
    Ragged red fibres in muscle biopsy or MTTK mutation

Neuronal ceroid lipofuscinosis
    Typical intracellular inclusions or mutation in TPP1, CLN3 and CLNS

Sialidoses
    Neuraminidase deficiency in leucocytes or fibroblasts

Familial autosomal dominant myoclonic epilepsy (FAME)

FAME has been described in several Japanese families. It starts during adulthood and is non-progressive. It is characterized by distal, rhythmic myoclonus, enhanced during posture maintenance (cortical tremor). The EEG shows generalized interictal spike and wave discharges, and photoparoxysmal response.[14]

Autosomal dominant cortical reflex myoclonus and epilepsy (ADCME)

The age of onset varies from 12 to 50 years. These patients have non-progressive cortical reflex myoclonus, expressed with semi-continuous rhythmic jerking. Generalized seizures are sometimes preceded by generalized myoclonic jerks.[15]

Progressive myoclonic epilepsies

The progressive myoclonic epilepsies (PMEs) are a group of symptomatic generalized epilepsies caused by rare disorders, most of which have genetic components, and they have a debilitating course and a poor outcome (Table 2). They are characterized by myoclonic seizures, tonic–clonic seizures and progressive neurological deterioration, typically accompanied with cerebellar signs and dementia.[1,6] Myoclonus in PME is typically multifocal and fragmentary, and often precipitated by posture, action or external stimuli such as light, sound or touch. The age of onset, presenting symptoms and predominance of symptoms (i.e. seizures, myoclonus, cerebellar signs and dementia) vary substantially across different disorders (Table 3). Each clinical myoclonic event may or may not be associated with EEG spikes or spike and wave discharges. Patients with PME may also have giant somatosensory-evoked potentials.[1]

- **Unverricht–Lundborg disease (ULD or Baltic myoclonus):** This is the most common type of

Table 3. The progressive myoclonic epilepsies: Salient features

Disease	Age (years)	Ataxia	Dementia	Other
NCL	2–10	+	+	Progressive blindness
Unverricht–Lundborg	8–12	+ (Slow)	+ / −	−
Lafora body	10–18	+	+	Rapid decline
Sialidosis	13–18	+	−	Progressive blindness with cherry-red spots
MERRF	Any age	+	+	+/− Myopathy, optic atrophy

PME worldwide. The age of onset is 6–15 years. The typical features include stimuli-sensitive myoclonus, generalized tonic–clonic seizures and progressive ataxia. With advances in antiepileptic drugs and due to the slow progression of the disease, patients now live into their sixties.[16] It is an autosomal recessive neurodegenerative disorder, caused by mutation in the cystatin B gene, which encodes for cysteine protease inhibitor. Due to loss of cysteine protease inhibition, apoptosis proceeds abnormally and neurodegeneration results.[17]

- **Lafora's disease:** First described by Lafora and Gluellcin in 1911, Lafora disease is characterized by epilepsy, myoclonus, dementia and Lafora bodies, which are periodic acid-Schiff-positive intracellular polyglucosar inclusion bodies found in neurons, the heart, skeletal muscle, liver and sweat gland duct cells.[18,19] Lafora body disease has a later onset than other PMEs, usually appearing between the ages of 10 and 18 years. Many patients appear to have a benign seizure disorder when they first present to the doctor and the diagnosis of PME is not considered. However, the emergence of myoclonus and rapidly progressive dementia differentiate it from benign conditions and identify it as one of the PMEs.[18] Most patients with Lafora body disease die within 10 years of diagnosis. Diagnosis is established by a skin biopsy that shows characteristic Lafora bodies

in the eccrine ducts of the sweat glands.[19] The narrow age of onset, progressive dementia, frequent occipital seizures, and rapid and relentless progression to death are clinical clues to the diagnosis.[1,18]

- **Myoclonic epilepsy with ragged red fibres (MERRF).** This is a typical PME characterized by myoclonus, tonic–clonic seizures, progressive ataxia and dementia. The additional presence of myopathy, neuropathy, hearing loss, short stature, optic atrophy, pigmentary retinopathy, ophthalmoparesis or diabetes may further point towards this mitochondrial disorder.[20] There may be elevated lactate levels in the serum and cerebrospinal fluid. A muscle biopsy typically reveals characteristic ragged red fibres in over 90% of patients.[21] Magnetic resonance imaging of the brain may show brain atrophy and basal ganglia calcification. The most common molecular defect is an adenosine to guanine substitution at nucleotide pair 8344 (8344 A–G) in the t–RNA gene (MTTK) of mitochondrial DNA. This is seen in more than 90% of cases.[22] As valproic acid causes inhibition of carnitine uptake, it must be used with caution and combined with L-carnitine supplementation.[23]

- **Neuronal ceroid lipofuscinoses (NCL):** These are characterized by the accumulation of large amounts of lipopigments in lysosomes. There are five types of NCL (Type 2 to Type 6) that can cause PME:

—Classic late infantile NCL (type 2) or Jansky–Bielschowsky disease, which, appears at the age of 2–5 years

—Juvenile NCL (type 3) or Spielmeyer–Vogt–Sjogren disease (also called Batten disease), the symptoms of which appear at the age of 4–10 years

—Adult NCL (type 4) or Kuf disease or Parry disease, which can make its appearance as late as 30 years of age

—Late infantile Finnish variant NCL (type 5), which appears at around 5 years of age

—Late infantile variant NCL (type 6), which starts at 5–7 years of age[24]

Except for the adult form, which is autosomal dominant, all other forms are autosomal recessive.[1] The clinical course is characterized by progressive mental and motor deterioration, blindness, seizures and premature death. Visual and ophthalmological abnormalities in the form of attenuated retinal vessels and the finding of macular degeneration on examination of the optic fundus point towards NCL.[1,6,24] Currently, the definitive diagnosis relies on the finding of typical intracellular inclusions in eccrine secretory cells by electron microscopy.[1,24]

- **Sialidosis (cherry-red spot myoclonus):** This is an autosomal recessive disorder caused by neuraminidase deficiency. The symptoms appear during adolescence and the patient presents with severe myoclonus and tonic–clonic seizures. This is followed by progressive visual loss, macular cherry-red spots and ataxia. Dementia does not usually occur.[25]

Treatment of myoclonic epilepsies

Treatment of myoclonic disorders, especially PMEs, consists essentially of managing the seizures and myoclonus, together with palliative, supportive and rehabilitative measures. The commonly used anti-epileptic drugs for the management of myoclonus include combinations of valproic acid, benzodiazepine and phenobarbital, and more recently, piracetam, levetiracetam and zonisamide.[26] Care must be taken to avoid anti-epileptic drugs that worsen myoclonus (Table 4). Lamotrigine has an unpredictable effect on myoclonus and must be used with caution.[27] Surgery, particularly corpus callostomy, may be beneficial in the treatment of children who have drop attacks as a result of myoclonus and suffer injuries. Vagal nerve stimulation has been used in the treatment of a variety of epilepsies, but there is a paucity of data on its use in myoclonic epilepsies.[6] Future methods of treatments, such as gene therapy and enzyme replacement, may help to modify and improve the course of these progressive disorders.

Table 4. Drugs in myoclonic epilepsies

Used for treatment
- Valproic acid
- Benzodiazepines
- Phenobarbital
- Piracetam
- Levetiracetam
- Zonisamide

May aggravate myoclonus
- Phenytoin
- Carbamazepine
- Gabapentin
- Vigabatrin
- Tiagabine

Use with caution
- Lamotrigine in all cases
- Valproic acid in MERRF

References

1. Leppik IE. Classification of the myoclonic epilepsies. *Epilepsia* 2003;**44** (Suppl 11):2–6.
2. Fahn S, Marsden CD, Van Woert MH. Definition and classification of myoclonus. *Adv Neurol* 1986;**43**:1–5.
3. Hallett M. Myoclonus: relation to epilepsy. *Epilepsia* 1985;**26** (Suppl 1):S67–77.
4. Commission on Pediatric Epilepsy of the International League Against Epilepsy. Myoclonus and epilepsy in childhood. *Epilepsia* 1997;**38**:1251–4.
5. Guerrini R, Dravet C, Genton P, *et al.* Epileptic negative myoclonus. *Neurology* 1993;**43**:1078–83.
6. Guerrini R, Bonanni P, Marini C, *et al.* The myoclonic epilepsies. In: Wyllie E (ed). *The treatment of epilepsy.* 4th ed. Philadelphia: Lippincot Williams and Wilkins; 2006:407–27.
7. Aicardi J. Early myoclonic encephalopathy. In: Roger J, Bureau M, Dravet C (eds). *Epilepsy syndromes in infancy, childhood and adolescence.* 2nd ed. London: John Libbey; 1992:13–23.
8. Dravet C, Bureau M, Genton P. Benign myoclonic epilepsy of infancy. *Epilepsy Res Suppl* 1992;**6**:131–5.
9. Tassinari CA, Rubboli G, Shibaksi H. Neurophysiology of positive and negative myoclonus. *Electroencephalogr Clin Neurophysiol* 1998;**107**:181–95.
10. Doose H, Lanau H, Castiglione E. Severe idiopathic

generalized epilepsy of infancy with generalized tonic–clonic seizures. *Neuropediatrics* 1998;**29**:229–38.

11. Pedersen SB, Petersen KA. Juvenile myoclonic epilepsy: Clinical and EEG features. *Acta Neurol Scand* 1998;**97**:160–3.

12. Kasteleijn-Nolst Trenite DG, Guerrini R, Binnie CD. Visual sensitivity and epilepsy: A proposed classification for clinical and EEG phenomenology. *Epilepsia* 2001; **42**:692–701.

13. Guerrini R, Carrozzo R, Rinaldi R. Angelman syndrome: Etiology, clinical features, diagnosis, and management of symptoms. *Pediatr Drugs* 2003;**5**: 647–61.

14. Okuma Y, Shimo Y, Shimura H. Familial cortical tremor with epilepsy: An under-recognised familial tremor. *Clin Neurol Neurosurg* 1998;**100**:75–8.

15. Guerrini R, Bonnani P, Patrignani A. Autosomal dominant cortical myoclonus and epilepsy (ADCME) with complex partial and generalized seizures. *Brain* 2001;**124**:2459–75.

16. Lehesjoki AE. Clinical features and genetics of Unverricht–Lundborg disease. *Adv Neurol* 2002;**89**: 193–7.

17. Berkovic SF, So NK, Andermann F. Progressive myoclonus epilepsies: Clinical and neurophysiological diagnosis. *J Clin Neurophysiol* 1991;**8**:261–74.

18. Busard BLSM, Renier WO, Gabreels FJM, *et al.* Lafora's disease. *Arch Neurol* 1986;**43**:296–99.

19. Carpenter S, Karpati G. Sweat gland duct cells in Lafora disease: Diagnosis by skin biopsy. *Neurology* 1981;**31**:1564-68.

20. Rosing HS, Hopkins LC, Wallace DC, *et al.* Maternally inherited mitochondrial myopathy and myoclonic epilepsy. *Ann Neurol* 1985;**17**:228–37.

21. DiMauro S, Hirano M, Kaufmann P, *et al.* Clinical features and genetics of myoclonic epilepsy with ragged-red fibers. *Adv Neurol* 2002;**89**:217–29.

22. Shoffner JM, Lott MT, Lezza A, *et al.* Myoclonic epilepsy and ragged-red fiber disease (MERRF) is associated with a mitochondrial DNA tRNALys mutation. *Cell* 1990;**61**:931–7.

23. Tein I, DiMauro S, Xie Z-W, *et al.* Valproic acid impairs carnitine uptake in cultured human skin fibroblasts: An *in vitro* model for pathogenesis of valproic acid-associated carnitine deficiency. *Pediatr Res* 1993;**34**:281–7.

24. Wisniewski KE, Zhong N, Philippart M. Pheno/genotypic correlations of neuronal ceroid lipofuscinoses. *Neurology* 2001;**57**:576–81.

25. Rapin I, Goldfisher S, Katzman R, *et al.* The cherry-red spot myoclonus syndrome. *Ann Neurol* 1978;**3**: 234–42.

26. Conry JA. Progressive myoclonic epilepsies. *J Child Neurol* 2002;**17** (Suppl 1):S80–S4.

27. Janszky J, Rasonyi G, Halasz P, *et al.* Disabling erratic myoclonus during lamotrigine therapy with high serum level, report of two cases. *Clin Neuropharmacol* 2000;**23**:86–9.

18

Women with epilepsy

ARABINDA MUKHERJEE

It is increasingly being realized that the varying hormonal milieu in women changes the natural history of many disorders, and epilepsy is no exception. The management of epilepsy in women encompasses a complex interplay between seizures, sex steroid hormones and anti-epileptic drugs (AEDs). The special issues which need to be addressed for managing epilepsy in women include:

- role of epilepsy in pregnancy and reproductive health
- impact of pregnancy on epilepsy
- effect of AEDs on pregnancy and foetal outcome
- role of AEDs in hormonal contraception
- impact of AEDs on bone health

Over the past decade, women's issues in epilepsy have received increasing attention from neurologists. With the advent of better diagnostic tests and the development of effective and safe AEDs, it is now possible for most women with epilepsy to have a normal reproductive life, including pregnancy.

This chapter aims to briefly address each of these issues and formulate guidelines to help ensure optimum management of epilepsy in women.

Contraception

Anti-epileptic medications may affect hormonal contraceptives. For instance, certain medications increase the metabolism of contraceptives, rendering them less effective. Women with epilepsy must take into account these known interactions while choosing a contraceptive. This is especially important because AEDs are teratogenic. Despite the known risks, these issues are not well understood by neurologists or obstetricians.

Currently, most oral contraceptives contain some combination of an oestrogen (often ethinyl oestradiol) and a progesterone. Other hormone-based contraceptive formulations include medroxy-progesterone (Depo-Provera) or levonorgestrel (Norplant). To avoid the potential thrombo-embolic or other complications of high-dose exogenous oestrogens, most modern oral contraceptives contain 35 mcg or less of oestrogen, unlike formulations popular in the 1970s that contained 50–100 mcg.

It is thought that hormonal contraceptives fail relatively more frequently among women on certain anti-epileptic medications primarily because of hepatic microsomal enzyme induction and increased metabolism of hormones. The hepatic enzyme-inducing AEDs (e.g. barbiturates, carbamazepine, oxcarbazepine, phenytoin, ethosuximide, and to some extent, topiramate) may reduce the hormone levels of oral contraceptives by as much as 40%–50%, and several reports have documented the increased risk of failure of oral contraceptives among women taking these medications. Mid-cycle breakthrough bleeding may herald contraceptive failure, but is not a reliable sign; contraceptive failure may occur without this warning. Another mechanism that may contribute to the failure of contraceptives is that these AEDs also increase sex hormone-binding globulins, leading to a fall in the level of free hormones. No evidence exists of increased failure rates in women taking newer generation AEDs or those which do not induce enzymes.

If women on hepatic enzyme-inducing AEDs wish to use oral contraceptives, formulations using the equivalent of 50–100 mcg of ethinyl oestradiol are recommended, ideally in conjunction with a barrier or other method of contraception. Despite the increased rate of failure of oral contraceptives among women taking enzyme-inducing AEDs, the success of pills with a higher oestrogen content is as good as or superior to barrier methods alone.

In spite of the known pro-convulsant effects of oestrogen, it has not been established that hormonal contraception has any definite adverse effects on seizure control, perhaps because of the concurrent administration of progesterones. Levonorgestrel is less effective if given concurrently with hepatic enzyme-inducing AEDs; intramuscular medroxyprogesterone may need to be administered more frequently, although this has not been studied carefully.[1–3]

Infertility and reproductive abnormalities

Epidemiological studies have demonstrated that women with epilepsy have only one-fourth to one-third as many children as women in the general population. A variety of hypotheses have been developed to explain this phenomenon. A direct effect of seizures or epileptiform discharges on the pituitary and hypothalamus could disrupt ovulation. Electroconvulsive therapy increases prolactin concentrations over five-fold within 15–20 minutes, and in pre-menopausal women there is an acute increase in luteinizing hormone

Table 1. Hormonal contraceptives affected by hepatic enzyme-inducing AEDs

ORAL	
Combined oestrogen/progesterone	Transdermal patch
Progestin only	Vaginal ring
Morning-after pill	Implant

(LH) and follicle-stimulating hormone (FSH). Generalized seizures lead to a threefold increase in the concentration of prolactin in the serum within 15–20 minutes. This fact has been used to assist physicians in differentiating epileptic from non-epileptic seizures.[4–6]

Women with epilepsy have higher rates of reproductive and endocrine disorders (RED) than expected. In a large clinical centre, 50% of women with epilepsy were found to have menstrual abnormalities. The incidence of anovulatory cycles in epileptic women is higher than normal. Though an increased incidence of anovulatory cycles is the most common in temporal lobe epilepsies, it has been reported in primary generalized epilepsies too. The REDs described include a relatively higher incidence of polycystic ovary disease (PCOD) and hypogonatropic hypogonadism.

Antiepileptic drugs may also interfere with the hypothalamic–pituitary axis. Amenorrhoea, oligomenorrhoea and prolonged or irregular cycles have been described in women with epilepsy. The incidence of PCOD is higher among women taking sodium valproate.

Women with epilepsy have more variation in LH pulse frequency and lower LH concentrations than controls. In addition, it has been found that women with left-sided ictal epileptiform foci have PCOD, while those with right-sided foci have hypogonadotropic hypogonadism.

There is a significant reduction in libido in one-third of men and women with epilepsy. Increasing frequency of seizures appears to decrease sexual desire, while there is no difference in libido between treated and untreated women with epilepsy. Hyposexuality and orgasmic dysfunction has been reported among 8%–68%

of women with epilepsy. Persons with localization-related epilepsies appear to have higher rates of sexual dysfunction than those with primarily generalized epilepsies. Shukla and colleagues[7] have demonstrated that 64% of women with partial epilepsies, compared to 8% with generalized epilepsies, report hyposexuality and sexual dysfunction.

The problem of infertility in women with epilepsy is, therefore, complex. There are multiple factors involved: the type and frequency of seizures, the site of ictal onset, as well as AEDs, which may affect an individual patient. Infertility in a couple deserves a careful evaluation of both partners. For women with epilepsy, ultrasonography to rule out PCOD, serum LH and FSH concentrations, and an evaluation of AED use will help one narrow the focus of treatment. There is evidence that valproate may have an adverse impact on fertility in some cases. If the patient's seizures have been brought under control, discontinuation of valproate is not warranted unless she develops PCOD or hypogondaotropic hypogonadism.[7,8]

Catamenial seizures

For many years, a connection has been observed between the timing of expression of seizures and menstruation, an observation validated by recent studies. Previously, catamenial seizures were defined as seizures occurring exclusively or primarily during the peri-menstrual period. Catamenial epilepsy is now defined more broadly as a pattern of increased seizures related to cyclical hormonal changes at various stages throughout the menstrual cycle.

Studies in animals have helped to define the neuro-endocrine basis of catamenial seizures. These studies generally support the proposition that oestrogen compounds are pro-convulsant (i.e. lower the seizure threshold), while progesterone compounds have anti-convulsant properties (i.e. raise the seizure threshold). However, these mechanisms are not well defined.

Neuro-active steroid sex hormones exert an influence on neural function by changing membrane excitability and influencing the regulation of gene expression in the nucleus. Intravenous administration of oestrogen to women with epilepsy increases interictal epileptiform discharges.

Several ways of tailoring AED therapy have been proposed for cases in which a catamenial pattern of seizures can be identified. These include a cyclic increase in AED doses or intermittent use of benzodiazepines during periods of vulnerability to seizures. Intermittent use of acetazolamide (Diamox) is supported by clinical experience and a small retrospective study. Specific hormonal manipulation has been examined in uncontrolled trials. There is theoretical as well as some clinical support for the use of oestrogen antagonists, such as clomiphene citrate, but concern about the long-term effects of oestrogen blockade has limited their use.

Synthetic and natural progesterone compounds have been studied. Preliminary clinical studies suggest that treatment with intermittent natural progesterone is beneficial in patients with well-defined catamenial seizures. In these studies, adverse effects, such as sedation, depression, tenderness of the breasts and breakthrough menstrual bleeding, were observed but it was only infrequently that therapy had to be stopped due to these causes. If hormonal therapies are to be considered, it is important to include the patient's gynaecologist in the planning stages and ensure adequate contraception. Randomized prospective clinical trials are needed before these therapies can be recommended more strongly.[9–11]

Pregnancy

The majority of women with epilepsy can conceive and bear normal, healthy children. While they do run a greater risk of facing complications of pregnancy, they are more likely to have difficulties during labour and there is a higher risk of adverse pregnancy outcomes.[12–14]

Epilepsy and maternal seizures

In about 25% of cases, the frequency of seizures increases during pregnancy. While most studies indicate that this increase tends to occur towards the last trimester of pregnancy, recent reports suggest that it occurs during the first trimester in a substantial number of women. The plasma concentration of AED steadily declines as pregnancy advances. Among the physiological changes associated with pregnancy, those that may alter the seizure threshold include the increase in sex hormone levels, and sodium and water retention. The physiological changes accompanying pregnancy can also destabilize the levels of AEDs in the blood. These include changes in absorption (either through changes in gastric motility or nausea and vomiting), changes in the volume of distribution of fluid, alterations in protein binding and an increase in hepatic metabolism. Physicians must be sensitive to the possibility that lower AED levels reflect non-compliance with medication due to a fear of the teratogenic effects of the drugs.

The levels of AEDs should be monitored more closely than usual during pregnancy. Pharmaco-kinetic changes demand the monitoring of free levels of highly protein-bound AEDs to avoid confusion with increased seizures (or symptoms of toxicity), despite therapeutic total serum drug levels. Drug levels should be monitored at least each trimester and for two to three months after delivery. If the dosage of a medication is increased during pregnancy, one should consider tapering it down in the postpartum period to avoid toxicity.

The occurrence of seizures during pregnancy increases the risk of an adverse outcome. While rare, isolated seizures carry uncertain risks, uncontrolled convulsive seizures place both mother and baby at risk. The mother runs a greater than usual risk of injury or other complications of seizures. As for the baby, there is an increased risk of bradycardia, placental abruption, pre-mature labour, intracranial haemorrhage, or even foetal death. This risk foetal death is particularly high if seizures progress to status epilepticus. The effects of non-convulsive seizures on developing foetuses are not well documented.[15–17]

Table 2. Increased risks related to pregnancy in women with epilepsy

Effects on epilepsy	Complications of pregnancy	Complications in offspring
Increased seizure frequency	Vaginal haemorrhage	Foetal malformations
		Low birth weight, hypoxia
Decline in level of AED	Anaemia of newborn	Haemorrhagic disease
	Hyperemesis graviderum	Drug withdrawal seizure
Alteration in drug pharmacokinetics	Toxaemia-induced labour	Delayed cognitive deficiency
	Premature membrane rupture	
	Stillbirth/Abortion	

Obstetrical complications

The reports regarding the risk of perinatal complications in children born to mothers with epilepsy are conflicting. Some studies suggest an increased incidence of eclampsia, vaginal bleeding, pre-term labour, low birth weight and perinatal mortality. Others have contradicted these reports. However, there is definite evidence of a relatively higher incidence of haemorrhage in the new-borns of mothers with epilepsy.

Haemorrhagic disease of the newborn

This syndrome consists of a neonatal bleeding diathesis (including intracranial haemorrhage of various types), typically appearing two to seven days postpartum, although early and late forms have also been described. Haemorrhagic disease of the newborns of women with epilepsy was first described in patients treated with phenobarbital and primidone; however, many AEDs have been implicated.

The putative mechanism is a deficiency of vitamin K-dependent clotting factors, possibly via hepatic microsomal enzyme induction in the foetal liver though the coagulation tests of the mother remain normal. The syndrome can be treated by maternal ingestion of vitamin K supplements in the last month of pregnancy, although transplacental transfer of vitamin K has been difficult to establish. Most clinicians recommend treating the mother with vitamin K (10 mg PO per day) during the last month of pregnancy, in addition to routine administration of 1 mg of vitamin K to the neonate at birth.[18,19]

Teratogenicity

The risk of having a child with major congenital malformations is twice as high among women taking AEDs than among the general population (i.e. 4%–6% for women with epilepsy versus 2%–3% for the general population). Foetal abnormalities can be classified as malformations (i.e. defects that lead to a significant functional impairment), or anomalies (i.e. minor variations of normal morphology without significant functional impact).

The malformations, which have been observed with all the older AEDs, commonly involve the cardiac, neurological and genito-urinary systems. Minor anomalies are usually noted in the facial features, most often in the mid-face structures, or digits (e.g. distal phalangeal hypoplasia and nail hypoplasia). Evidence regarding medication-specific syndromes (e.g. 'foetal hydantoin syndrome') is lacking; perhaps more striking is the similarity of defects caused by the use of different AEDs. An exception is neural tube defects (NTDs), which are more common with maternal use of valproate or carbamazepine.

While genetic influences or other factors such as socioeconomic status may contribute to the increased incidence of foetal malformations, several lines of evidence suggest that AEDs play a primary role. The rate of occurrence of foetal malformations is higher in the case of pregnant women treated with AEDs than those who are not treated. Higher AED levels are associated with higher rates of malformation, and polytherapy carries a higher risk than monotherapy. One report showed that malformations were more common when the dosage of valproate was more than 1000 mg/day or the plasma concentration higher than 70 µg/ml.

The mechanisms underlying the teratogenicity of AEDs are still poorly defined. It is suspected that interference with the absorption or activation of folate could produce NTDs. Reactive products of oxidative metabolism have been implicated, but not all AEDs produce these intermediate products. Nonetheless, similar types and rates of malformation appear with different antiepileptic medications, including the newer AEDs, which do not induce hepatic enzymes and do not undergo oxidative metabolism. This is suggestive of a common risk to women with epilepsy, independent of the type of medication used. Since all the major AEDs are teratogenic, the best therapy is generally that which is appropriate for the type of epilepsy and which controls seizures the most effectively. However, the use of valproate and carbamazepine should be avoided in women who have a family history of NTDs in the offspring or who themselves have had offspring with NTDs in the past.

Like all women of childbearing age, women with epilepsy should take folate supplementation. The dose recommended by the Centers of Disease Control, of 400 µg/day, may not be high enough for many women who do not metabolize folate effectively. Even with folate supplementation, a prenatal diagnostic ultrasound is necessary for women taking valproate or carbamazepine to rule out NTDs. The role of folate deficiency in the pathogenesis of teratogenicity is complex and poorly understood. A few recent reports have raised doubts regarding the efficacy of folate supplementation in the prevention of NTDs.[20–28]

Pregnancy registry

In recent years, several registries have been created to keep track of the adverse effects of AEDs on foetal growth and development. The North American AED registry, which had approximately 4500 enrollees in July 2005, reported on its findings over a period of six years (1997–2002)—major malformations were found in 6.5% of infants exposed to phenobarbitone, as compared to 1.6% of infants who were not exposed. Among the infants exposed to valproic acid, 10.7% had major birth defects (spina bifida, heart defects, multiple anomalies), while only 1.62% of those not exposed had non-genetic major malformations.

The U.K. Pregnancy Registry had 2829 reports that contained full data on outcomes spanning the period 1996–2003. The key findings were that the risk of major malfomations was 6.6% with polytherapy, 3.7% with monotherapy and 3% in the absence of the use of AEDs.

A Swedish birth registry study which reviewed 1398 infants exposed to AEDs found that the odds ratio for malformations in infants exposed to AEDs was 1.86 (95% CI:1.4–2.4). The rates of malformation for specific AEDs in monotherapy were: 4.0% for carbamazepine; 4.4% for lamotrigine; 6.8% for phenytoin; and 9.7% for valproic acid.

The European and International Registry of Anti-epileptic Drugs in Pregnancy (EURAP) is a prospective registry, which currently includes 38 countries in Europe, Australia, Asia and South America. The registry, which had data on 2238 pregnancies in May 2004, found that 126 cases had major malformations, including 13 induced abortions, 2 stillbirths and 2 perinatal deaths. The rate of malformation was 6%. With monotherapy, it was 5% and with polytherapy, 8%.

A recent publication from the North American Registry suggested that infants exposed to lamotrigine had an increased risk of non-syndromic cleft lip and cleft lip. The risk was 8.9%, compared to 0.6% for infants who were not exposed. However, this has not been confirmed by other registries.[29,30]

Management of pregnancy

The management of pregnancy for women with epilepsy should begin with pre-pregnancy counselling. All women with childbearing potential and who are on AEDs should be counselled on pregnancy and contraception to enable them to make informed decisions, regardless of when they plan to have children. If medications require adjustments, ideally this should be done at least six months before pregnancy is attempted. This will allow stabilization of seizure control and avoid the risk of exposure to multiple AEDs. Discontinuation of AEDs prior to pregnancy is the best option, but must be done when it is safe and there is a minimal risk of the recurrence of seizures. However, the majority of women will need to continue medication and the goal is then low-dose monotherapy. The control of seizures cannot be sacrificed in this effort and patients must be told about the importance of complying with medication.

Pre-conception counselling should address the importance of folic acid. There is strong evidence of the effectiveness of folic acid supplementation in preventing NTDs in the general population. The optimal dose and effectiveness

Table 3. Types of major congenital malfomations (U.K. Pregnancy Registry, 2006)

Malformations	CBZ (*n*=900)	Valproate (*n*=751)	LTG (*n*=647)	PHT (*n*=82)
NTD	2 (0.2%)	7 (1.0%)	1 (0.2%)	0 (0.0%)
Facial clefts	4 (0.4%)	11 (1.5%)	1 (0.2%)	1 (1.2%)
Cardiac	6 (0.7%)	5 (0.7%)	4 (0.6%)	1 (1.2%)
Hypospadius	2 (0.2%)	9 (1.3%)	6 (0.9%)	0
Skeletal	3 (0.3%)	8 (1.1%)	2 (0.3%)	0
Gastrointestinal	3 (0.3%)	2 (0.3%)	3 (0.5%)	1 (1.2%)
Others	1 (0.1%)	2 (0.3%)	4 (0.6%)	0

CBZ carbamazepine; LTG lamotrigine; PHT phenytoin; NTD neural tube defects of folic acid have not been established in the case of women with epilepsy. Pregnancy registries tracking the use of folic acid supplements have not demonstrated a protective effect. At present, it is recommended that women taking AEDs should take 0.4–5 mg folic acid supplementation throughout pregnancy. In the case of patients who visit the physician only after they are already pregnant, there is little sense in attempting to change the prescription of AEDs. Rather, the emphasis must be on preventing maternal seizures during pregnancy. Patients and physicians can be assured that most women have uneventful pregnancies and healthy babies.

Intrapartum management

Intrapartum management should focus on the prevention of maternal seizures, optimization of the AED dosage and early detection of foetal abnormality. To achieve this goal, the guidelines recommend that the level of AEDs in the serum should be estimated at the 12th, 24th and 36th weeks of gestation. The level of alpha foetoprotein in the serum should be estimated at the 16th week to detect NTDs. Ultrasound by experts to assess foetal growth and organ formation is indicated at the 16th and 36th weeks of gestation.

Lactation

Breastfeeding has many benefits for the infant and the mother-child relationship. The concentration of anti-epileptic medications in breast milk depends upon the degree of lipophilicity, protein binding and the level of the drug in the mother's serum. Transmission via breast milk depends on protein binding; highly protein-bound AEDs are present in low concentrations in breast milk. The infant's exposure to anticonvulsants from breast milk is lower than exposure *in utero*. However, in the case of some medications, the drug level may reach the therapeutic range in the infant and this could theoretically place the infant at risk for dose-related or idiosyncratic side-effects of the AED, though these problems have not been widely reported. The children of women taking sedating AEDs, such as barbiturates, should be monitored for sedation, poor feeding, or behavioural changes. In general, maternal use of anticonvulsants is not a contraindication to breastfeeding, and the risks and benefits should be discussed so that each mother can make an informed decision based on the available information.[31–34]

Bone health in women on anti-epileptic medication

It is now well established that the use of AEDs may promote bone loss and osteoporosis. This is an active area of research, growing in magnitude as the population on AEDs ages and the number of older women with epilepsy increases. The importance of this topic is compounded by the fact that seizures increase the risk of falls and other injuries.

Several AEDs are implicated in the production of accelerated bone loss: phenobarbital, primidone, phenytoin, carbamazepine and valproate. Long-term data on most of the newer AEDs are too limited to make definite recommendations; however, many of these have more favourable pharmacological properties and may prove safer with respect to bone health.

The mechanism or mechanisms of accelerated osteoporosis secondary to AED use are under active investigation. There are likely to be multiple mechanisms. Hepatic microsomal enzyme induction, producing vitamin D catabolism, is a major mechanism. However, additional mechanisms (e.g. direct effects on bone cells, impaired calcium absorption) must be considered to explain bone loss from non-enzyme-inducing medications such as valproate.

Bone mineral density studies (dual energy X-ray absorptiometry [DEXA] scans) should be obtained in individuals at risk, especially patients who are institutionalized and older women taking AEDs. The optimal strategies for the prevention and treatment of bone loss related to AEDs remain to be defined.

Vitamin D and calcium supplementation are recommended for patients taking the older AEDs (phenobarbital, primidone, phenytoin, carbamazepine, valproate). The recommended dosages of calcium and vitamin D for premenopausal women are at least 1000 mg and 400 IU, respectively, and for postmenopausal women, 1500 mg and 600 IU respectively. Some authorities recommend even higher dosages. Whether this supplementation strategy is adequate in the face of strong hepatic enzyme inducers, such as phenytoin, is not clear. Crossing over to one of the newer AEDs that do not induce enzymes may be an advisable strategy, especially as we come to learn more about the effects of these medications on the bones. For patients with known osteoporosis, treatment with bisphosphonates should be considered, although in the case of young patients, some questions are still unanswered about the effects of the long-term use of these medications.[35,36]

References

1. Guberman A. Hormonal contraception and epilepsy. *Neurology* 1999;**53** (Suppl 1):38–40.
2. Haukkamaa M. Contraception by Norplant subdermal capsules is not reliable in epileptic patients on anticonvulsant treatment. *Contraception* 1986;**33**:559–65.
3. Krauss GL, Brandt J, Campbell M, *et al.* Antiepileptic medication and oral contraceptive interactions: A national survey of neurologists and obstetricians. *Neurology* 1996;**46**:1534–9.
4. Cogen PH, Antunes JL, Correll JW. Reproductive function in temporal lobe epilepsy: The effect of temporal lobectomy. *Surg Neurol* 1979;**12**:243–6.
5. Cummings LN, Giudice L, Morrell MJ. Ovulatory function in epilepsy. *Epilepsia* 1995;**36**:355–9.
6. Schupf N, Ottman R. Reproduction among individuals with idiopathic/cryptogenic epilepsy: Risk factors for reduced fertility in marriage. *Epilepsia* 1996;**37**:833–40.
7. Shukla GD, Srivastava ON, Katiyar BC. Sexual disturbances in temporal lobe epilepsy: A controlled study. *Br J Psychiatry* 1979;**134**:288–92.
8. Webber MP, Hauser WA, Ottman R, *et al.* Fertility in persons with epilepsy: 1935–1974. *Epilepsia* 1986;**27**:746–52.
9. Lim LL, Foldvary N, Mascha E, *et al.* Acetazolamide in women with catamenial epilepsy. *Epilepsia* 2001;**42**:746–9.
10. Herzog AG, Klein P, Ransil BJ. Three patterns of catamenial epilepsy. *Epilepsia* 1997;**38**:1082–8.
11. Herzog AG. Progesterone therapy in women with complex partial and secondary generalized seizures. *Neurology* 1995;**45**:1660–2.
12. Fedrick J. Epilepsy and pregnancy: A report from the Oxford Record Linkage Study. *Br Med J* 1973;**2**:442–8.
13. Hiilesmaa VK, Bardy A, Teramo K. Obstetric outcome in women with epilepsy. *Am J Obstet Gynecol* 1985;**152**:499–504.
14. Yerby M, Koepsell T, Daling J. Pregnancy complications and outcomes in a cohort of women with epilepsy. *Epilepsia* 1985;**26**:631–5.
15. Morrell MJ. Guidelines for the care of women with epilepsy. *Neurology* 1998;**51** (Suppl 4):S21–S27.
16. Morrell MJ. Epilepsy in women: The science of why it is special. *Neurology* 1999;**53** (Suppl 1):S42–S48.
17. Olafsson E, Hallgrimsson JT, Hauser WA, *et al.* Pregnancies of women with epilepsy: A population-based study in Iceland. *Epilepsia* 1998;**39**:887–92.
18. Minkoff H, Schaffer RM, Delke I, *et al.* Diagnosis of intracranial hemorrhage *in utero* after a maternal seizure. *Obstet Gynecol* 1985;**65** (3 Suppl):22S–24S.
19. Cornelissen M, Steegers-Theunissen R, Kollée L, *et al.* Supplementation of vitamin K in pregnant women receiving anticonvulsant therapy prevents neonatal vitamin K deficiency. *Am J Obstet Gynecol* 1993;**168** (Pt 1):884–8.
20. Robert E, Guibaud P. Maternal valproic acid and congenital neural tube defects. *Lancet* 1982;**2**:937.
21. Battino D, Binelli S, Caccamo ML, *et al.* Malformations in offspring of 305 epileptic women: A prospective study. *Acta Neurol Scand* 1992;**85**:204–7.
22. Kaaja E, Kaaja R, Hiilesmaa V. Major malformations in offspring of women with epilepsy. *Neurology* 2003;**60**:575–9.
23. Kaneko S, Battino D, Andermann E, *et al.* Congenital malformations due to antiepileptic drugs. *Epilepsy Res* 1999;**33**:145–58.
24. Lindhout D, Hoppener RJ, Meinardi H. Teratogenicity of antiepileptic drug combinations with special emphasis on epoxidation (of carbamazepine). *Epilepsia* 1984;**25**:77–83.

25. Milunsky A, Jick H, Jick SS, *et al.* Multivitamin/folic acid supplementation in early pregnancy reduces the prevalence of neural tube defects. *JAMA* 1989;**262:** 2847–52.

26. Nakane Y, Okuma T, Takahashi R, *et al.* Multi-institutional study on the teratogenicity and fetal toxicity of antiepileptic drugs: A report of a collaborative study group in Japan. *Epilepsia* 1980;**21:**663–80.

27. Nau H. Valproic acid-induced neural tube defects. *Ciba Found Symp* 1994;**181:**144–52; discussion 152–60.

28. Yerby MS, Collins SD. Teratogenicity of antiepileptic drugs. In: Engel J, Pedley T (eds). *Epilepsy: A comprehensive textbook*, Vol 2. Philadelphia, Pa: Lippincott-Raven; 1997:1195.

29. Hunt S, Morrow J, Russel A, *et al.* Levetiracetam therapy in human pregnancy; Preliminary experience from UK epilepsy and pregnancy register. *Neurology* 2006;**67:**1867–69.

30. Holmes LB. Increased risk of non syndromic cleft palate among infants exposed to lamotrigine during pregnancy. Birth Res (part A). *Clini Mol Teratol* 2006;**76:**318.

31. Report of the Quality Standards, Subcommittee of the American Academy of Neurology. Practice parameter: Management issues for women with epilepsy (summary statement). *Neurology* 1998;**51:** 944–8.

32. El-Sayed YY. Obstetric and gynecologic care of women with epilepsy. *Epilepsia* 1998;**39** (Suppl 8): S17–S25.

33. Zahn C. Neurologic care of pregnant women with epilepsy. *Epilepsia* 1998;**39** (Suppl 8):S26–S31.

34. Zahn CA, Morrell MJ, Collins SD, *et al.* Management issues for women with epilepsy: A review of the literature. *Neurology* 1998;**51:**949–56.

35. Stephen LJ, McLellan AR, Harrison JH, *et al.* Bone density and antiepileptic drugs: A case–controlled study. *Seizure* 1999;**8:**339–42.

36. Pluskiewicz W, Nowakowska J. Bone status after long-term anticonvulsant therapy in epileptic patients: Evaluation using quantitative ultrasound infants of women treated with carbamazepine during pregnancy. *N Engl J Med* 1991;**324:**674–7.

19

Rational use of antiepileptic drugs

DEBASIS BASU, RIVU BASU

'This human ritual of suppliant and provider of balm is deeply rooted, extending back thousands of years.'[1]

Epilepsy is a socioeconomic problem that has a tremendous medical and sociofinancial impact on the personal and social life of the patient, his family and society in general. Epilepsy is still treated by traditional medicines and judged according to primitive conceptions, and the patient's failure to opt for proper medical consultation reflects the ignorance and social stigma attached to it. When it comes to the pharmacological treatment of epilepsy, it has been observed that even with the use of modern medical facilities and antiepileptic drugs (AEDs), about 30% of patients are medically refractory. Even when moderate-to-good control of the disease is achieved, the patient has to carry a heavy economic burden and face side-effects, leading to occasional loss of compliance with drugs. Given this scenario, finding a rational approach to the use of AEDs might at least help in reducing the inherent problems associated with their use.

How rational is the word RATIONAL?

When speaking of the rational use of a drug, we must consider at least two very important limiting factors. First, we often concentrate only on the efficacy of the AED and whether the medicine will be effective for a particular type of epilepsy and seizure pattern, often ignoring totally, or at least partially, other important parameters of rational drug therapy, e.g. the patient's compliance, pharmacological parameters and different co-morbid conditions. Second, and more important, is that we try to prescribe AEDs in a knee-jerk or dogmatic fashion, depending heavily on the commonly called principle of evidence-based medicine (EBM). It must be emphasized that EBM stands on two legs. While the first is the hierarchy of different clinical trials, what is more important is the second, i.e. the insufficiency of evidence alone. Evidence should always be integrated with the clinical expertise of the decision-maker, as also the patients' expectations and values. This corroborates the concept of the cognitive continuum spectrum, as postulated by Hamm.[2] On one end are Hammond[3] and his co-workers, who believed that it is evidence which is the most important, and at the other end is Hubert Dreyfus,[4] who argued in favour of experience—in fact, they are not mutually exclusive, but additive.

Overview of treatment strategies

First, we should make the diagnosis at three fundamental levels:

- The aetiological diagnosis
- The seizure diagnosis
- The epilepsy syndrome diagnosis

Having achieved this, we should set up our treatment variables, keeping the following in mind:

- The patient's quality of life (aiming for the best)
- Principles of drug treatment
- Strategies of pharmacotherapy
- Special therapeutic considerations, if any

Treatment should be tailored to match individual patients, taking into account their medical, social and psychological needs. They should be consulted on and apprised of the treatment protocol at each step.

The factors influencing rational AED therapy may be summarized as follows:

- Factors that are the concern mainly of the treating physician
- Factors that are especially relevant to the patient

Physician-related factors
- Efficacy of therapy (discussed at the end)
- When to start therapy
- Role of polytherapy
- When to stop therapy
- Pharmacological factors
  —Pharmacokinetics (what the body does to the drug)
  —Pharmacodynamics (what the drug does to the body)—toxicity and drug interaction
- Clinical situations, for example, epileptic emergencies and situation-related epilepsy.

Patient-related factors
- Cost of therapy
- Side-effects of therapy
- Phases of life, ability to work
- Co-morbid conditions

When to start therapy

Opinion remains divided on whether to treat patients who have had a single seizure, since only about 25% of patients will have a recurrence within two years in the absence of factors that predict a high probability of recurrence (e.g. epileptiform activity detected in an EEG, a known cause such as remote head injury). Even in the presence of risk factors, the probability of recurrence in two years is no more than 40%. In many such cases, seizures will not recur if the patient is left untreated and treatment after the first seizure does not improve the long-term prognosis.

By definition, epilepsy must have recurrence. In general, however, the first seizure does not warrant the institution of therapy,[5] except in the following conditions:

- If the patient has a structural lesion—brain tumour, arterio-venous malformations, MRI-proven cortical dysplasia, etc.
- If the patient does not have a structural lesion, but a sibling has epilepsy, there is a history of previous symptomatic seizure, previous stroke or major brain injury, patients presenting with status epilepticus, etc.[6]

Provided the epileptic nature of the seizures has been established, patients with recurrent seizures generally require AED therapy. However, there are exceptions, such as when the seizures are rare, mild and brief, and occur only during sleep, provided that they do not interfere with cognition, the person's daily activities and occupation. Pharmacological treatment is also contraindicated in some benign childhood epilepsies which have a self-limiting course. In such cases, the side-effects would be more detrimental than the seizures themselves. An example is benign rolandic epilepsies, unless they are frequent and occur during the daytime as well.

Role of polypharmacy

In general, it is widely accepted that one should start with a single AED, which is known to be efficacious for the given seizure pattern, and gradually build up the dose till the seizures come under control or side-effects appear, when another add-on AED may be started. Monotherapy is preferable and is usually sufficient to control seizures. There is little evidence that AEDs act synergystically. Common causes of the failure of monotherapy include selection of the wrong AEDs and suboptimal serum levels of the drug.

The hazards of polytherapy include greater incidence and severity of side-effects, drug interaction, poor compliance and higher economic costs. For those who truly need polytherapy after trying optimal monotherapy, two AEDs should be sufficient. While prescribing these, their individual drug dynamic and kinetic properties must be kept in mind.[7,8]

When to consider withdrawal of therapy

There is considerable uncertainty as to when AEDs can be discontinued. Studies show that when AEDs are withdrawn after two years of a seizure-free period, the incidence of recurrence is between 12% and 66%. The risk factors for recurrence are adolescent-onset epilepsy, remote symptomatic epilepsies, especially with mental retardation, and EEG abnormalities.[5] The specific epilepsy syndrome is thought to be the single most important prognostic factor. Recurrence is rare in benign rolandic epilepsy. The chance of recurrence of childhood absence seizures is 5%–25%, while that of cryptogenic or symptomatic partial seizures is 25%–75%. The figure is very high (85%–95%) in cases of juvenile myoclonic epilepsy.[5]

Withdrawal of AEDs should be gradual, depending on the molecule, to prevent acute seizures, and status epilepticus. Individual preferences of the patient should also be taken into account. The patient's occupation and preference are other important considerations.

Pharmacokinetics

The components of drug pharmacokinetics are absorption, distribution and elimination, and the resultant bioavailability, volume of distribution, clearance and half-life. AEDs are absorbed via the oral, rectal or parenteral (intramuscular or intravenous) route. The oral route is the one used most commonly and it has been observed that, in general, syrups are absorbed better than tablets. It has also been observed that sometimes the same formulation, when produced by different manufacturers using different processes, may have a different bioavailability and may cause either dose-dependent side-effects or result in poor control of seizures.[9] Sustained-release preparations may cause attenuation of excessive fluctuations in the plasma level of the drug, depending on the plasma half-life of the AED. Absorption is rapid through the rectal route, which is especially useful in the case of lipophilic drugs, when it is not feasible to use the oral route. This is especially relevant to the administration of diazepam in the emergency management of febrile seizure. It also reduces the first-pass effect and can be administered by a non-medical person. The intramuscular route is highly unpredictable,[10] and the solubility and pharmaceutical character of the formulation, as well as the local blood flow, play an important role. Intramuscular AEDs are better absorbed in the deltoids than in the buttocks; thus intramuscular AEDs should preferably be given in the deltoids. Intramuscular absorption of diazepam is poor, but that of midazolam is good, making it a better choice in the domiciliary management of acute seizures.[11]

Metabolism of AEDs should ideally be linear, i.e. the plasma level of the drug should have a uniform relationship with bioavailability at all dosages. However, in the case of some common AEDs, it may be non-linear at therapeutic doses, leading either to sub- or supra-optimal response, depending on age, genetic factors and concurrent drug administration. Typical examples are phenytoin, carbamazepine and sodium valproate.

Drug–drug interaction

With the recent introduction of newer AEDs as

add-on drugs and the persistence of the old practice of unnecessary polytherapy, physicians should try to rationalize combinations of AEDs. Moreover, patients, especially the aged, may have other concurrent illnesses which require other medications. Therefore, to prevent either toxicity or a low drug level in the body, treating physicians should develop a working knowledge of drug interactions.

Pharmacodynamic interaction is discussed at two levels, i.e. in terms of the clinical effects and in terms of the neurotoxic effects. Usually, the clinical effect is additive (one AED at full dosage has the same effect as two AEDs at half doses). Only the combination of valproate and carbamazepine, besides that of valproate and phenytoin, has a supra-additive effect (potentiation). Neurotoxic interaction is usually additive or hypoadditive.[12,13]

Pharmacokinetic drug interactions may be numerous, at least theoretically, but their clinical relevance may be a matter of conjecture. Antacids may hamper the absorption of phenytoin and gabapentin. Regarding metabolism, the important factor is the induction or inhibition of enzymes by a drug. The metabolizing enzymes include cytochrome P450 and glucuronyl transferase. Some drugs are enzyme inducers and some inhibitors, and this becomes clinically relevant when a drug is added in the presence of an inducer, or an inducer is added to the existing therapy, or an inducer is removed from chronic therapy.

Regarding drug displacement due to variable protein binding, the interaction between warfarin and phenytoin is a well-known example.

AEDs in special situations— convulsive status epilepticus

It is desirable that drugs acting in status epilepticus should have a rapid and prolonged duration of action. An ideal AED used in status epilepticus should have no active metabolites (diazepam and midazolam do); should not react with other medications; should not have saturable metabolism (phenytoin has saturable metabolism at the therapeutic dose); should not be affected by renal or hepatic blood flow; and should be stable in solution and unreactive to sets. Rapidly acting drugs are usually lipid-soluble and rapidly redistribute to lipid stores outside the brain after the first injection, and are thus short-acting. However, after the repeat injection, they tend to get stored in the brain compartment, thus causing side-effects such as hypotension. Phenytoin is a widely used drug in status epilepticus, but has some inherent problems. For example, its action is relatively delayed. Further, if added to solutions with a pH lower than its own, e.g. 5% dextrose, it may precipitate in the bag or tubing.[14] Midazolam has the advantage that it can be given intramuscularly, but it has a relatively short duration of action and there is a chance of recurrence of seizures. Chlormethiazole has a rapid onset of action, which, however, is short-lived. It, therefore, qualifies for continuous intravenous administration and the rate can be titrated to balance its action and side-effects.[15] Thiopentone has saturable pharmacokinetics and a tendency to accumulate. It is incompatible with polyvinyl bags and tubings. Both the parent drug and its metabolite, phenobarbitone, are active. Propofol is highly suitable for continuous drip and has a rapid onset of action.

Remembering basic pharmacology helps in rationalizing and planning AED therapy in status epilepticus.

The cost factor

In settings where resources are limited, as in developing countries, the cost of therapy has an important bearing on compliance with drugs. The cost of any medicine is fixed primarily by the industry. In general, newer AEDs are priced high, while the older ones are relatively cheap, sometimes due to the interference of the government. In several welfare societies, including some South American countries, certain AEDs are distributed free of cost or at a subsidized rate. Our country has no uniform rule on this, though some state-run hospitals often distribute AEDs, provided that they get their supplies regularly. Thus, those depending solely on free distribution cannot afford to do so as the supply of AEDs is erratic. It is, therefore, logical to think of using cheaper AEDs, whenever possible. Industry, the administration and different professional bodies should sit together regularly to try and solve this problem. The recent reduction in the price of levetiracetam has helped to foster better drug compliance among many patients.

Side-effect profile

Treatment options are often restricted by the serious side-effects of medication. Polytherapy, which leads to drug interactions, can cause toxicities. Proper knowledge and clinical and drug-level monitoring may, in the long run, prevent dose-dependent drug reactions, while slow build-up, e.g. doses of AEDs, may prevent common, less serious side-effects. The common side-effects of more or less all AEDs are drowsiness, fatigue, ataxia and sedation, as also blurred vision and sometimes diplopia. Mild weight gain is common with carbamazepine, gabapentin and sodium valproate, while some of the side-effects of topiramate are weight reduction, difficulty finding words and paraesthesias. Phenobarbitone causes sedation, as well as hyperirritability in children. Both topiramate and zonisamide may cause oligohydrosis in children and may result in the formation of renal stones.[16–18]

The serious side-effects of AEDs can be enumerated as follows.

- *Carbamazepine:* Agranulocytosis, aplastic anaemia, allergic reaction and Steven–Johnson syndrome, hyponatraemia
- *Oxcarbazepine:* Rash, Steven–Johnson syndrome, toxic epidermal necrolysis (TEN), hyponatraemia
- *Phenytoin:* Conduction block, pseudolymphomas, skin rash, lupus syndrome
- *Phenobarbitone:* Rare
- *Topiramate:* Metabolic acidosis, renal calculi, acute glaucoma
- *Valproate:* Hepatic failure (mainly in children), pancreatitis, hyperammonimia
- *Zonisamide:* Renal calculi, skin rash, aplastic anaemia

In general, proper monitoring of therapy and attention to the choice and combination of AEDs prescribed may, to a great extent, prevent side-effects.

Co-morbid conditions and special situations

A knowledge of pharmacokinetics and associated relevant factors, e.g. age and different disease conditions, can help us make the right choice regarding which AEDs to prescribe and at what dosage. The following examples may serve as a guide.

- *Carbamazepine:* Enzyme induction may lead to drug interactions. Special caution must be exercised in the case of patients with hepatic disease, blood dyscrasias, arrhythmias and hyponatraemia. Asian patients have a relatively greater risk of developing skin rash. Carbamazepine reduces free thyroxine levels.
- *Phenytoin:* This is an enzyme inducer. Caution is required in cases of liver disease. It worsens heart block or arrhythmias, causes hypotension and may mask hypoglycaemic symptoms in diabetics.
- *Phenobarbitone:* This is an enzyme inducer. Caution must be exercised in those with hepatic and renal disease.
- *Valproate:* This is an enzyme inhibitor. One must be careful about prescribing it to those with hepatic disease and bleeding disorders.
- *Zonisamide:* This can cause renal calculi. A reduced dose should be prescribed to those with renal or hepatic disease.

- *Lamotrigine:* One should be careful in the case of patients with known hypersensitivity to other AEDs. A reduced dose should be prescribed to those with hepatic disorders.
- *Topiramate:* This can cause renal calculi. A reduced dose should be prescribed to those with renal disorders and one should be careful in the case of patients prone to develop metabolic acidosis.

The increased incidence of epilepsy in the elderly population demands a special knowledge of the effects of AED therapy on the elderly. Carbamazepine causes increased sedation, and the dosages of phenobarbitone, sodium valproate, topiramate and zonisamide have to be reduced. For non-linear kinetics with phenytoin, the toxicity profile is not good.

AED and phases of life

An epileptic patient, like any other person, engages in various activities and passes through different phases of life in which he has to fulfil different demands and commitments. The choice and dosage of AEDs should be adjusted according to the phase and activities of life.

Schooling

Anti-epileptic drugs that are known to affect scholastic performance are better avoided during the school-going years. Phenobarbitone is known to affect cognition and causes hyper-irritability, especially in children, and is to be avoided. Often, the epileptic process itself causes cognitive dysfunction, but drug-induced problems should be avoided as far as possible.

Leisure

No specific AED is known to hinder leisure activities, but sedating AEDs are better avoided, depending upon the type of leisure activity the patient prefers.

AEDs and women

Patients having sodium valproate are prone to develop polycystic ovarian syndrome (PCOS), though it should be kept in mind that about 20% of the normal population has features of PCOS. It has been shown that those developing PCOS due to sodium valproate usually revert to normalcy on withdrawal of the medicine.

Oral contraceptives usually contain a mixture of oestrogens and progesterones. Earlier, oral contraceptive pills (OCP) contained 50 mcg of oestrogens, but now pills containing 35 mcg of oestrogens are available. Antiepileptic drugs induce hepatic P450 enzymes, which potentiate the metabolism of OCPs. Sometimes AEDs such as phenytoin and carbamazepine increase the level of steroid hormone-binding globulin, causing a further fall in the level of free OCPs. So naturally, AEDs can cause OCP failure. Patients should be counselled on this and pills with a higher oestrogen content should be prescribed. Sodium valproate and gabapentin may help in this respect, provided they are useful in the type of epilepsy the patient is suffering from.[19,20]

Regarding teratogenicity, a multicentric study[21] has shown that the teratogenic risk to the foetus with sodium valproate, phenytoin, carbamazepine and phenobarbitone is 11.1%, 9%, 5.7% and 5.1%, respectively. Among the newer AEDs, lamotrigine and gabapentin have been shown to be relatively safe in this regard, followed closely by topiramate, but further studies are required before a final judgement can be made on their safety.

Efficacy of AEDs

The efficacy, or rather, relative efficacy of different AEDs is difficult to assess under several parameters, although some general observations and dictums have emerged in this context on the basis of day-to-day clinical practice. Our general experience vis-à-vis the efficacy of different drugs has given rise to the concept of using first-

and second-line AEDs in different subtypes of epilepsy and the idea of prescribing add-on AEDs in some chronic patients.

Among the relatively older AEDs, sodium valproate is thought to be effective in all types of seizures, whereas phenobarbitone and primidone are not effective in absence seizures but in all other types. Carbamazepine, phenytoin and oxcarbazepine are effective mainly in partial seizures and generalized tonic–clonic seizures, while ethosuximide is effective in absence seizures.[22] These generalizations and observations were at least partially challenged in the recommendations made by the recent World Congress of Epilepsy held in Helsinki, which concluded that the efficacies of the drugs are at different levels of statistical significance.

Another problem in assessing the relative efficacy of different AEDs arises when we try to evaluate the level of actual gain achieved. There is little doubt regarding the fact that complete control of seizures is the optimal result that can be achieved, simply because this can make a great difference to the patient's quality of life. Still, sometimes we make a compromise in selected difficult cases, where we talk in terms of relative seizure control and balance this with restricting the side-effects within an acceptable limit.

Over the past one or two decades, many new AEDs have been introduced in the market.[23] There is no doubt that these drugs definitely improve the outcome in chronic epilepsies, but the physician needs to familiarize himself with these new drugs so far as their indications, contra-indications and pharmacology are concerned. At present, many of them are best used as add-on therapy in chronic epilepsies that are difficult to treat. In a few countries, however, some of them are being used as initial therapy in specific types of epilepsy.

The million dollar question is whether the newer AEDs are therapeutically better than the older ones. Many clinical trials are being conducted on the use of newer versus older AEDs, but it is unfortunate that these trials are often biased in favour of the newer AEDs. For example, in a trial aimed at comparing the clinical efficacy of lamotrigine and carbamazepine, both drugs were used at a dosage of twice daily, which is acceptable in the case of lamotrigine but not carbamazepine. A fluctuating serum level is often the result of using carbamazepine twice daily, which leads to the failure of therapy.[24] A study on the relative efficacy of older and newer AEDs showed that their efficacies are more or less comparable, but the newer ones are definitely tolerated better.[25] Vigabatrine is beneficial in infantile spasms due to tuberous sclerosis, and lamotrigine in older-onset epilepsies.

One of the studies assessing the efficacy of newer AEDs showed that when the drug was introduced, there was total freedom from seizures in 16% cases and a 50%–99% reduction in the frequency of seizures in 21% of cases.[23] The factors that made for a better prognosis were fewer previously used AEDs, idiopathic epilepsy and short duration of epilepsy.

Levetiracetam has been the subject of the widest trials on the newer AEDs. Most of these have shown it to be effective and safe. It is also useful in status epilepticus, which has resulted in the introduction of parenteral formulations of the drug. According to the preliminary results of the large, multinational SKATE Trial, there was a median reduction of seizure frequency in 47.8% of cases and a seizure-free rate of 17.2% in all those with partial seizures.[26]

Another trial showed that with rational use of the new drug, zonisamide, the frequency of seizures was reduced by 50% or more in 75.4% of patients.[27] The effect of topiramate in the reduction of partial seizures has been shown to be acceptable.[28]

Any algorithm or table attempting to show the relative efficacy of AEDs for different types of seizures may seem to be an exercise in over-simplification, but may sometimes be useful (Table 1).

The rational selection and use of AEDs requires an understanding of the patient's requirements, a sound knowledge of the pharma-cological parameters of AEDs and, above all,

Table 1. Efficacies of antiepileptic drugs (AEDs)[22]

Effective or possibly effective in all seizure types	Effective in all except absence seizures	Effective in partial and GTCS	Effective in absence seizures
Valproic acid	Phenobarbital	Carbamazepine	Ethosuximide
Lamotrigine	Primidone	Phenytoin	
Topiramate		Oxcarbazepine	
Benzodiazepine		Gabapentin	
Zonisamide		Tiagabine	
Levetiracetam		Vigabatrine	
Felbamate			

GTCS generalized tonic–chronic seizures

proper judgement of the social factors guiding the outcome. Knowledge is essential for prescribing AEDs, but it should be supplemented with wisdom.

References

1. Caveness WF, Gallop GH. A survey of public attitudes towards epilepsy in 1979 with an indication of trends over the past thirty years. *Epilepsia* 1980;**21**:509–51.
2. Hamm RM. Clinical intuition and clinical analysis; expertise and cognitive continuum. In: Dowie J, Elstein A (eds). *Professional judgment.* Chapter 3; Cambridge University Press; 1988.
3. Hammond KR, Mcclettand GH, Mumpower J. *Human judgment and decision making.* New York: Hemisphere; 1980.
4. Dreyfus HL, Dreyfus SE. *Mind over machine: The power of human intuition and expertise in the era of the computer.* Oxford Blackwell; 1998.
5. Beghi E, Perucca E. The management of epilepsy in 1990s: Acquisitions, uncertainties and perspectives for future research. *Drugs* 1995;**49**:680–94.
6. Leppik IE. *Contemporary diagnosis and management of patients with epilepsy.* 2nd ed. In: Newtown PA (ed). Handbooks in Healthcare; 1996.
7. Perucca E. Clinical pharmacology and therapeutic use of new antiepileptic drugs. *Fund Clin Pharmacol* 2001;**15**:405–17.
8. Perucca E. The new generation of antiepileptic drugs: Advantages and disadvantages. *Br J Clin Pharmacol* 1996;**42**:531–43.
9. Gilman JT, Alvarez LA, Duchowny M. Carba-mazepine toxicity resulting from generic substitution. *Neurology* 1993;**43**:2696–7.
10. Hoyumpa AM, Schenker S. Is glucuronidation truly preserved in patients with liver disease. *Hepatology* 1991;**13**:786–95.
11. Bebisa M, Bleck JP. New anticonvulsant drugs: Focus on flunarizine, fosphenytoin, midazolam and stiriputol. *Drugs* 1994;**48**:153–71.
12. Bourgeois BFD. Anticonvulsant potency and neurotoxicity of valproate alone or in combination with carbamazepine and phenobarbital. *Clin Neuropharmacol* 1988;**11**:348–59.
13. Morris JC, Dodsin WF, Ferrendalli JA. Phenytoin and carbamazepine alone and in combination; anticonvulsant and neurotoxic effect. *Neurology* 1087;**37**:1111–18.
14. Wallis W, Kutt H, Mcdowell F. IV diphenyl-hydantoin in treatment of acute repetitive seizures. *Neurology* 1968;**18**:513–25.
15. Lingam S, Bertwistle H, Elliston H, *et al.* Problems with intravenous chlormethiazole (Heminervin) in status epilepticus. *BMJ* 1980;**i**:155–6.
16. Isojarvi JI, Rattya J, Myuya VV. Valproate, lamotrigine and insulin mediated risks in women with epilepsy. *Ann Neurol* 1998;**43**:446–51.
17. Mordis GP, Gibbard FB, Hut HA. Plasma activity of hepatic enzymes in patients with anticonvulsant therapy. *Seizure* 1993;**2**:319–23.
18. Sheth RD. Metabolic concerns associated with antiepileptic medication. *Neurology* 2004;**63** (Suppl 4):S24–S29.
19. Crawford P. Interactions between antiepileptic drugs and hormonal contraception. *CNS Drugs* 2002;**16**:263–72.
20. Vessey M, Painter R, Yates D. Oral contraception

and epilepsy: Findings of a large cohort study. *Contrception* 2002;**66:**77–9.

21. Kaneko S, Battino D, Andermann E, *et al.* Congenital malformation due to antiepileptic drugs. *Epilepsy Res* 1999;**33:**145–58.

22. Gatti G, Bonomi I, Jannuzzi G, *et al.* The new anti-epileptic drugs: Pharmacological and clinical aspects. *Curr Pharm Des* 2000;**6:**617–38.

23. Luciano AL, Shorvon SD. The results of treatment changes in patients with apparently drug resistant chronic epilepsy. *Ann Neurol* (in press) from Shorvon SD. The treatment of chronic epilepsy: A review of recent studies of clinical efficacy and side-effects. *Curr Opin Neurol* 2007;**20:**159–63.

24. Brodie MJ, Richens A, Yuen AW. Double blind comparison of lamotrigine and carbamazepine in newly diagnosed epilepsy. *Lancet* 1995;**345:**476–9.

25. Perucca E. Clinical pharmacology and therapeutic uses of new antiepileptic drugs. *Fund Clin Pharmacol* 2001;**15:**405–17.

26. Genton P, Sadzot B, Fejerman N, *et al.* Levetiracetam in a broad population of patients with refractory epilepsy: Interim results of the international SKATE trial. *Acta Neurol Scand* 2006;**113:**387–94.

27. Kothare SV, Kaleyia J, Mostafi N, *et al.* Efficacy and safety of zonisamide monotherapy in a cohort of children with epilepsy. *Paediatr Neurol* 2006;**3:**351–4.

28. van Passel L, Arif H, Hirsch LJ. Topiramate in the treatment of epilepsy and other nervous system disorders. *Expert Rev Neurother* 2006;**6:**19–31.

20

Pre-surgical evaluation in intractable epilepsy

M.V. PADMA SRIVASTAVA

Over the past 20 years, epilepsy surgery has been recognized increasingly as a viable treatment option for patients with medically refractory seizures. However, it often takes 20 years before patients are evaluated and referred for epilepsy surgery. This delay is probably because of the physician's perception of surgical intervention being a 'last resort' procedure.

Most epilepsy centres define intractability as a failure of at least two or three first-line antiepileptic medications. A conservative estimate is that one-half of patients with medically refractory seizures are potential candidates for epilepsy surgery. Because patients and their primary care providers are unwilling to accept surgery as an option, many patients, who could otherwise become seizure-free with surgery, undergo treatment with multiple medications over several years. These patients suffer from adverse effects of recurrent seizures, short- and long-term effects of antiepileptic drugs (AEDs), and psychosocial, interpersonal and occupational consequences of recurrent seizures. Hence, in assessing intractability, these quality-of-life factors should also be taken into account.

Studies underscore the fact that patients with partial epilepsy who do not become seizure-free after trying two first-line AEDs are less likely to become seizure-free after medication with additional or alternative AEDs.[1–7] Consequently, it is crucial to identify patients who would benefit from early surgical intervention, the success rate of which has been shown to be 70%–80% in well selected cases.[1]

Recent evidence indicates that the prototype surgically remediable syndrome, viz. medial temporal lobe epilepsy (TLE), can have prolonged periods of remission before becoming intractable.[2–7] For example, the Yale Multicenter Epilepsy Surgery Study found that in the group with TLE, the average time taken to develop intractable epilepsy, defined as failure of two AEDs, was 9 years.[2] Often, medial TLE begins in childhood but does not become refractory until adolescence or early adulthood. Thus, it appears that medial TLE can have a period of prolonged remission before becoming intractable.

Whereas in some cases a delay occurs from onset to intractability, the time from medical intractability to surgery is also prolonged. Intractable epilepsy following initial remission may lead to unnecessarily prolonged AED trials in the hope of once again attaining remission, and the misconceptions of the risks of epilepsy surgery by physicians and patients are the main causes of prolonged delays in surgical referral.

Definition of terms

- *Epileptogenic lesion:* This is a lesion that is capable of producing seizures. It needs to be resected for the patient to become seizure-free.
- *Epileptogenic zone:* This is an area of the cortex that needs to be resected to make the patient seizure-free. This zone usually includes the epileptogenic lesion.
- *Irritative zone:* This is an area of the cortex that generates epileptiform discharges. Its resection does not necessarily make the patient seizure-free. However, the irritative spikes often cease after surgical resection of the epileptogenic lesion and/or zone. This region is usually larger than the epileptogenic lesion.
- *Symptomatic zone:* This is the region of the cortex that produces clinical symptoms, but whose surgical removal does not necessarily result in the patient becoming seizure-free. Cortical stimulation studies have shown that the region producing auras is often much larger than the epileptogenic zone.
- *Functional deficit zone:* This zone of hypometabolism is seen on fluorodeoxyglucose-positron emission tomography (FDG-PET) to be much larger than the epileptogenic lesion and zone. In medial TLE, the area of abnormality on FDG-PET includes both the medial and lateral temporal lobe cortices. Some areas of hypometabolism may also be seen in remote areas of the cortex that are not connected to the primary areas of interest. These remote areas have been seen to disappear with good seizure control post-surgery.

Seizure semeiology[8–20]

Obtained through history: Observation and by video-electroencephalography (VEEG) monitoring. Patients are admitted to the long-term epilepsy monitoring unit, where seizures are recorded with video and simultaneous electroencephalogram (EEG) monitoring. The dose of antiepileptic medications is tapered and the patients may need to be sleep-deprived to induce seizures. Recorded seizures are reviewed, and the information regarding clinical semeiology the interictal and ictal EEG will be analysed to help localize and/or lateralize the seizure focus.

The clinical features are correlated with the EEG findings to determine if the patient has a single seizure type with consistent localization. Occasionally, the recorded events are not representative of the patient's commonly occurring events. At times, the patient's commonly occurring disabling event is determined to be non-epileptic, whereas the epileptic seizures are controlled adequately with medications.

Certain clinical features and semeiology of the seizures can have both a lateralizing and localizing value. Some of the common patterns seen are as follows:

- *Ictal speech:* This is usually associated with non-dominant temporal lobe seizures, as is also preserved responsiveness with unilateral manual automatisms.
- *Dystonic limb posturing:* This usually involves flexion of the arm at the elbow with internal or external rotation of the forearm, flexion at the wrist and extension of the fingers, and is contralateral to the side of temporal lobe seizure.
- *Post-ictal nose wiping:* This is defined as wiping of the nose with one hand twice in the post-ictal period which is usually ipsilateral to the temporal lobe of onset.
- *Post-ictal dysnomia:* This lasts for >2 min and suggests that the onset of seizure is in the dominant temporal lobe.
- *Postictal thirst, peri-ictal urinary urge* and ictal spitting are lateralized to the non-dominant hemisphere.
- *Auras:* Many patients with TLE experience auras, which are simple partial seizures that precede most or all of their complex partial seizures and which often occur in isolation. These auras consist of the following types: autonomic phenomena, such as epigastric

rising sensation, nausea; olfactory auras, such as strange taste and odour; and psychic auras, such as fear, déjà vu, jamais vu, depersonalization or derealization.

- *Hippocampal origin:* Seizures originating in this area are characterized by behavioural arrest, wide-eyed stare with papillary dilatation, and oral or alimentary automatisms, such as repetitive chewing and lip-smacking.
- *Elementary visual aura:* This has an occipital lobe origin.
- *Complex visual hallucination involving faces:* This has a fusiform or an inferior temporal gyrus origin.
- *Auditory aura:* This has a superior temporal gyrus origin.
- *Asymmetrical tonic limb posturing:* This is also known as the 'figure of four' sign, and is defined as the extension of one arm at the elbow and flexion of the other arm at the elbow during the tonic phase of a secondarily generalized tonic–clonic seizure. The extended limb is usually contralateral to the hemisphere of onset.
- Asymmetric ending of the late clonic phase of a secondarily generalized tonic–clonic seizure is ipsilateral to the hemisphere of onset in 80% of cases.
- Forced head, eye and body version suggests onset in the dorsolateral frontal lobe. It is usually contralateral to the hemisphere of onset.
- *Gyratory seizures:* These are defined as a rotation around the body axis of at least 180° during the seizure. Gyratory seizures that begin with forced head version are usually contralateral, whereas gyratory seizures without forced head turning are usually ipsilateral to the hemisphere of onset.
- *Hypermotor seizure:* These seizures are characterized by agitation with prominent motor activity and thrashing, suggesting an orbitofrontal onset.
- Asymmetric tonic posturing of bilateral limbs, monotonous vocalization and variable preservation of consciousness are seen in seizures arising from the supplementary motor region of the medial frontal lobe, anterior to the motor strip (area 6).
- Seizures arising from the frontal operculum consist of unilateral facial clonic twitching and profuse salivation immediately followed by tonic posturing of all limbs.

Interictal EEG[21–25]

A baseline 30 min recording and random awake and sleep samples need to be reviewed. Patients with TLE have epileptiform activity consisting of spikes and/or sharp waves that are usually maximal at the anterior temporal (F7 and F8 electrodes) and the mid-temporal regions (T3 and T4 electrodes). Nearly 20%–30% of patients with intractable TLE have bilaterally independent temporal epileptiform activity. However, most of them have a single, or dominant, localization for their habitual seizures. Occasionally, patients with extratemporal epilepsy of occipital or frontal lobe origin have interictal epileptiform activity at the temporal region, even though seizures do not localize to that region because of propagation of the interictal epileptiform discharges.

EEG characteristics that help in lateralization of secondary bilateral synchrony include:

- Consistent phase reversal over one region
- Higher amplitude of generalized or bilaterally synchronous interictal epileptiform activity over one hemisphere
- A consistent lead in one hemisphere
- Persistent lateralized interictal slowing.

Many patients with extratemporal neocortical epilepsy have no interictal epileptiform discharges.

Ictal scalp sphenoidal EEG

An EEG recording taken during an epileptic seizure (an ictal recording) displays a variety of patterns depending on the seizure type and pathways of spread. The recordings are usually sustained, rhythmic and clearly different from the interictal record. They evolve in frequency and/or amplitude in partial epilepsies, sometimes being followed by flattening of the trace and/or slow activity. Simple partial seizures are often not associated with any discernible change in the scalp EEG. Frontal lobe attacks often have prominent motor components that obscure the EEG, but even when readily visible, few if any changes are seen. Focal spikes may propagate to produce bilaterally synchronous discharges mimicking generalized epilepsy. This is most likely to occur with extratemporal epilepsy, especially if it is caused by parasagittal lesions or cortical dysgenesis.

In temporal lobe epilepsy, interictal spikes are usually maximal over the temporal or fronto-temporal regions. Even in patients with unilateral temporal lobe lesions or hippocampal sclerosis, who are good candidates for surgery, the interictal spikes are often bilateral and independent, especially during sleep. The ictal scalp EEG often shows rhythmic beta activity, which at the onset may be localized to the affected temporal lobe, or it could be bilateral.

In frontal lobe epilepsy, the scalp EEG is extremely variable, reflecting the heterogeneity of syndromes and the difficulties in recording from the frontal cortex. The interictal EEG often shows no epileptiform activity, bilaterally synchronous spikes or widespread spiking. Localized unifocal spikes are relatively uncommon. The ictal scalp EEG is often obscured by muscle and movement artefacts; localized changes are rare because of rapid seizure propagation.

In parieto-occipital lobe epilepsy, interictal spikes may be localized posteriorly, but there are often more anterior discharges, either over the temporal regions, or bilateral, synchronous, widespread discharges. The latter may be the most apparent feature, presumably because of rapid propagation. Similarly, ictal scalp recordings may show greater anterior changes than would be expected.

Magnetic resonance imaging (MRI)[26–37]

The basic epilepsy MRI protocol that is employed currently is as follows:

- Volume acquisition T1-weighted coronal dataset that covers the whole brain in 1.5–3 mm thick slices. This sequence produces approximately cubic voxels, allowing for reformatting in any orientation, subsequent measurement of hippocampal morphology and volumes, and 3-D reconstruction and surface-rendering. The sequences used are IRPF-SPGR and MPRAGE
- An oblique coronal inversion recovery sequence that is heavily T1-weighted and oriented perpendicular to the long axis of the hippocampus, which best demonstrates the internal structure and T1-weighted signal intensity of the hippocampus
- An oblique coronal spin echo or double-echo STIR sequence that is heavily T2-weighted and oriented perpendicular to the long axis of the hippocampus, to demonstrate any increase in T2-weighted signal intensity
- Software advances include the development of new imaging sequences that may identify abnormalities that are not visible using standard methodologies, such as fluid-attenuated inversion recovery (FLAIR), which gives images that are heavily T2-weighted, but in which the signal from the cerebrospinal fluid (CSF) is suppressed and so appears black.
- Diffusion-weighted imaging, obtained with echoplanar techniques, and magnetization transfer imaging, promise to be highly sensitive methods for the identification of neuronal injury.
- Co-registration of data from different imaging modalities, such as MRI, single-photon emission computed tomography (SPECT) and positron emission tomography (PET), is now becoming commonplace and allows precise structure-function correlations to be made, greatly enhancing the interpretation of both sets of data.

High-resolution structural MRI using T1-weighted spoiled gradient-recall sequences, with contiguous slices perpendicular to the long axis of the temporal lobe, has the highest sensitivity (85%) for detecting unilateral hippocampal atrophy. Hippocampal atrophy on MRI correlates with the presence of hippocampal sclerosis, which is the pathological substrate of medial TLE in 70% of cases. Hippocampal sclerosis is defined as >30% cell loss in hippocampal regions CA1 and CA3, with relative sparing of the CA2 region. Approximately 20%–30% of patients with hippocampal sclerosis have dual pathological lesions, with the concurrent presence of haematomas, cortical dysplasia and heterotopic grey matter.

An increased signal in the hippocampus can be seen on conventional spin echo T2-weighted imaging. MR FLAIR sequences are even more sensitive for detecting signal changes within the abnormal sclerotic hippocampus. A visually evident increase in hippocampal T2-weighted signal intensity generally has been reported in up to 60% of cases of hippocampal sclerosis. Similar to the quantification of hippocampal atrophy by volumetric analysis, T2-weighted signal intensity may be quantified reproducibly by measuring T2 relaxation time. Surface coil MRI and 3-D surface rendering increase the sensitivity for identifying subtle cortical malformations, by using multichannel phased array head coils, and T1-weighted and T2-weighted inversion recovery sequences. 3T phased-array MRI can further increase the signal-to-noise ratio six- to eight-fold, compared with a non-phase array coil of 1.5T MRI.

Prediction of surgical outcome

3-D preoperative maps of the hippocampi can help predict surgical outcome. Voxel-based morphometry involves the voxel-based comparison of a whole-brain grey matter between the patient and the control group. This method is useful for demonstrating enhanced sensitivity, and in identifying subtle grey matter abnormalities in patients with focal cortical dysplasia.

Minor anomalies of the morphology and arrangement of cortical gyri can only be visualized if the data are processed after acquisition and reformatting. At present, such detailed analysis is operator-dependent; it requires experienced personnel and is time-consuming. A focal area of polymicrogyria, for example, may not be evident on conventional sagittal, coronal or axial scans. This may be visible only on a reformatted tangential slice that cuts across the affected area, or on a 3-D reconstruction of the surface of the brain.

MR spectroscopy[38–39]

Patients with TLE have reductions in the N-acetyl aspartate:choline:creatinine ratio. This reduction has been shown to correlate with the presence of hippocampal sclerosis and to correctly lateralize the side of seizure onset in 97% of patients. Approximately 20%–40% of patients have bilateral metabolic disturbances; preliminary evidence suggests that this finding is associated with a higher probability of surgical failure.

Functional MRI[33,35]

Functional MRI (fMRI) uses the blood oxygen level-dependent (BOLD) contrast technique for evaluating the cerebral blood flow, by examining the difference between venous oxyhaemoglobin and deoxyhaemoglobin. Cortical activation results in a relative decrease of the lowered signal intensity produced by the decreased concentration of deoxyhaemoglobin, which in turn leads to a relative increase in signal in the activated cortex relative to the contiguous cortex. fMRI has been used mainly to map language, motor function and interictal spikes. It may also help in seizure localization. However, capturing seizures with fMRI is difficult because they are unpredictable, and complex partial seizures are usually associated with movement that obscures the fMRI image.

Positron emission tomography[40–54]

18-F-fluorodeoxyglucose PET (FDG-PET)

FDG-PET reveals an interictal zone of hypometabolism in the epileptogenic region in nearly 85% of TLE patients. This zone of hypometabolism is usually larger than the epileptogenic area, as defined electrophysiologically or pathologically. Use of an asymmetry index, calculated by comparing the quantitative metabolism of each temporal lobe, prevents the partial volume averaging artefacts and improves the sensitivity of the test. In patients with TLE, unilateral hippocampal atrophy on MRI and concordant EEG data, the use of FDG-PET is redundant. However, it provides valuable information in patients with substrate-negative MRI or when the EEG and MRI findings are discordant.

Newer techniques, such as statistical parametric mapping (SPM) and 3-D stereotactic surface projection (3-DSSP) images may be more sensitive than conventional FDG-PET analysis. Co-registration with MRI will also improve the sensitivity and specificity of FDG-PET by correcting for partial volume effects.

[11]C-flumazenil PET

[11]C-flumazenil (FMZ) PET binds with the central benzodiazepine/gamma amino butyric acid (cBZR/GABA) receptors. Early studies showed a reduction in FMZ binding in the temporal lobe of patients with intractable TLE, which is more restricted than the region of hypometabolism seen with FDG-PET. The reduction in FMZ binding correlates with neuron loss in the hippocampus. Newer techniques using SPM have shown that the reduction in FMZ binding is greater than would be expected from volume loss alone. This suggests that in addition to neuronal loss, GABA binding in the epileptogenic hippocampus is reduced. FMZ-PET also shows enhanced sensitivity in localizing cortical dysplasias and neuronal migration disorders.

Alpha methyl L-tryptophan and serotonin receptor PET imaging

Alpha methyl L-tryptophan PET (AMT-PET), like L-tryptophan, is a serotonin precursor that can help measure brain serotonin synthesis rates. Like tryptophan, AMT is metabolized to serotonin, but unlike tryptophan, it is not converted into protein. AMT is converted to alpha methyl serotonin, but unlike serotonin it is not metabolized by monoamine oxidase. Chugani and colleagues used AMT in patients with tuberous sclerosis and found reduced AMT uptake in cortical tubers compared with the normal cortex. However, epileptogenic tubers, confirmed by the region of ictal onset, demonstrated an increased uptake of AMT. Fedi and colleagues evaluated patients with either cortical dysplasia on MRI or a normal MRI. Increased AMT uptake was identified in 60% of patients with cortical dysplasia and in 30% with normal MRI. Serotonin 5-HT1A receptor binding has also been studied with the PET ligands, [18F]CWAY and [11C]WAY. Toczek *et al.* found reduced 5-HT1A binding in the medial and lateral temporal regions, ipsilateral to the epileptogenic temporal lobe.

Single-photon emission computed tomography[55–60]

Ictal and interictal SPECT, with hexamethyl-propyleneamine oxime (HMPAO), is performed during the ictal period to help delineate the epileptogenic zone. It is particularly helpful in patients with substrate-negative (normal) MRI and when there is discordance between the MRI and electrophysiological localization. As seizures are associated with increased glucose metabolism, which is closely coupled to cerebral blood flow, ictal SPECT scans show increased perfusion in the region of seizure onset. Ictal SPECT when superimposed and subtracted from the interictal SPECT, should show a hypo-perfused area (SISCOS technique), and clearly identifies the epileptogenic region. Ictal SPECT scans can also be superimposed on MRI (SISCOM) to obtain a structurally better defined area of epileptogenesis. Postictal subtraction SPECT co-registered with MRI has been studied as a method of localizing the epileptogenic zone. Newer methods include statistical parametric mapping, in which a control database of interictal SPECT scans are subtracted from the patient's ictal perfusion pattern and a z-score is generated; this is subsequently co-registered to the MRI. In TLE, ictal SPECT has >90% sensitivity in localizing seizures, with good interobserver reliability. However, the timing of the injection of the radio tracer is of paramount importance. In the immediate postictal period (60 sec), hyper-perfusion of the medial temporal lobe with hypoperfusion of the lateral temporal lobe are noted. In the late postictal period (up to 20 min postictally), perfusion in both the medial and lateral temporal lobes may be decreased. Ictal SPECT is of little value in patients with bitemporal lesions. However, it has a sensitivity of 90% in localizing extratemporal lobe seizures-such as frontal and parietal lobe seizures-provided ictal injection is administered shortly after ictal onset (i.e. within 20 sec).

Magnetoencephalography[61–67]

Magnetoencephalography (MEG) detects the magnetic fields produced by the electrical currents of neuronal activity. Unlike the electrical currents of neuronal activity, which are extra-cellular, magnetic fields are produced by the intracellular currents of apical dendrites, which are recorded from the scalp by MEG. Magnetic fields are minimally affected by intervening tissue layers. This is unlike conventional EEG, which detects radially oriented electrical activity that is attenuated in strength and spatially distorted by tissues between the brain and scalp surface. MEG also measures a subset of neuronal activity that is tangential to the scalp. These magnetic dipoles generated by MEG are then superimposed on structural MRI, creating magnetic source imaging (MSI). Numerous studies have shown that this technique is helpful in mapping inter-ictal epileptiform activity in patients with neo-cortical epilepsies which, in conjunction with other non-invasive structural and imaging data, guide the placement of the intracranial subdural grid to improve surgical outcome.

The objectives of MSI are as follows:

- To confirm the epileptogenic zone along with other functional imaging data
- To aid in the identification of a subtle cortical abnormality on MRI
- To provide localizing information not obtain-able with other imaging modalities.

Thus, MSI has the potential to obviate the need for invasive monitoring in cases with a structural lesion without localizing ictal EEG data or guide intracranial subdural electrode placement to improve localization of the epi-leptogenic zone and improve seizure-free out-come post-surgery. MSI is at present available in very few centres in the world.

Intracranial EEG monitoring[68–71]

With the advent of newer, more sophisticated and sensitive neuroimaging techniques to localize the epileptogenic region, the need for invasive monitoring is diminishing. At present, only 10%–20% of all surgical candidates require this type of evaluation, whereas 10 years ago, 50%–60% of surgical candidates required invasive monitoring.

Clinical indications for intracranial EEG monitoring are as follows:

- Bilaterally independent temporal lobe seizures

- Extratemporal lobe onset seizures with rapid propagation to the medial temporal lobe.
- Temporal lobe seizures of localized onset, but with normal MRI and FDG-PET scans.
- Discordant EEG localization and imaging findings.
- To distinguish neocortical epilepsy from medial temporal lobe epilepsy.
- Lateralization of seizures to a particular lobe in the absence of abnormalities on structural or functional imaging.
- Epileptogenic zone located in or near the eloquent cortex, usually confirmable by extensive extraoperative cortical stimulation studies.

The types of electrodes used for intracranial electrode monitoring include depth electrodes, subdural strips and subdural multicontact grid electrodes. Depth electrodes are useful for sampling deep structures, such as the hippocampus, amygdala and subcortical heterotopias, but are useful only in a restricted area. For sampling the temporal lobe, depth electrodes may be implanted orthogonal to it, from medial to lateral. In other centres of the brain, depth electrodes are implanted along the antero-posterior axis of the hippocampus, with the most anterior contact in the amygdala and the most posterior contact in the posterior temporo-occipital lobe. Subdural electrodes, on the other hand, record from the cortical surface and can sample larger areas. However, they are incapable of adequately sampling the cortical gyri within the depth of a sulcus. Neocortical seizures propagate rapidly. So, if the onset of a seizure is deep within a sulcus, only propagated seizure activity is recorded. For this reason, cortical resections based on invasive EEG data without an MRI abnormality, are associated with seizure-free outcome in only 20% of patients.

In patients with TLE who are monitored with depth electrodes, propagation of the seizure discharges to the contralateral temporal lobe in >5 sec correlates with hippocampal neuron cell loss and seizure-free outcome. Lieb *et al.* showed that contralateral propagation in <5 sec correlates with surgical failure. In TLE, the typical depth electrode onset of seizure activity consists of either a hypersynchronous discharge with periodic sharp and slow waves followed by low-voltage fast activity, or low-voltage fast activity as the initial change. A less common ictal-onset pattern consists of cessation of ongoing interictal activity. Neocortical EEG onset has the following features:

- Cessation of ongoing interictal activity
- Slow periodic discharges
- Low-voltage fast activity consisting of beta (13–15 Hz) or gamma activity (>35 Hz).

Although more sensitive than surface EEG, invasive recordings provide a limited view of cerebral activity because information is obtained only from areas where electrodes are placed. In cases where the epilelptogenic zone is located in or near eloquent areas, cortical stimulation for mapping language and the somatosensory cortex can be performed extra- or intraoperatively. The use of tailored resections based on intraoperative electrocorticography (ECoG) is generally used for excising the epileptogenic area without damaging the eloquent cortex.

The carotid amytal test[72–73]

WADA testing, also known as the carotid amytal test, is performed primarily to determine which cerebral hemisphere is dominant for language, and also to see whether the contralateral hemisphere can sustain basic memory function. If the contralateral hemisphere is unable to support basic memory function, a temporal lobectomy would not be carried out; in some cases, a more selective procedure would be performed. A subsidiary role is to find confirmatory evidence of impaired memory function in the temporal lobe proposed for resection. Considerable patient cooperation is required.

Functional MRI techniques have largely replaced carotid amytal testing for investigating lateralization of language and memory functions in patients considered for surgical treatment of epilepsy.

Pre-surgical neuropsychological evaluation[74–77]

A detailed neuropsychological evaluation is fundamental when considering patients for epilepsy surgery, particularly when a temporal lobe resection is being contemplated. In this setting, evidence is sought for dysfunction of that part of the brain from which seizures are believed to arise, when the remainder of the brain is functionally intact. Concordance of neuropsychological deficit with clinical features, imaging and EEG data and the lack of evidence for a widespread cerebral dysfunction is favourable for a good post surgical outcome in terms of seizure control as well as in avoiding functional deficits after surgery. The finding of global or multifocal neuropsychological deficits is an adverse prognosis for surgical intervention, because the cerebral pathology would persist even after resection of the putative focus. In general, the dominant temporal lobe primarily undertakes verbal memory processing and the non-dominant temporal lobe undertakes non-verbal memory processing. Memory test scores and tests of other cognitive functions contribute in lateralizing and localizing disturbed cerebral function.

References

1. Engel J Jr. Update on surgical treatment of the epilepsies. Summary of the Second International Palm Desert Conference on Surgical Treatment of the Epilepsies (1992). *Neurology* 1993;**43**:1612–17.
2. Agency for Healthcare Research and Quality. Management of treatment-resistant epilepsy. Agency for Healthcare Research and Quality. AHRQ Publication No.: 03-0028; 2003:1–8.
3. Benbadis SR, Heriaud L, Tatum WO. Epilepsy surgery, delays and referral patterns—are all your epilepsy patients controlled? *Seizure* 2003;**12**:167–70.
4. Berg AT, Kelly MM. Defining intractability: Comparisons among published definitions. *Epilepsia* 2006;**47**:431–6.
5. Berg AT. Understanding the delay before epilepsy surgery: Who develops intractable focal epilepsy and when? *CNS Spectr* 2004;**9**:136–44.
6. Berg AT, Langfitt J, Shinnar S. How long does it take for partial epilepsy to become intractable? *Neurology* 2003;**60**:186–90.
7. Cendes F. Progressive hippocampal and extrahippocampal atrophy in drug resistant epilepsy. *Curr Opin Neurol* 2005;**18**:173–7.
8. Dobesberger J, Walser G, Embacher N. Gyratory seizures revisited: A video-EEG study. *Neurology* 2005;**64**:1884–7.
9. Fakhoury T, Abou-Khalil B. Association of ipsilateral head turning and dystonia in temporal lobe seizures. *Epilepsia* 1995;**36**:1065–70.
10. Geyer JD, Payne TA, Faught E. Postictal nose-rubbing in the diagnosis, lateralization and localization of seizures. *Neurology* 1999;**52**:743–5.
11. Kernan JC, Devinsky O, Luciano DJ. Lateralizing significance of head and eye deviation in secondary generalized tonic-clonic seizures. *Neurology* 1993;**43**:1308–10.
12. Kotagal P, Luders H, Morris HH. Dystonic posturing in complex partial seizures of temporal lobe onset: A new lateralizing sign. *Neurology* 1989;**39**:196–201.
13. Katagal P, Bleasel A, Geller E. Lateralizing value of an asymmetric tonic limb posturing observed in secondarily generalized tonic–clonic seizures. *Epilepsia* 2000;**41**:457–62.
14. Manford M, Fish DR, Shorvon SD. An analysis of clinical seizure patterns and their localizing value in frontal and temporal lobe epilepsies. *Brain* 1996;**119**:17–40.
15. Privitera MD, Morris GL, Gilliam F. Postictal language assessment and lateralization of complex partial seizures. *Ann Neurol* 1991;**30**:391–6.
16. Rheims S, Demarquay G, Isnard J. Ipsilateral head deviation in frontal lobe seizures. *Epilepsia* 2005;**46**:1750–3.
17. Risinger MW, Engel J Jr, Van Ness PC. Ictal localization of temporal lobe seizures with scalp/sphenoidal recordings. *Neurology* 1989;**39**:1288–93.
18. Schulz R, Luders HO, Tuxhorn I. Localization of

epileptic auras induced on stimulation by subdural electrodes. *Epilepsia* 1997;**38**:1321–9.

19. Serles W, Pataraia E, Bacher J. Clinical seizure lateralization in mesial temporal lobe epilepsy: Differences between patients with unitemporal and bitemporal interictal spikes. *Neurology* 1998;**50**:742–7.

20. Siegel AM, Williamson PD, Roberts DW. Localized pain associated with seizures originating in the parietal lobe. *Epilepsia* 1999;**40**:845–55.

21. Bautista RE, Spencer DD, Spencer SS. EEG findings in frontal lobe epilepsies. *Neurology* 1998;**50**:1765–71.

22. Blum WT, Pillay N. Electrographic and clinical correlates of secondary bilateral synchrony. *Epilepsia* 1985;**26**:636–41.

23. Burnstine TH, Vining EP, Uematsu S. Multifocal independent epileptiform discharges in children: Ictal correlates and surgical therapy. *Neurology* 1991;**41**:1223–8.

24. Ebersole JS, Pacia SV. Localization of temporal lobe foci by ictal EEG patterns. *Epilepsia* 1996;**37**:386–99.

25. Pataraia E, Lurger S, Series W. Ictal scalp EEG in unilateral mesial temporal lobe epilepsy. *Epilepsia* 1998;**39**:608–14.

26. Chan S, Chin SS, Nordli DR. Prospective magnetic resonance imaging identification of focal cortical dysplasia, including the non-balloon cell subtype. Prospective magnetic resonance imaging identification of focal cortical dysplasia. *Epilepsia* 1998;**44**:749–57.

27. Colliot O, Bernasconi N, Khalili N. Individual voxel-based analysis of grey matter in focal cortical dysplasia. *Neuroimage* 2006;**29**:162–71.

28. Colliot O, Antel SB, Naessens VB. *In vivo* profiling of focal cortical dysplasia on high-resolution MRI with computational models. *Epilepsia* 2006;**47**:134–42.

29. Detre JA, Sirven JI, Alsop DC. Localization of subclinical ictal activity by monitoring. *Ann Neurol* 1995;**38**:618–24.

30. Grant PE, Barkovich AJ, Wald LL. High-resolution surface-coil MR of cortical lesions in medically refractory epilepsy: A prospective study. *Am J Neuroradiol* 1997;**18**:291–301.

31. Jack CR Jr, Sharbrough FW, Cascino GD. Magnetic resonance image-based hippocampal volumetry: Correlation with outcome after temporal lobectomy. *Ann Neurol* 1992;**31**:138–46.

32. Jack CR Jr, Rydberg CH, Krecke KN. Mesial temporal sclerosis: Diagnosis with fluid-attenuated inversion-recovery versus spin-echo MR imaging. *Radiology* 1996;**199**:367–73.

33. Jackson GD, Connelly A, Cross JH. Functional magnetic resonance imaging of focal seizures. *Neurology* 1994;**44**:850–6.

34. Knake S, Triantafyllou C, Wald LL. 3T phased array MRI improves the presurgical evaluation in focal epilepsies: A prospective study. *Neurology* 2005;**65**:1026–31.

35. Krakow K, Woermann FG, Symms MR. EEG-triggered functional MRI of interictal epileptiform activity in patients with partial seizures. *Brain* 1999;**122**(Pt.9):1679–88.

36. Kuzniecky RI, Bilir E, Gilliam F. Multimodality MRI in mesial temporal sclerosis: Relative sensitivity and specificity. *Neurology* 1997;**49**:774-8.

37. Sisodiya SM, Stevens JM, Fish DR. The demonstration of gyral abnormalities in patients with cryotogenic partial epilepsy using three-dimensional MRI. *Arch Neurol* 1996;**53**:28–34.

38. Kuzniecky RI, Hugg JW, Hetherington H. Relative utility of 1H spectroscopic imaging and hippocampal volumetry in the lateralization of mesial temporal lobe epilepsy. *Neurology* 1998;**51**:66–71.

39. Kuzniecky RI, Bilir E, Gilliam F. Multimodality MRI in mesial temporal sclerosis: Relative sensitivity and specificity. *Neurology* 1997;**49**:774–8.

40. Engel J Jr, Henry TR, Swartz BE. Positron emission tomography in frontal lobe epilepsy. *Adv Neurol* 1995;**66**:223–38.

41. Fedi M, Reutens DC, Andermann F. Alpha-[11C]-methyl-L-tryptophan PET identifies the epileptogenic tuber and correlates with interictal spike frequency. *Epilepsy Res* 2003;**52**:203–13.

42. Fedi M, Reutens D, Okazawa H. Localizing value of alpha-methyl-L-tryptophan PET in intractable epilepsy of neocortical origin. *Neurology* 2001;**57**:1629–36.

43. Henry TR. Functional neuroimaging with positron emission tomography. *Epilepsia* 1996;**37**:1141–54.

44. Juhasz C, Chugani DC, Muzik O. Alpha-methyl-L-tryptophan PET detects epileptogenic cortex in children with intractable epilepsy. *Neurology* 2003;**60**:960–8.

45. Juhasz C, Chugani DC, Padhye UN. Evaluation with alpha-[11C]methyl-L-tryptophan positron emission tomography for reoperation after failed epilepsy surgery. *Epilepsia* 2004;**45**:124–30.

46. Kagawa K, Chugani DC, Asano E. Epilepsy surgery outcome in children with tuberous sclerosis complex

evaluated with alpha-[^{11}C]methyl-L-tryptophan positron emission tomography (PET). *J Child Neurol* 2005;**20**:429–38.

47. Knowlton RC. The role of FDG-PET, ictal SPECT and MEG in epilepsy surgery evaluation. *Epilepsy Behav* 2006;**8**:91–101.

48. Koepp MJ, Richardson MP, Labbe C. ^{11}C-flumazenil PET, volumetric MRI and quantitative pathology in mesial temporal lobe epilepsy. *Neurology* 1997;**49**: 764–73.

49. Koepp MJ, Hand KS, Labbe C. *In vivo* ^{11}C-flumazenil-PET correlates with *ex vivo* ^{3}Hflumazenil autoradiography in hippocampal sclerosis. *Ann Neurol* 1998;**43**:618–26.

50. Richardson MP, Koepp MJ, Brooks DJ. ^{11}C-flumazenil PET in neocortical epilepsy. *Neurology* 1998;**51**:485–92.

51. Savic I, Thorell JO, Roland P. ^{11}C-flumazenil positron emission tomography visualizes frontal epileptogenic regions. *Epilepsia* 1995;**36**:1225–32.

52. Spencer SS. The relative contributions of MRI, SPECT and PET imaging in epilepsy. *Epilepsia* 1994;**35**(Suppl 6):S72–S89.

53. Aswartz BW, Khonsari A, Vrown C. Improved sensitivity of 18FDG-positron emission tomography scans in frontal and 'frontal plus' epilepsy. *Epilepsia* 1995;**36**:388–95.

54. Theodore WH, Sato S, Kufta CV. FDG-positron emission tomography and invasive EEG: Seizure-focus detection and surgical outcome. *Epilepsia* 1997;**38**:81–6.

55. Harvey AS, Hopkins IJ, Bowe JM. Frontal lobe epilepsy: Clinical seizure characteristics and localization with ictal 99mTc-HMPAO SPECT. *Neurology* 1993;**43**:1966–80.

56. Ho SS, Berkovic SF, Newton MR. Parietal lobe epilepsy: Clinical features and seizure localization by ictal SPECT. *Neurology* 1994;**44**:2277–84.

57. Ho SS, Berkovic SF, Berlangieri SU. Comparison of ictal SPECT and interictal PET in the presurgical evaluation of temporal lobe epilepsy. *Ann Neurol* 1995;**37**:738–45.

58. Knowlton RC, Lawn ND, Mountz JM. Ictal SPECT analysis in epilepsy: Subtraction and statistical parametric mapping techniques. *Neurology* 2004;**63**: 10–15.

59. O'Brien TJ, So EL, Mullan BP. Subtraction ictal SPECT co-registered to MRI improves clinical usefulness of SPECT in localizing the surgical seizure focus. *Neurology* 1998;**50**:445–54.

60. O'Brien TJ, So EL, Mullan BP. Subtraction SPECT co-registered to MRI improves post-ictal SPECT localization of seizure foci. *Neurology* 1999;**52**: 137–46.

61. Baumgartner C, Pataraia E, Lindinger G. Magnetoencephalography in focal epilpesy. *Epilepsia* 2000;**41** (Suppl):S39–S47.

62. Ebersole JS. Magnetoencephalography/magnetic source imaging in the assessment of patients with epilepsy. *Epilepsia* 1997;**38** (Suppl):S1–S5.

63. Fischer MJ, Scheler G, Stefan H. Utilization of magnetoencephalography results to obtain favorable outcomes in epilepsy surgery. *Brain* 2005;**128**:153–7.

64. Knowlton RC, Laxer KD, Aminoff MJ. Magnetoencephalography in partial epilepsy: Clinical yield and localization accuracy. *Ann Neurol* 1997;**42**: 622–31.

65. Knowlton RC, Shih J. Magnetoencephalography in epilepsy. *Epilepsia* 2004;**45**(Suppl 4):61–71.

66. Mamelak AN, Lopez N, Akhtari M. Magnetoencephalography-directed surgery in patients with neocortical epilepsy. *J Neurosurg* 2002;**97**:865–73.

67. Minassian BA, Otsubo H, Weiss S. Magnetoencephalographic localization in pediatric epilepsy surgery: Comparison with invasive intracranial electroencephalography. *Ann Neurol* 1999;**46**:627–33.

68. Hamer HM, Morris HH, Mascha EJ. Complications of invasive video-EEG monitoring with subdural grid electrodes. *Neurology* 2002;**58**:97–103.

69. Lee SA, Spencer DD, Spencer SS. Intracranial EEG seizure-onset patterns in neocortical epilepsy. *Epilepsia* 2000;**41**:297–307.

70. Pacia SV, Ebersole JS. Intracranial EEG substrates of scalp ictal patterns from temporal lobe foci. *Epilepsia* 1997;**38**:642–54.

71. Pacia SV, Ebersole JS. Intracranial EEG in temporal lobe epilepsy. *J Clin Neurophysiol* 1999;**16**:399–407.

72. Acharya JN, Dinner DS. Use of the intracarotid amobarbital procedure in the evaluation of memory. *J Clin Neurophysiol* 1997;**14**:311–25.

73. Buchtel HA, Passaro EA, Selwa LM. Sodium methohexital (brevital) as an anesthetic in the WADA test. *Epilepsia* 2002;**43**:1056–61.

74. Herman BP, Wyler AR, Richey ET. Wisconsin card sorting test performance in patients with complex partial seizures of temporal-lobe origin. *J Clin Exp Neuropsychol* 1988;**10**:467–76.

75. Kanner AM, Palac S. Depression in epilepsy: A common but often unrecognized comorbid malady. *Epilepsy Behav* 2000;**1**:37–51.

76. Oyegbile TO, Dow C, Jones J. The nature and course of neuropsychological morbidity in chronic temporal lobe epilepsy. *Neurology* 2004;**62:** 1736–42.

77. Williamson PD, French JA, Thadani VM. Characterisitics of medial temporal lobe epilepsy-II. Interictal and ictal scalp electroencephalography, neuropsychological testing, neuroimaging, surgical results, and pathology. *Ann Neurol* 1993; **34:**781–7.

21

The surgical treatment of temporal lobe epilepsy in children*

P. DAVID ADELSON

Introduction

Epilepsy affects approximately 0.5%–1.0% of the population in the United States and Canada,[1] and most often begins in childhood during the first decade. Up to 50% of the cases of epilepsy begin before the age of 5 years.[1–3] Although not the most common etiology of seizures in children, temporal lobe epilepsy (TLE) has historically been the most common surgically treated form.[1] Since the seizures of temporal lobe onset usually arise focally, and are accessible for surgical extirpation, temporal lobe seizures remain the single most important 'subtype of epilepsy' for successful surgical treatment.[4] The temporal lobe and its medial structures, the amygdalohippocampal complex, have a higher susceptibility to seizure-induced brain injury and incidence of epileptic activity. As a result, they are the most common sources of medically intractable complex partial seizures in the adult population,[1] and occur in children in approximately 30% of cases.[1] Surgically, though, the number of temporal lobe resections in most pediatric series is upwards of 56%.[5,6]

The successful use of temporal lobectomy specifically for the treatment of epilepsy in children was described now over 40 years ago[7,8] and despite the overwhelming evidence of the improvement in development and quality of life for patients seizure free following surgery, there had been a reluctance to consider surgical resection in children with intractable seizures. Whether due to the possible morbidity/mortality of surgery or the ongoing hope that the children would 'outgrow' the seizures or be medically controlled, many children who may have benefited from a surgical intervention continued to grow and develop with intractable seizures. It is clear now in both adults and children that TLE surgery is superior to prolonged medical therapy.[9] Through our better understanding of seizures and seizure subtypes, it has become clear that consequences of intractable seizures in children have a 'malignant' natural history which negatively impacts on both intellectual and behavioral functions. As well, the duration of seizures negatively impacts on the potential for a good long-term seizure-free outcome following surgery.[10,11]

Presently, the evaluation and the determination

of intractability in children can be done in a systematic and effective way to identify earlier the patients who would benefit from surgical treatment and an intervention proposed once the affected child has truly failed medical management.[12] With improved surgical expertise, excellent surgical and seizure outcomes are now possible with little morbidity and virtually no mortality in children.[13] As well, epilepsy surgery is a more cost-effective option than continued medical therapy.[14] In this chapter, the evaluation and the surgical treatment of children with medically intractable seizures of the temporal lobe will be reviewed.

Natural history

Of particular importance for the clinician involved with treating children with seizures is that the natural history for medically-intractable temporal seizures has been well documented and shown to be particularly poor.[15,16] These children can be affected in all areas of neurocognitive function including intelligence and cognition, behavior and language, as well as psychosocial competence.[17] In one long-term study of patients with poorly controlled temporal lobe seizures, follow-up revealed that only one-third of patients with medically-intractable seizures improved and became seizure free on medication; the other two-thirds of patients continued to suffer from seizures even on medication.[15] Only half of these patients with continued seizures were able to be self-supporting, while the other half remained dependent for their day-to-day needs. Many of these children can end up with a multitude of psychosocial problems and social isolation into adulthood.[17,18] While complex partial seizures that develop in adulthood may substantially impact the adult patient's choice of vocation and psychosocial interaction, in children, the consequences of intractable seizures on brain development can be catastrophic. It was originally believed that seizure intractability had a direct effect on intellectual and psychosocial

development.[15] More recently, others have postulated that in young children with intractable seizures, the adverse effects on cognitive and behavioral function are more likely due to a combination of factors. These may include: The prolonged use of anti-convulsant medication, the frequent need for multiple medications and medication regimens, at times the need for toxic levels of medication with difficult to control seizures, and/or the constant seizures and the electrophysiologic abnormalities themselves throughout the period of brain development and maturation which may contribute to the aberrant development of intellectual pathways and abnormal social behaviors.[13,16,19–22]

Whether singly or due to a combination of insults, the young brain is affected in its long-term outcome by the impact of these factors throughout the developmental period. It has been postulated that the intractability of the electrophysiologic disturbance and/or antiepileptic drug toxicity in these children interferes with the normal critical periods for the development of higher functions.[16,22] The use of anti-epileptic medication even at 10 levels has been shown to significantly impact the normal brain development and function in animal models,[23,24] and cognitive and behavioral function in children.[25–27] One can also envision though that besides structural changes, that since these children are often on multiple medications at often supranormal levels, or suffer significant periods of abnormal electrophysiologic states, they spend a significant portion of their 'awake' time with an altered perception of surrounding stimuli. The effect of this intrusion into the child's normal developmental schema blurs and therefore affects the normal processing of information necessary for the normal functional development for cognition and other neuropsychological abilities. Numerous studies using full range IQ scoring[28,29] have shown that intellectual function is depressed in these children and many have debilitating behavioral problems that include temper tantrums, aggression, attention deficit disorders and hyperactive states, particularly while they continue to have medically intractable seizures.[16,22,30,31] Lower intelligence (IQ) scores are seen in children with epilepsy compared to normal children[28] and more often have problems with school secondary to learning difficulties or behavioral problems.[16,32] These difficulties have contributed to overall decreased academic achievement.[17]

Poor long-term prognostic features of children with seizures include age, particular types of seizure syndromes, and poor psychosocial development.[16,22] An early onset of the intractable seizures, specifically in children less than 3 years old, have a particularly poor prognosis and exhibit early and marked motor features including tonic and myoclonic features and spasms.[33] Seizure control in these children, even with multiple medication regimens is unlikely to have any long-term benefit. Further prognostic factors for good seizure outcome are short duration of epilepsy and when electroencephalography (EEG) shows pattern in only one particular location.[34] Other adverse prognostic features include daily complex partial seizures, a hyperkinetic syndrome, an IQ less than 90, an episode of status epilepticus, or a total of greater than five grand mal attacks. Other factors that carry a poor prognosis for normal intellectual and behavioral development in children include a long duration of seizures prior to control, e.g. multiple episodes of status epilepticus, abnormal neurologic or radiologic findings, frequent seizures, clusters of seizures and auras, and/or psychotic episodes. These factors portend a poor outcome even with surgical intervention. Overall, it is believed that of the 10%–20% of children with medically intractable seizures, 15% might benefit from surgery.[4,35–37]

While young children have a greater potential for seizure-induced brain injury, young children also have a much greater potential for recovery. In the young child, during the period of brain maturation and synaptogenesis, and unlike the mature brain, the developing nervous system is able to reconfigure for a better outcome lost secondary to injury. As a result, the young child that becomes seizure free has greater potential than adults to improve intellectual, motor and/or behavioral functions impaired as a result of surgery or seizure-induced injury.[31,38] The indications for consideration of a surgical option for intractable temporal lobe seizures in children therefore include: (a) a significant number and high frequency of seizures that are affecting or by natural history will affect cognitive and functional development, (b) intractability to medical management requiring 3 or more medications that have failed singly or in combination, and (c) localization of a focal onset in the temporal lobe. These indications are often determined through the standard seizure evaluation and are not limited by age.

Surgical evaluation

Many children with new onset idiopathic seizure or epilepsy are often and adequately treated in community practice once a lesional source has been excluded. Since the medical treatment and natural history for children with intractable seizures of temporal lobe origin remain unsatisfactory with the new generation of antiepileptic medications now available, it becomes necessary to identify those patients who are most likely to fail further medical interventions and consider a surgical option.[39,40] The advantages, as mentioned earlier, of operating on these children with temporal lobe epilepsy at an earlier age, is to not only have the benefit of better recovery potential from morbidity but also to lessen the impact of drug toxicity and ictal events on functional development.[2,8,19]

The initial epilepsy evaluation may be useful for many children with intractable seizures and has multiple purposes which include characterization of the seizures and seizure syndromes and optimization of the medication regimens. The further evaluation when considering a surgical intervention includes the regional lateralization and localization of the seizure focus or epileptogenic zone, and determination of its proximity to eloquent cortex. With the improved evaluative and neuroimaging techniques available, many pathologic and physiologic changes that were previously undetectable can now be identified earlier and facilitate the decision for surgical intervention.[41] Even in very young children who would have previously had a prolonged observation period, modern neuroimaging techniques are able to delineate a cytoarchitectural, neoplastic, or metabolic abnormality that when correlated with the electrophysiologic abnormality and seizure syndrome, may warrant a focused surgical resection.[19,42] There are as many selection criteria for surgical candidacy as there are different epilepsy centers. The evaluative techniques described below have different advantages and disadvantages in regard to the information that is provided which the author has found to be successful for the identification of surgical candidates. (The different types of evaluation and descriptions are explained in further detail in a preceding chapter and will be presented as an overview in the next sections.)

Noninvasive evaluation

When a child presents with intractable seizures of temporal lobe origin and is to undergo evaluation, the initial phase of the evaluation is a noninvasive characterization of the child's seizure syndrome and optimization of the medical management. For those children who have previously failed multiple medication trials, this formalized evaluation permits the physician the focused time to strictly monitor medication administration and its serum levels, compliance, and correlate the EEG (the electrophysiologic function) to the semiology to confirm the seizure syndrome. Often this will include multiple outpatient visits and EEG's in an attempt to identify the origin of the seizures but may include an in-hospital observation for particularly difficult cases.[43] Other outpatient studies include a neuropsychologic battery and anatomic and

functional imaging. Baseline neurologic and neuropsychologic studies preoperatively of the motor function, developmental competence and adaptive functioning of the individual, and the behavioral/psychosocial functions provide a better understanding of the impact of the seizures on the child's neurocognitive development as well as provide data for comparison to the postoperative outcome assessment. Anatomic and functional imaging in conjunction with the electrophysiology may be adequate to define the seizure syndrome and its etiology. If necessary, further evaluation may include EEG/video telemetry for further definition of the seizure semiology and syndrome, and amobarbital (Wada) testing when needed for language and memory localization.

Imaging

Neuroimaging modalities, specifically magnetic resonance imaging (MRI), have revolutionized the evaluation and localization of previously idiopathic cases. Since epilepsy is a *functional* disorder of the brain, defining the anatomic abnormalities may not be sufficient to completely define the epileptic focus. In these instances, *functional* neuroimaging has been shown to detect the generalized and focal functional abnormalities and to define their relationship to the electrophysiologic dysfunction by EEG[44] and anatomical abnormalities visualized on the MRI. Functional imaging has utilized MRI technology, e.g. functional (fMR) and MR spectroscopy (MRS), as well as other modalities such as positron emission tomography (PET) and single photon emission computerized tomography (SPECT); all have had a major impact on the evaluation of the patients with intractable temporal lobe seizures as well as extratemporal lobe epilepsy. Additionally, with the advent of technology to co-register the structural (MR) and functional images, as well as utilize subtraction images of ictal and interictal data or comparisons to normative data sets, can increase the reliability of these functional imaging modalities in the pre-surgical evaluation.[45] These new imaging technologies have decreased the need for invasive monitoring with intracranial electrodes in some adult studies by 50%,[46] and in children in over 90%[47] by identifying more patients who would have had a previously undetectable focal lesion that now might benefit from a focal surgical resection.

MRI (Magnetic resonance imaging)

Now well established as the imaging modality of choice, standard MRI revolutionized the discovery of pathophysiologic substrates within the intracranial space, particularly with each improvement in the imaging hard and software packages. As with the other modalities of evaluation, MRI cannot detect all abnormalities but it has become both sensitive and specific for cerebral 'lesions' that may be causing or contributing to an epileptic syndrome. The imaging capability has improved such that MRI can detect even subtle anatomical changes and abnormalities, such as cortical dysplasia that even a few years ago were undetectable. In the early studies using MRI for the detection of medial temporal *foci*, T2 weighted imaging was able to identify only 91% of patients with mesial temporal sclerosis,[48] but was more accurate than other conventional images such as proton-density (72%) or T2 weighted-fast spin (84%). Since that study, improved MR resolution along with new sequence acquisitions such as fluid attenuated inversion recovery (FLAIR) have contributed markedly to the improved identification and definition of subtle structural differences of normal and abnormal areas of cortex as well as the subtle changes in hippocampal signal intensity with increased sensitivity[49,50] with increased accuracy and improved specificity and sensitivity particularly of the medial structures and in areas of white matter changes. FLAIR images are a mixture of TI and T2 weighted images that has heavy T2 weighting with suppression of the cerebrospinal fluid signal. Because of the increased tissue free water in the hippocampus with medial temporal sclerosis (MTS), these images have become incorporated into the standard imaging protocols for patients with epilepsy.[49] With the improvement in the technology, intraoperative MR has recently been used as an adjunct to standardize the extent of hippocampal resection in patients undergoing temporal lobe surgery.[51]

As well as an adjunct to the standard imaging, hippocampal volumetrics have been utilized to evaluate the differences between the medial structures of the two temporal lobes. Serial thin cut coronal sections using T1 images with software to outline the hippocampus and calculate the volume of the medial structures, as well as the grey matter concentrations of the medial structures, facilitate the comparative analysis and differences in volume of an affected structure. As expected with MTS, significant degeneration and therefore differences in hippocampal volumes have been shown to lateralize and localize the temporal seizure focus when correlated with the other anatomic images and electrophysiologic findings.[50]

Long-term seizure outcome is enhanced when neuroimaging is concordant with the electrophysiologic EEG findings. In one study by Blume *et al.*,[52] all patients with EEG abnormality and neuroimaging (MR) findings congruent with the clinical data were made seizure-free following surgical intervention. Though this is a selected group of patients, neuroimaging has enhanced the ability of the clinician to elucidate the pathologic substrate in over 90% of cases.[48,49] MTS and cortical dysplasia can often be identified[19,48–49,52–53] preoperatively which facilitates the intervention. Interestingly, MTS can exist in a setting without temporal lobe epilepsy. In a series of 204 non-epileptic patients, Benbadis *et al.*[54] showed that hippocampal atrophy or unilateral MTS was seen in 14%.

Functional imaging using MRI

Other imaging modalities that use MR technology include MRS and fMR. These functional imaging modalities have also been utilized in conjunction with the standard MRI to further define and delineate 'abnormal tissue'. MRS is capable of identifying the different chemical metabolites within different regions of interest and is based on the concept that every chemically distinct nucleus resonates at a slightly different frequency. A variety of proton signals can be detected and identified during one scanning period for both anatomic and spectroscopic data. Since seizures typically produce alterations in energy metabolism with interictal periods of glucose hypometabolism, MRS in patients of temporal lobe epilepsy has shown that the affected temporal lobe is alkaline compared to the unaffected side.[55] Additionally, using [31p] Phosphorus NMR spectra, there is increased inorganic phosphate (Pi) concentration in the affected temporal lobe. These findings reflect the differences in energy metabolism with the differences of the metabolites of ATP consumption.[55] Recently, other spectra, e.g. N-acetylaspartate, have been found to be particularly useful in lateralizing to the affected side in temporal lobe epilepsy since the subtle 'chemical profile' differs in normal neural tissue compared to sclerotic or 'lesional' areas of the temporal lobe.[56] At the present time, MRS can only give regional information which is useful in lateralization but its poor spatial resolution does not yet allow for the further delineation of the epileptogenic zone.

During specific tasks or functional use of regional areas of brain, there is an increase in metabolic need and a resultant increase in cerebral blood flow. FMR is a modality sensitive enough to detect changes in cerebral load flow and deoxyhemoglobin from baseline images compared to images obtained during a repetitive language or functional task, and then used to identify regions of eloquent cortex. Overlay of these *functional* changes on the abnormal regions obtained with conventional anatomical images would then aid in the preoperative planning of an anatomically 'safe' operation. In regard to its use in the pediatric population, the acquisition of images is time intensive and task dependent; thus, functional imaging has been found to be difficult and inconsistent in young children but is possible in older or mature children. As well, eloquent areas, e.g. language, may be represented in more than just one area in children and even in adults. With improved speed and registration of the images, fMR may become more useful in the pediatric group in the future. As well in the future, with the improvement of the resolution in fMR, it may become more readily available than PET since existing MRI machines can readily be upgraded to perform both and MRS and fMR.

Positron emission tomography (PET)

Functional neuroimaging with PET has long been used in conjunction with the anatomic studies such as CT and MRI in detecting generalized and focal areas of abnormality in patients with epilepsy,[47] and has become an important adjunct in evaluating patients with temporal lobe epilepsy.[5,57] PET can quantify the differences in either glucose uptake or oxygen consumption for different regions of brain and differentiate between 'normal' areas of functionality or metabolism. Glucose utilization or metabolism within intracerebral structures is determined by the extent of the uptake of the radionuclide [18F] deoxyglucose (FDG) and the regional detection of positron emissions. Because of its relatively high resolution, even previously undetectable anatomic abnormalities have been found to have metabolic or functional abnormalities that correlated with the intraoperative electrophysiologic findings.[44] These regional areas of glucose hypometabolism, particularly in the temporal lobe, have been shown to correlate with both the electrophysiologic or EEG abnormality[44] as well as with the pathologic abnormality.[58] This has further facilitated the selection of both adult and pediatric patients with temporal lobe epilepsy for surgery by supplanting the need for an operation for invasive monitoring with either depth or surface electrodes and allowed them to go directly to surgery for a focal resection.[19,58] In one series, 40% of adult patients with temporal lobe epilepsy were able to avoid invasive monitoring and proceed directly to surgery.[58]

Children, too, with focal epilepsy have been shown by PET to have focal metabolic abnormalities that have correlated with the electro-physiologic and the pathologic findings,[44] particularly when the temporal lobe is involved.[19] In children, the anatomic abnormality may be subtle and eMRI may not be sensitive enough to detect a cortical abnormality. This is unlike the situation seen in adults where the vast majority of patients have medial temporal sclerosis which can be visualized with MRI. PET is useful in identifying the functional abnormalities, even in temporal neocortical regions, which may more closely correlate with the EEG findings and define the seizure focus.[47] As well, this type of functional imaging may serve to define the extent of cerebral abnormalities along the neocortex and define the relationship of epileptic *foci* to neoplasms.[19,59–62] With our further understanding of the pharmacokinetics and mechanics of receptor binding in patients with temporal lobe epilepsy, a variety of bioactive pharmaceuticals can be labeled that may be able to image more sensitively and specifically functional abnormalities. Presently, benzodiazapine or opiate receptor differences in functionally abnormal tissue are being investigated.

Single photon emission computerized tomography (SPECT)

SPECT is another radionuclide study that images the regional differences of cerebral blood flow. Biotracers such as [^{99m}Technetium] HMPAO and IMP have a high first pass uptake in the brain parenchyma and behave like 'chemical micro-spheres' creating a 'snapshot' of CBF. Though these tracers have improved the resolution of SPECT so as to make anatomical and electro-physiologic correlations possible, SPECT still does not have the resolution of PET. Interictal SPECT studies have not been particularly helpful except when there are clear instances of interictal hypoperfusion.[63–65] The efficacy of ictal or postictal SPECT has been shown to be more correlative and superior to interictal SPECT and, in some centers, SPECT (HMPAO) has also been useful in bypassing the need for invasive monitoring with good surgical outcomes in both adults[66,67] and in children.[68,69] In temporal lobe epilepsy, ictal SPECT often shows hyperper-fusion in the region of the onset of the epileptic focus, particularly in the medial temporal lobe. Postictal SPECT though may be more variable but most often has continued hyperperfusion in the area of seizure onset, namely the medial temporal lobe, and decreased perfusion in the lateral temporal cortex on the side of the seizure. By using subtraction software of the ictal and interictal SPECT studies and co-localizing to the MR images, the particular locus can often be better defined.

Intracarotid amobarbital or Wada testing

Wada testing has long been the mainstay for the determination of the lateralization or the dominant hemisphere and, in particular, the dominant temporal lobe and is often performed in the perioperative evaluation phase to determine language dominance and memory dependence so as to avoid resections of these eloquent areas. Through the selective intra-arterial injection of amobarbital, the language and memory ability in a functionally sedated hemisphere as well as the capacity of the contralateral side to support those functions after resection can be determined. This type of evaluation, though, requires cooperation through a long and arduous exam and, rarely performed in children <9–10 years old, can be done in children as young as 5 years old.[45]

Preliminary studies using fMR during language and memory tasks have been promising and fMR may eventually be used to identify these eloquent functions for the younger age groups. It is important to again note that the extent of language and memory dominance remain unclear in the younger child. Since these functions may be bilaterally represented until 9–10 years of age, it is questionable whether there is any interference of function after a resection of the 'dominant' side in the young child when dominance may not yet be lateralized. Wada memory performance was prognostic of seizure outcome with asymmetries consistent with the lateralization of the seizure focus having an increased incidence of seizure relief postoperatively.[45]

Magnetoencephalography (MEG)

MEG imaging utilizes the principle that magnetic fields are created by the electrical activity of nerve cells, both cortical and subcortical. From these magnetic fields, MEG 'images' the brain by providing real time assessment of this activity and co-localizes the dipoles to the MR anatomy. MEG is now being tested for clinical usefulness in the surgical treatment of TLE. Early findings have shown that if there is spike localization on the MEG to the anterior temporal lobe or to a lesion, prognosis for a seizure-free outcome is good.[71] Further work though is necessary to identify those who would potentially benefit from pediatric surgical intervention.

Guidelines for patient selection following the non-invasive evaluation

Following the initial comprehensive evaluation, a discussion and decision is made by the multi-disciplinary epilepsy group regarding intervention. A decision to proceed directly to surgery for temporal lobectomy is usually reserved for the patient who has medically intractable seizures that are localized to the temporal lobe, with

concordance between the different data obtained, based on the clinical data (seizure semiology on video/EEG and neuro-psychological testing), EEG (ictal and/or interictal spikes), and neuroimaging-anatomical (MR) and/or functional (PET, SPECT). Patients with a higher degree of concordance of seizure focus localization, e.g. if the seizure semiology, scalp EEG and neuroimaging are correlative, are more likely to have a better seizure outcome.[73] In patients with unclear abnormalities or longer degree of concordance on the noninvasive evaluation, further investigation may be necessary prior to a recommendation for surgical resection, e.g. further functional imaging. If the data remain unclear as to the origin of the epileptic focus or there is evidence of bitemporal involvement either by imaging or EEG,[72] the recommendation to the family is to undergo further electro-physiologic evaluation using chronic invasive monitoring to obtain a higher degree of concordance.[73]

Chronic invasive monitoring

Previously, there was concern whether children could tolerate a chronic hospital stay with indwelling electrodes with little morbidity. Studies utilizing either depth and/or surface electrodes for chronic invasive monitoring in the evaluation of epileptic *foci* in children have shown that both may be underutilized modalities that are effective and safe in children.[59] Chronic invasive monitoring with indwelling electrodes, at present, may include multi-contact depth and/or surface electrodes such as grid and strip electrodes and has been widely discussed in the literature with regard to the evaluation of temporal lobe epilepsy.[58,70] Depth electrodes have historically been utilized most often and can be placed stereotactically with low morbidity. Since the majority of temporal lobe epilepsy in adults is secondary to medial temporal sclerosis,[74] depth electrodes have been the most efficacious for direct study of the medial structures in order to ascertain the extent and location of the pathologic process in these patients.[75] Depth electrodes can also be considered as an option in the evaluation of the temporal lobe in children and have been shown to be a safe modality, particularly when medial temporal lobe pathology is suspected.[76]

Invasive monitoring decisions are often more complicated in children than in adults since many young children, particularly below 12 years of age, have epileptic *foci* that are cortical and/or extra-temporal.[1,77] Pathologically, the epileptogenic zone results from an architectural abnormality rather than medial temporal sclerosis[6,19,42] and may not adequately defined with depth electrodes. Surface electrodes, such as grid and strip electrodes, can more precisely localize seizure *foci* of the lateral cortex and still adequately map the medial structures as well. They are placed through a craniotomy or a burr hole in the area that most likely represents the epileptogenic zone, as well as in contralateral sites if there is a question of lateralization. Another important benefit for children with surface electrodes is that following the localization and mapping of the seizure focus, cortical stimulation protocols can be performed in the patients with surface electrodes to define eloquent areas of cortex and their relationship to the epileptic focus. In selected patients, MR images are acquired following electrode placement and a 3-dimensional (3D) reconstruction of the data performed so as to provide an anatomic correlation of electrophysiologic and functional mapping.

Epidural grids have also been used to localize seizure *foci* in children.[78] Without interference of bone and scalp, these electrodes can further evaluate the cortical surface of the lateral neocortex of the temporal lobe through the dura with low morbidity. This monitoring is not useful for studying the amygdalohippocampal complex or orbitofrontal regions since medial propagation of electrical abnormalities from the contralateral side may confuse the lateralization and location of the seizure focus.

Guidelines for surgical intervention following invasive monitoring

The decision to proceed to surgical intervention, again, depends on the concordance and consistency of the collected data. If the invasive monitoring documents the initiation and propagation of a seizure focus and lateralizing and localizing unilaterally, the outcome for surgical intervention is enhanced. While, in the majority of cases, the seizure focus will lateralize to one side, bilateral *foci* occur in 20%–35% of patients with temporal lobe epilepsy.[79] While previously temporal lobectomy in these instances was contraindicated, more recently some have advocated an intervention if one side is the predominant seizure focus (>80% of the seizures are unilateral) with a resultant excellent outcome in approximately 50%.[80] This study, though, was performed in adults and there is presently no data in children. Whether seizure reduction alone is adequate for good overall outcome in children remains unclear.

At times, localization can be unresolved, particularly when the psychomotor manifestations precede the electrophysiologic abnormalities indicating a distant focus. Often, imaging can provide a clue that there is widespread abnormality including the temporal lobe. Orbitofrontal, cingulate, occipital epilepsies all may spread to the temporal lobe resulting in semiology that is temporal lobe specific. In these instances, further study of the suspected extratemporal regions using surface electrodes is required prior to a decision of surgical intervention.

Histopathology of temporal lobe epilepsy

The histopathologic findings in children with temporal lobe epilepsy are variable and may include congenital, neoplastic, vascular, inflammatory, traumatic, and/or infectious etiologies.[19,42] It is useful in these patients to understand how the different possible etiologies of epileptic *foci* may affect the decision for surgical intervention. In TLE, there are three major categories of pathologic findings.[81] The first is when the epileptogenic focus resides in the temporal neocortex and most often is due to cortical dysplasia.[82] Neocortical abnormalities are more commonly found in children and also include other congenital anomalies of cerebral development such as microgyria and heterotopias that result in architectural or structural anomalies. These anomalies may occur alone or in combination with other pathologies, e.g. mesial temporal sclerosis.[83] The seizures that arise in these children are most often medically intractable. The successful surgical intervention in these patients depends on adequately defining the extent of the 'abnormal' tissue. Noninvasive evaluation in conjunction with high resolution MRI and functional neuroimaging such as with PET or SPECT has had an increasing role in defining the seizure focus for this subpopulation of children.[47,84] Invasive monitoring with surface electrodes to map out the abnormal regions may still be used when the noninvasive evaluation is unable to adequately define the functional abnormality.

The second histopathologic category is termed 'lesion-related epilepsy' and occurs as a result of an intracranial mass. The pathologic substrates most often include low grade gliomas, gangliogliomas, hamartomas, vascular malformations, or, in rare cases, middle fossa arachnoid cysts with brain tumors being the most common pathology.[85] Scalp EEG localization and anatomic imaging are usually concordant and sufficient to lateralize the seizure focus. It is controversial in these patients whether the optimal treatment is a lesionectomy or whether a more standard, complete temporal lobectomy is required. It has been argued that it is not the lesion itself that is the source of seizures, but the margins around the lesion that may be the epileptogenic zone.[86] Many patients continue to have seizures after surgical resection of their lesion[87] and as a result, it remains unclear how to

best define the margins necessary to excise the lesion and control the seizures. Most agree that cortical mapping through invasive monitoring or electrocorticography (ECoG) has been useful, but obviously will not be necessary in the majority of patients. Noninvasive measures have been sought to best define the lesion and its seizure focus. Usually in these patients, there is no anatomic or functional hippocampal abnormality, yet it also remains unclear whether the medial structures can become altered by the abnormal electrical activity to become an alternate seizure focus. One approach is that if a lesion is discovered as part of the evaluation of new onset seizures, then lesionectomy alone is probably sufficient. If the patient suffers significant or intractable seizures more long-term prior to the discovery of the lesion, e.g. greater than one year, then more formal approach and mapping of the lesion and its surrounding tissue may be indicated. Electrophysiologic study of the lesional margins and the hippocampus is often performed intra- or extraoperatively to determine the epileptogenicity of these structures.

The last histopathologic category is MTS which is believed to cause seizures that originate in the medial structures, the hippocampus and/or amygdala. There is often a history of aberrant neurologic insult such as febrile seizures in early childhood with the subsequent development of complex partial seizures in later childhood or as an adult,[88] rather than a consequence of recurrent temporal lobe seizures.[50] Within the hippocampus, there is diffuse neuronal loss and gliosis and loss of the normal architecture, particularly in Sommer's sector (CA1 and prosubiculum), the end-folium (CA4 and hilus) and CA3 regions.[74,75] The other areas such as granule cell layer and CA2 are also severely damaged. The only region not as badly affected is the subiculum though there is some damage. The neuroimaging anomalies are as noted earlier and include increased signal on T2 or FLAIR MRI within the medial structures and/or decreased hippocampal volumes as well as functional abnormalities, e.g. unitemporal hypometabolism on PET scan).[58] There are often deficits on neuropsychological testing with generalized cognitive impairment as compared to lesional epilepsy[89] or failure of the memory portion on Wada testing.[90] MTS tends to be less common in children than in adults,[19,53,77,91] but occurs frequently in combination with cortical dysplasias in this population.[83] This dual pathology has also been hypothesized as a cause for early onset and high seizure frequency in children.

Surgical management

There are several techniques that have been used for temporal lobectomy for epilepsy. The original description by Penfield[92] which was later modified by Falconer and used in children[58] consisted of an *en bloc* resection of the temporal lobe and the medial structures. The procedure has undergone multiple changes in the past 30 years and for the most part, reflects different philosophies as to the etiology of the seizures and the further understanding of the histopathologic substrates. The differences in the techniques described are variations of the extent of the lateral resection and the approach to the medial temporal structures.

Surgical anatomy of the temporal lobe

As discussed above, anatomically there are two different regions that may be a source for temporal lobe seizures in children; the medial basal portion and the lateral neocortex. The medial basal portion includes the fusiform and the parahippocampal gyri as well as the amygdalohippocampal complex. Anteromedially the parahippocampal gyrus curves in front of the midbrain to form the uncus; immediately posterolateral to the uncus is entorhinal cortex. Medial to these structures lies the hippocampal formation; when approached from lateral to medial, the subiculum is the initial structure and

arises from the parahippocampal gyrus. Directly medial to the subiculum are the fields of the cornu ammonis (CA1–CA4) and the dentate gyrus. At the medial aspect of the temporal horn of the lateral ventricle, the body of the hippocampus is covered by the alveus which posteriorly, in the tail of the hippocampus, merges into the fimbria of the fornix. Within the ventricle and superomedial is the choroidal fissure and the choroid plexus which lies in the roof of the temporal horn and obtains its vascular supply from the anterior choroidal artery. The lateral neocortex consists of the superior and medial temporal gyri, and the anterior part of the inferior temporal gyrus. Though these cortical regions may be the source of the seizure focus, adjacent areas may contain eloquent or functionally important tissue, especially in the dominant hemisphere. The vascular supply to the temporal lobe consists of multiple perfusing vessels. There is a lateral and superolateral supply (the anterior temporal artery) from the middle cerebral artery as it enters from the sylvian fissure. The inferior surface of the temporal lobe is supplied by the posterior cerebral artery. The P2 and P3 segments traverse the posterior portion of the ambient cistern to reach the inferior part of the temporal lobe. The P2 segment also supplies the medial temporal structures, specifically part of the hippocampus and parahippocampal gyrus via the small Ammon's horn arteries. The anterior choroidal artery also contributes to the medial vasculature as it extends posteriorly from the internal carotid through the choroid plexus within the temporal horn and supplies part of the cascade of microvessels to the hippocampus and parahippocampal gyrus. Cranial nerves III and IV extend from the brainstem within the ambient cistern anteriorly along the edge of the tentorium. Injury to these nerves during a temporal lobectomy can be minimized by maintaining the integrity of the pia arachnoid border of the superior compartment, staying superior to the tentorial edge.

En-bloc or one stage removal

The original procedure for temporal lobectomy was developed and modified by Falconer in children[8] to remove the temporal lobe and medial structures safely and yet maintain the anatomical relationships. This allowed comprehensive study of the pathophysiology of the medial temporal structures and the detailed neuropathologic histology for patients with temporal lobe epilepsy.[74,75] The procedure consists of a subpial dissection along the sylvian fissure through the superior border of the superior temporal gyrus and sectioning medially through the isthmus of the temporal lobe and its origin. Following identification of the medial structures, the entire specimen is reflected laterally avoiding damage to the perforating vessels of the hippocampus or 'Ammon's horn' vessels which can be stretched or avulsed, causing damage to the parent artery. The final specimen includes the anterior temporal lobe and the amygdalohippocampal complex which is removed *en bloc*. This particular procedure is more difficult than the two phase removal since the gross specimen may be a hindrance to anatomical identification.

Two phase removal

The two phase resective procedure described by Spencer,[93] involves an initial anterolateral cortical resection, followed by a separate medial resection. The subpial dissection is initiated through the middle temporal gyrus at the level of the superior temporal sulcus and carried anteriorly across the superior temporal gyrus beyond the sphenoid wing. The resection is deepened posteriorly and superiorly until entry into the temporal horn of the lateral ventricle, and the anterolateral temporal lobe resected using suction aspiration through the white matter. The medial structures (the amygdalo-hippocampal complex) are removed as part of the second phase using microscopic magnification. Following unroofing of the temporal horn, the hippocampus is resected subpially, maintaining the integrity of the arachnoidal border between the middle and posterior fossae. The perforating arteries are selectively coagulated as they arise from the anterior choroidal and posterior cerebral arteries and pass through the pia arachnoid into the hippocampal complex. The amygdala can be removed along with the hippocampus or suction-aspirated along its medial extent. The two phase removal still allows for a complete removal of the temporal lobe but maintains the anatomic landmarks for pathologic confirmation and further examination of the resection specimens.

Tailored temporal lobectomy

This procedure, advocated by Ojemann and his colleagues at the University of Washington,[94] 'tailors' each resection of the lateral neocortex to avoid eloquent areas such as language. Using this approach, the abnormal cortex is resected based on the patient's interictal epileptiform activity and adjacent regions of eloquent cortex determined intraoperatively. Localization is achieved by mapping the electrical abnormalities using ECoG and the language areas are defined in awake patients using intraoperative cortical stimulations and language paradigms. Once the mapping is completed, the anterior temporal lobectomy can be performed so as to avoid the functional areas and safely resect the abnormal regions. The hippocampus is removed as necessary depending on the pre- and intra-operative studies. This method has not been strongly advocated in children since it is difficult to perform the awake studies or surgery in preadolescent children. As well, the issue of hemispheric dominance in pre-teenage children remains unclear. This methodology is therefore more useful in older adolescent children with dominant temporal lobe epilepsy.

Amygdalohippocampectomy

The method of selective amygdalohippo-campectomy has been advocated for patients with non-lesional temporal lobe epilepsy by Yasagil *et al.*[95] In this approach, the amygdalo-hippocampal complex is resected via a trans-Sylvian approach which avoids an anterolateral temporal lobectomy completely. This methodology is obviously not used for patients with suspected lesional or temporal neocortical abnormalities. The sylvian fissure is opened, exposing the middle cerebral artery branches (M2 segments) and the anterior one-third of the insula. The temporal horn is then entered at the base of the superior temporal gyrus and through the anterior temporal stem which allows access to the amygdala and the hippocampus. The amygdalo-hippocampal complex is then removed *en bloc* dissection via a subpial dissection. Though more technically difficult, this resection allows for the focal removal of the etiologic epileptogenic zone leaving the rest of the temporal lobe untouched. This approach, in Dr Yasargil's hands, has comparable results to the other more standard temporal lobectomy series.[95]

Radiosurgical treatment of temporal lobe epilepsy

The more recent introduction of radiosurgery in the treatment of TLE in children raises the possibility of 'minimally' invasive treatment for epilepsy. It has previously been reported that radiosurgical treatment of lesions, (e.g.) arterio-venous malformations, in patients with seizures has resulted in relief of seizures in many.[96] The antiepileptic effect of the radiosurgery in both adults and children remain unknown, but is believed to be both an indirect effect through the obliteration of the lesion, and a direct effect of the radiation on the epileptic tissue.[97,98] It has been postulated that 'radiosurgical' resection of the amygdalohippocampal complex would be a noninvasive method for the treatment of medial temporal epilepsy.[99] While radiosurgical dosing had been developed, for an *in situ* resection, others have been interested in using lower dosing of the radiation in order to 'modulate' hippocampal function. In one study, low dose radiosurgery (50% isodose level at 18 Gray) though failed to control seizures in patients with temporal lobe epilepsy.[100] There is only limited data in this area,[98,100] and further studies are needed not only in regard to dosage and conformational strategies, but efficacy in children where radiation may be contra-indicated.

Complications

At the present time, major morbidity for elective temporal lobe resections is infrequent. In early series', there was a less than 0.5% chance of mortality[101] with the most recent randomized control trial having a 0% mortality,[9] with a morbidity rate for surgical complications in the range of 2%–8%.[9,85,102] The most common that have been described are neurologic injuries as a direct result of the resection of eloquent cortex or interruption of white matter tracts or indirectly through a vascular injury with the resultant ischemic complication. The most common adverse effect is a homonymous superior quadrantanopsia which occurs when there is interruption of the optic tract and/or its radia-tions via Meyer's loop during the medial or posterior resection of the temporal lobe.[103] The risk can be reduced by limiting the posterior and superior extent of the anterolateral resection. Language or verbal deficits occur when language areas of the dominant hemisphere are resected. Though this is often not a problem in children less than 9 years of age and often transient[2,103] avoidance of these areas can be achieved via the tailored approach or limiting the resection posteriorly and inferior to the superior temporal gyrus on the dominant side. Manipulation hemiplegia occurs when there is manipulation and possible vasospasm of the Sylvian vessels following *en bloc* resections.[104] A similar neurologic injury can occur with interference of the perforating vessels to the internal capsule from the anterior choroidal artery or posterior cerebral artery which may induce stroke or ischemia to the posterior limb of the internal capsule or corticospinal tract within the brainstem. Careful dissection of the medial structures and the identification of the Ammon's horn arteries prior to coagulation and sectioning of the vessels can help to avoid this complication. Complications of infection and postoperative meningitis, both infectious and non-infectious, have also been known to occur following temporal lobectomy in both adults[105] and in children.[2,7,19]

Outcome

A postoperative evaluation of these patients is routinely performed at 6 months after surgery in addition to a 1 and 2 year follow-up. The final outcome assessment consists of a battery of radiologic, EEG, and neuropsychologic testing. Seizure outcome is mainly dependent on diagnosis and clinical factors. The optimal outcome for epilepsy surgery is usually achieved when a specific seizure focus has been localized preoperatively. This has been especially true in patients with temporal lobe epilepsy where seizure control following temporal resection, ranges between a 60%–90% marked reduction and/or complete elimination of seizures. Other preoperative factors associated with good seizure outcome and control include low seizure frequency, absence of status epilepticus, concordant lateralizing memory deficit, clear abnormality on MR images, suspected ganglioglioma or dysembryoplastic neuroepithelial tumor (DNET), and absence of dysplasia on MR images.[106] Good outcome was also seen more frequently in patients with a shorter interval from seizure onset to surgery and operated on at an earlier age.[107] A good outcome is thought to be dependent on the extent of mesiobasal resection or, in instances of temporal neocortical resection, the complete removal of the epileptogenic zone.[93,108] In the pediatric series, there are similarly high range of good outcomes with over 75% having improvement in seizure frequency or complete control; less than 5%–10% show no improvement. Davidson and Falconer[7] reported an 85% seizure free/marked reduction in seizure outcome in 40 children who underwent temporal lobectomy. Similarly, Adelson *et al.*[19] had an 87% good or excellent outcome in 33 patients. Others have reported similar results.[42,85,109,110] Recently, Blume *et al.*[52] reported 100% seizure-free outcomes in patients selectively chosen for surgery with only EEG and neuroimaging criteria. No specific reports have looked at the outcome differences between temporal lobectomy techniques in children. There is little evidence that outcomes differ with the different surgical approaches and it is most likely that patient selection correlates best with outcome.[52,94] Children with MTS or lesional epilepsy often have better postoperative seizure control than atypical TLE.[89] With longer term follow-up, even in children who were seizure-free, seizure recurrence can occur in 25% of cases even upwards of 15 years.[111,112] Again, prognostic factors of good, long-term outcome is focal EEG discharge and MR finding of low grade tumor. Poor prognostic factors include generalized EEG discharges and normal MR.[111,113]

Improvements in seizure outcome have not been the sole beneficial effect of temporal lobe resections in children. Earlier surgery has been advocated in children in order to avoid the long-term complications of epileptic drug toxicity and intractable seizures on intellectual and behavioral development and psychosocial maturation.[8,19,85] The effect of improving behavior, function and neuropsychologic outcomes has been shown in multiple studies,[2,15,35] but was first noted by Falconer[8] in the early 1970's. Rausch *et al.*[114] reported improvement in intellectual function and psychosocial adjustment in many patients following temporal lobe surgery with a reduction or elimination of seizure frequency. They found in their series of children a ten point gain on average on full scale IQ mostly in the area of performance IQ rather than verbal IQ[115] which can facilitate rehabilitation to an age appropriate psychosocial development following surgery and seizure control. The best outcomes in children occur when surgery was performed in or prior to adolescence.[114,116,117] As well, the shorter interval between onset and surgical control of the seizures has been shown to have the greatest likelihood of postoperative improvement in IQ.[2] It remains controversial whether improvements in IQ are due to the surgical intervention or lessened medication needs, but clearly better and complete seizure control has been shown to reverse adverse behavioral and intellectual declines and may even, more importantly, enhance the quality of life of these children.[116,118] Neuropsychological results are improved after resection if the resection is limited to an epileptic focus and lesion.[106] In a study by Gleissuer *et al.*,[119] left temporal resection showed an increased decline in learning and delayed recall and performed significantly lower than right-sided resection. These declines were associated with a higher preoperative performance, but were also reversible by 1 year following surgery in the majority of children.

Summary

Most often seizures in childhood are self limited and/or controllable with medical therapy. Because intractable seizures and prolonged anticonvulsant medication can adversely affect intellectual development and psychosocial maturation in children, it is important to identify those children who will not respond to medical therapy. Temporal lobectomies for complex partial seizures of temporal lobe origin in children have been recommended since they can be performed with minimal morbidity. With improvement in our neuroimaging capabilities and evaluative procedures, more children can be identified earlier who might benefit from a resective procedure. Temporal lobectomy in carefully selected children can have a significant impact and benefit with gains in both intellectual and behavioral function with seizure control and lessened medication needs thus improving overall quality of life. Children with temporal lobe epilepsy with intractable seizures should have early evaluation and surgical intervention in order to maximize their long-term improvement in seizure control and psychosocial development. Different techniques exist for temporal lobe resections in children, but any operation must specifically address the particular pathologic process and extent of the temporal epileptogenic zone.

Pearls

1. Intractable seizures in children have a 'malignant' natural history, with eventual declines in both intellectual and behavioral functions.
2. Children with imaging abnormalities rarely 'outgrow' their seizures. The addition of further medication regimens beyond second-line medications in children with temporal lobe imaging abnormalities concordant with the EEG will not likely lead to a seizure-free state.
3. In children, the pathologic substrate may vary, but the epileptogenic zone is usually either lateral neocortical or mediobasal.
4. Early surgery in children with MTS leads to an overall improved chance of seizure-free state and improved outcome with regard to cognitive and neuropsychologic measures.
5. If a patient has had seizures for less than a year and is found to have a lesion, they can be treated for the lesion alone with excision with a high likelihood of curing the seizures. If the seizures have been occurring for more than a year, in children with lesions, then they are less likely to be cured with lesional resection alone and may need to be additionally evaluated and treated for their epilepsy.
6. Surgery remains superior to continued

medical therapy with regard to outcome, morbidity and mortality in children with intractable temporal lobe epilepsy. With the advent of minimally invasive approaches with improved surgical techniques and the possibility of radiosurgical options in the future, further improvements in outcome with less likelihood of complications from surgery are likely.

References

1. Hauser WA. Seizure disorders: The changes with age. *Epilepsia* 1992;**4**:S6–S14.
2. Meyer FB, Marsh WR, Laws ER, *et al.* Temporal lobectomy in children with epilepsy. *J Neurosurg* 1986;**64**:371–6.
3. Cowan LD, Bodensteiner JB, Leviton A, *et al.* Prevalence of the epilepsies in children and adolescents. *Epilepsia* 1989;**30**:94–106.
4. National Commission for the Control of Epilepsy and its Consequences: Plan for a Nationwide Action on Epilepsy, *DHEW Publications* No. (NIH) 1977:78–276.
5. Peacock WJ, Comair Y, Chugani HT, *et al.* Epilepsy surgery in childhood. In: Luders H (ed). *Epilepsy Surgery*. New York: Raven Press; 1991:589–98.
6. Rasmussen T. Results of cortical resection in focal epilepsy. Advances in epileptology. 15th Epilepsy International Symposium. New York: Raven Press; 1984:449–55.
7. Davidson S, Falconer MA. Outcome of surgery in 40 children with temporal lobe epilepsy. *Lancet* 1973;**1**:1260–3.
8. Falconer MA. Neurosurgery (Volume 14). In: Logue V (ed). *Operative Surgery*. Philadelphia: Lippincott; 1971:142.
9. Wiebe S, Blume WT, Girvin JP, Eliasziw M. A randomized, controlled trial of surgery for temporal-lobe epilepsy. *N Engl J Med* 2001;**345**:311–18.
10. Westerveld M, Sass KJ, Chelune GJ, *et al.* Temporal lobectomy in children: Cognitive outcome. *J Neurosurg* 200;**92**:24–30.
11. Hennessy MJ, Elwes RD, Honavar M, Rabe-Hesketh S, Binnie CD, Polkey CE. Predictors of outcome and pathological considerations in surgical treatment of intractable epilepsy associated with temporal lobe lesions. *J Neurol Neurosurg Psychiatry* 2001;**70**:450–8.
12. Adelson PD. The surgical management of epilepsy in childhood: A review. *Neurosurg Q* 1996;**6**:1–20.
13. Adelson PD. Temporal lobectomy in children with intractable seizures. *Pediatr Neurosurg* 2001;**34**:268–77.
14. Rao MB, Radhakrishna K. Is epilepsy surgery possible in countries with limited resources? *Epilepsia* 2000;**41** (Suppl 4):S31–S34.
15. Lindsey J, Ounsted C, Richards P. Long-term outcome in children with temporal lobe seizures: Social outcome and childhood factors. *Dev Med Child Neurol* 1979;**21**:630–6.
16. Holmes GL. The long-term effects of seizures on the developing brain: Clinical and laboratory issues. *Brain Dev* 1991b;**13**:393–409.
17. Jalava M, Sillanpaa M, Camfield C, *et al.* Social adjustment and competence 35 years after onset of childhood epilepsy: A prospective controlled study. *Epilepsia* 1997;**38**:708–15.
18. Duchowny M, Levin B, Iayakar P, *et al.* Neurobiologic considerations in early surgery for epilepsy. *J Child Neurol* 1994;**9**:42–49.
19. Adelson PD, Peacock WJ, Chugani HT, *et al.* Temporal and extended temporal resections for the treatment of intractable seizures in early childhood. *Pediatr Neurosurg* 1992;**18**:169–78.
20. Blume WT, Girvin JP, Kaufmann JC. Childhood brain tumors presenting as chronic uncontrolled focal seizure disorders. *Ann Neurol* 1982;**12**:538–41.
21. Gerris F. Clinical aspects and long-term prognosis of intracranial tumors in infancy and childhood. *Dev Med Child Neurol* 1976;**18**:145–59.
22. Holmes GL. Do seizures cause brain damage? *Epilepsia* 1991a;**32**:514–28.
23. Diaz J, Schain RJ, Bailey BG. Phenobarbital-induced brain growth retardation in artificially reared rat pups. *Biol Neonate* 1977;**32**:77–82.
24. Diaz J, Schain RJ. Phenobarbital: Effects of long-term administration on behavior and brain of artificially reared rats. *Science* 1978;**199**:90–91.
25. Camfield CS, Chaplin S, Doyle AB, *et al.* Side-effects of phenobarbital in toddlers; behavioral and cognitive aspects. *J Pediatr* 1979;**95**:361–5.
26. Vining EP, Mellitis D, Dorsen MM, *et al.* Psychological and behavioral effects of antiepileptic drugs in children: A double blind comparison between phenobarbital and valproic acid. *Pediatrics* 1987;**80**:165–74.
27. Herranz JL, Armijo JA, Artega R. Clinical side-effects of phenobarbital, primidone, phenytoin,

carbamazapine, and valproate during monotherapy in children. *Epilepsia* 1988;**29**:794–804.

28. Farwell JR, Dodrill CB, Batzel LW. Neuropsychological abilities of children with epilepsy. *Epilepsia* 1985;**26**:395–400.

29. Rodin EA, Schmaltz S, Twitty G. Intellectual functions of patients with childhood-onset epilepsy. *Dev Med Child Neurol* 1986;**28**:25–33.

30. Shields WD, Peacock WJ, Roper SN. Surgery for Epilepsy: Special pediatric considerations. In: Silbergeld DL, Ojemann GA (eds). *Epilepsy Surgery. Neurosurgery Clinics of North America* 1993;**4**: 301–10. Philadelphia: W.B. Saunders.

31. Shewmon DA, Shields WD, Chugani HT, *et al.* Contrasts between pediatric and adult epilepsy: Rational and strategy for focal resection. *J Epilepsy* 1990;**3**:141–55.

32. Holmes GL. Epilepsy in the developing brain: Lessons from the laboratory and clinic. *Epilepsia* 1997;**38**:12–30.

33. Fogarasi A, Jokeit H, Faveret E, Janszky J, Tuxhorn I. The effect of age on seizure semiology in children temporal lobe epilepsy. *Epilepsia* 2002;**43**:638–43.

34. Holmes MD, Born DE, Kutsy RL, Wilensky AJ, Ojemann GA, Ojemann LM. Outcome after surgery in patients with refractory temporal lobe epilepsy and normal MRI. *Seizure* 2000;**9**:407–11.

35. Brown WI. Structural substrates of seizure *foci* in the human temporal lobe: A combined electrophysiological optical microscopic and ultrastructural study. In: Brazier MAB (ed). *Epilepsy: Its phenomena in man.* New York: Academic Press, 1973:339–74.

36. Cavanagh JB, Meyer A. Aetiological aspects of Ammon's horn sclerosis associated with temporal lobe epilepsy. *Br Med J* 1956;**44**:1403–7.

37. National Institutes of Health. Surgery for epilepsy. *Consensus Statement* 1990;**8**:1–20.

38. Holmes GL. Surgery for intractable seizures in infancy and early childhood. *Neurology* 1993;**43**: 28–37.

39. Mattson RH, Cramer JA, Collins JF, *et al.* Comparison of carbamazepine, phenobarbital, phenytoin, and premadone in partial and secondarily generalized tonic–clonic seizures. *N Engl J Med* 1985; **313**:145–51.

40. Penry JK. Perspectives in complex partial seizures. *Adv Neurol* 1975;**11**:1–11.

41. Rich KM, Goldring S, Gado M. Computed tomography in chronic seizure disorder caused by glioma. *Arch Neurol* 1985;**42**:26–27.

42. Jay V, Becker LE, Otsubo H, *et al.* Pathology of temporal lobectomy for refractory seizures in children: Review of 20 cases including some unique malformative lesions. *J Neurosurg* 1993;**79**:53–61.

43. Blume WT, Hwang PA. Pediatric candidates for temporal lobe epilepsy surgery. *Can J Neurol Sci* 2000;**27** (Suppl 1):S14–S19; discussion S20–S21.

44. Olson DM, Chugani HT, Shewmon DA, *et al.* Electrocorticographic confirmation of focal positron emission tomographic abnormalities in children with intractable epilepsy. *Epilepsia* 1990;**31**:731–9.

45. Henry TR, Van Heertum RL. Positron emission tomography and single photon emission computed tomography in epilepsy care. *Semin Nucl Med* 2003; **33**:88–104.

46. Laxer KD, Garcia PA. Imaging criteria to identify the epileptic focus. In: Silbergeld DL, Ojemann GA (eds). *Epilepsy Surgery. Neurosurgery Clinics of North America* 1993;**4**:199–209. Philadelphia: W.B. Saunders.

47. Chugani HT. PET in preoperative evaluation of intractable epilepsy. *Ped Neurol* 1994;**9**:411–13.

48. Jack CR, Krecke KN, Luetmer PH, *et al.* Diagnosis of mesial temporal sclerosis with conventional versus fast spin-echo MR imaging. *Radiology* 1994;**192**: 123–7.

49. Jack CR, Rydberg CH, Krecke KN, *et al.* Mesial temporal sclerosis: Diagnosis with fluid-attenuated inversion-recovery versus spin-echo MR imaging. *Radiology* 1996;**199**:367–73.

50. Keller SS, Wieshmann UC, Mackay CE, Denby CE, Webb J, Roberts N. Voxel-based morphometry of grey matter abnormalities in patients with medically intractable temporal lobe epilepsy: Effects of side of seizure onset and epilepsy duration. *J Neurol Neurosurg Psychiatry* 2003;**73**:648–55.

51. Schwartz TH, Marks D, Pak J, *et al.* Standardization of amygdalohippocampectomy with intraoperative magnetic resonance imaging: preliminary experience. *Epilepsia* 2002;**43**:430–6.

52. Blume WT, Girvin JP, McLachlan RS, *et al.* Effective temporal lobectomy in childhood without invasive EEG. *Epilepsia* 1997;**38**:164–67.

53. Duchowny M, Levin B, Jayakar P, *et al.* Temporal lobectomy in early childhood. *Epilepsia* 1992;**33**: 298–303.

54. Benbadis SR, Wallace J, Reed Murtagh F. MRI evidence of mesial temporal sclerosis in subjects without seizures. *Seizure* 2002;**11**:340–3.

55. Hubesch B, Marineier DS, Hetherington HP, *et al.*

Clinical MRS studies of the brain. *Invest Radiol* 1989; **24**:1039–42.

56. Connelly A, Jackson GD, Duncan JS, *et al.* Magnetic resonance spectroscopy in temporal lobe epilepsy. *Neurology* 1994;**44**:1411–17.

57. Abou-Khalil BW, Siegel GI, Sackellares JC, *et al.* Positron emission tomography studies of cerebral glucose metabolism in chronic partial epilepsy. *Ann Neurol* 1987;**22**:480–6.

58. Engel J, Kuhl DE, Phelps ME. Comparative localization of epileptic *foci* in parietal epilepsy by PET and EEG. *Ann Neurol* 1982;**12**:529–37.

59. Adelson PD, Black PMcL, Kramer U, *et al.* The use of grid and strip electrodes to identify a seizure focus in children. *Pediatr Neurosurg* 1997;**22**:174–180.

60. Chugani HT, Phelps ME, Shewmon DA, *et al.* Cerebral glucose utilization in intractable neonatal seizures and the developing brain. In: *Neonatal Seizures.* New York: Raven Press; 1990a.

61. Chugani RT, Shewmon DA, Peacock WJ, *et al.* Surgical treatment of intractable neonatal-onset seizures: The role of positron emission tomography. *Neurology* 1988;**38**:1178–88.

62. Theodore WR, Sato S, Kufta C, *et al.* Temporal lobectomy for uncontrolled seizures: The role of positron emission tomography. *Ann Neurol* 1992;**32:**789–94.

63. Franck G, Sadzot B, Salmon E, *et al.* Regional cerebral blood flow and metabolic rates in human focal epilepsy and status epilepticus. *Adv Neurol* 1986;**44**:935–48.

64. Roman RW, Devous MD, Stokely EM, *et al.* Correlation of EEG findings and cerebral blood flow in patients with partial seizures. *Neurology* 1984;**34** (Suppl 1):124–5.

65. Ochs RF, Yamamoto L, Gloor P, *et al.* Correlation between positron emission tomography measurement of glucose metabolism and oxygen utilization with focal epilepsy. *Neurology* 1984;**34** (Suppl 1):125.

66. Rowe CC, Berkovic SF, Austin MC, *et al.* Patterns of post-ictal cerebral blood flow in temporal lobe epilepsy: Qualitative and quantitative analysis. *Neurology* 1991;**41**:1096–1103.

67. Rowe CC, Berkovic SF, Sia ST, *et al.* Localization of epileptic *foci* with post-ictal single photon emission computed tomography. *Ann Neurol* 1989;**26**:660–8.

68. Harvey AS, Bowe JM, Hopkins IJ, *et al.* Ictal [99mTc]-HMPAO single photon emission computed tomography in children with temporal lobe epilepsy. *Epilepsia* 1993;**34**:869–77.

69. Lynch BJ, O'Tuama L, Holmes GL, *et al.* Correlation of [Tc99-m]HMPAO SPECT with EEG monitoring: prognostic value for outcome of epilepsy surgery in children. *Ann Neurol* 1992;**32**:433–4.

70. Sperling MR, O'Connor MJ. Comparison of depth subdural electrodes in recording temporal lobe seizure. *Neurology* 1989;**39**:1497–1504.

71. Iwasaki M, Nakasato N, Shamoto H, *et al.* Surgical implications of neuromagnetic spike localization in temporal lobe epilepsy. *Epilepsia* 2002;**43**:415–24.

72. Diehl B, Luders HO. Temporal lobe epilepsy: When are invasive recordings needed? *Epilepsia* 2000;**41** (Suppl 3):S61–S74.

73. Labiner DM, Weinand ME, Brainerd CJ, Ahern GL, Herring AM, Melgar MA. Prognostic value of concordant seizure focus localizing data in the selection of temporal lobectomy candidates. *Neurol Res* 2002;**24**:747–55.

74. Babb TL, Brown WJ. Pathological findings in epilepsy. In: Engel JE (ed). *Surgical Treatment of the Epilepsies.* New York: Raven Press; 1987:511–40.

75. Scheibel ME, Scheibel AB. Hippocampal pathology in temporal lobe epilepsy: A Golgi Survey. In: Brazier MAB (ed). *Epilepsy: Its phenomena in man.* New York: Academic Press; 1973:311–37.

76. Adelson PD, Albright AL, Gerszten PC, *et al.* Seizure focus localization using stereotactic depth electrodes in children. *Surg Neurol* 1997; in revision.

77. Duchowny MS. Surgery for intractable epilepsy: Issues and outcome. *Pediatrics* 1989;**84**:886–94.

78. Goldring S. A method for surgical management of focal epilepsy, especially as it relates to children. *J Neurosurg* 1978;**49**:344–56.

79. So NK. Depth electrode studies in mesial temporal epilepsy. In: Luders H (ed). *Epilepsy Surgery.* New York: Raven Press; 1991:371–84.

80. So NK, Olivier A, Andermann F, Gloor P, Quesney LF. Results of surgical treatment in patients with bitemporal epileptiform abnormalities. *Ann Neurol* 1989;**25**:432–39.

81. Fried I. Anatomic temporal lobe resections for temporal lobe epilepsy. In: Silbergeld DL, Ojemann GA (eds). *Epilepsy Surgery. Neurosurgery Clinics of North America* 1993;**4**:233–43. Philadelphia: W.B. Saunders.

82. Kuzniecky R. Neuroimaging in pediatric epilepsy. *Epilepsia* 1996;**37**:S10–S21.

83. Bocti C, Robitaille Y, Diadori P, *et al.* The pathological basis of temporal lobe epilepsy in childhood. *Neurology* 2003;**60**:191–5.

84. Chugani HT, Shields WD, Shewmon DA, *et al.* Infantile spasms: I. PET identifies focal cortical dysgenesis in cryptogenic cases for surgical treatment. *Ann Neurol* 1990b;**27:**406–13.

85. Sinclair DB, Aronyk K, Snyder T, *et al.* Pediatric temporal lobectomy for epilepsy. *Pediatr Neurosurg* 2003;**38:**195–205.

86. Drake J, Hoffman HJ, Kobayashi J, Hwang P, Becker L. Surgical management of children with temporal lobe epilepsy and mass lesions. *Neurosurgery* 1987;**21:**792–7.

87. Pollack IF, Claassen D, Al-Shboul Q, *et al.* Low grade gliomas of the cerebral hemispheres in children: An analysis of 71 cases. *J Neurosurg* 1995;**82:**536–47.

88. Taylor DC, Ounsted C. Age, sex, and hemispheric vulnerability in the outcome of seizures in response to fever. *Clin Dev Med* 1991;**40:**266–273.

89. York MK, Rettig GM, Grossman RG, *et al.* Seizure control and cognitive outcome after temporal lobectomy: A comparison of classic Ammon's horn sclerosis, atypical mesial temporal sclerosis, and tumoral pathologies. *Epilepsia* 2003;**44:**387–98.

90. Rausch R, Babb TL, Engel JE. Memory following intracarotid amobarbital injection contralateral to hippocampal damage. *Arch Neurol* 1989;**46:**783–8.

91. Wyllie E; Chee M, Granstrom ML, *et al.* Temporal lobe epilepsy in early childhood. *Epilepsia* 1993;**34:**859–68.

92. Penfield W, Flanigin H. Surgical therapy of temporal lobe seizures. *Arch Neurol* 1950;**64:**491–500.

93. Spencer DD, Spencer SS, Mattson RH, *et al.* Access to the posterior medial temporal lobe structures and the surgical treatment of temporal lobe epilepsy. *Neurosurgery* 1984;**15:**667–70.

94. Silbergeld DL, Ojemann GA. The tailored temporal lobectomy. In: Silbergeld DL, Ojemann GA (eds). *Epilepsy Surgery. Neurosurgery Clinics of North America* 1993:273–82. Philadelphia: W.B. Saunders.

95. Yasargil MG, Wieser HG, Valavanis A, *et al.* Surgery and results of selective amygdalohippocampectomy in one hundred patients with nonlesional epilepsy. In: Silbergeld DL, Ojemann GA (eds). *Epilepsy Surgery. Neurosurgery Clinics of North America* 1993;**4:**243–61.

96. Gerszten PC, Adelson PD, Kondziolka D, *et al.* Seizure outcome in children treated for arteriovenous malformations using gamma knife radiosurgery. *Pediatr Neurosurg* 1996;**24:**139–44.

97. Heikkinen ER, Konnov B, Melnikov L, *et al.* Relief of epilepsy by radiosurgery of cerebral arteriovenous malformations. *Stereotact Funct Neurosurg* 1989;**53:**157–66.

98. Barcia-Salorio IL, Barcia JA, Hernandez G, *et al.* Radiosurgery of epilepsy. Long-term results. *Acta Neurochir* 1994;**62** (Suppl):111–13.

99. Elomaa E. Focal irradiation of the brain: An alternative to temporal lobe resection in intractable focal epilepsy? *Med Hypotheses* 1980;**6:**501–3.

100. Kawai K, Suzuki I, Kurita H, Shin M, Arai N, Kirino T. Failure to low-dose radiosurgery to control temporal lobe epilepsy. *J Neurosurg* 2001;**95:**883–7.

101. Van Buren JM. Complications of surgical procedures in the diagnosis and treatment of epilepsy. In: J Engel (ed). *Surgical Treatment of the Epilepsies.* New York: Raven Press; 1987:465–75.

102. Pilcher WH, Rusyniak WG. Complications of epilepsy surgery. In: Silbergeld DL, Ojemann GA (eds). *Epilepsy Surgery. Neurosurgery Clinics of North America* 1993;**4:**311–25. Philadelphia: W.B. Saunders.

103. Buchhalter JR, Jarrar RG. Therapeutics in pediatric epilepsy, Part 2: Epilepsy surgery and vagus nerve stimulation. *Mayo Clin Proc* 2003;**78:**371–8.

104. Penfield W, Lende, Rasmussen T. Manipulation hemiplegia. *J Neurosurg* 1961;**18:**760.

105. Girvin JP. Complications of epilepsy surgery. In: Luders H (ed). *Epilepsy Surgery.* New York: Raven Press; 1991:653–60.

106. Clusmann H, Schramm J, Kral T, *et al.* Prognostic factors and outcome after different types of resection for temporal lobe epilepsy. *J Neurosurg* 2002;**97:**1131–41.

107. Prevedello DM, Sandmann MC, Ebner A. Prognostic factors in mesial temporal lobe epilepsy surgery. *Arq Neuropsiquiatr* 2000;**58:**207–13.

108. Awad IA, Katz A, Hahn JF, *et al.* Extent of resection in temporal lobectomy for epilepsy. I. Interobserver analysis and correlation with seizure outcome. *Epilepsia* 1989;**30:**756–62.

109. Morrison G, Duchowny M, Resnick T, *et al.* Epilepsy surgery in childhood. *Pediatr Neurosurg* 1992;**18:**291–7.

110. Fish DR, Smith SI, Quesney LF, *et al.* Surgical treatment of children with medically intractable frontal or temporal lobe epilepsy: Results and highlights of 40 years experience. *Epilepsia* 1993;**34:**244–7.

111. Sotero de Menezes MA, Connolly M, Bolanos A, Madsen J, Black PM, Riviello JJ Jr. Temporal lobectomy in early childhood: The need for long-term follow-up. *J Child Neurol* 2001;**16:**585–90.

112. Jarrar RG, Buchhalter JR, Meyer FB, Sharbrough FW, Laws E. Long-term follow-up of temporal lobectomy in children. *Neurology* 2002;**59**:1635–7.

113. Hennessy MJ, Elwes RD, Rabe-Hesketh S, Binnie CD, Polkey CE. Prognostic factors in the surgical treatment of medically intractable epilepsy associated with mesial temporal sclerosis. *Acta Neurol Scand* 2001;**103**:344–50.

114. Rausch R, Crandall PH. Psychological status related to surgical control of temporal lobe seizures. *Epilepsia* 1982;**23**:191–202.

115. Miranda C, Smith ML. Predictors of intelligence after temporal lobectomy in children with epilepsy. *Epilepsy Behav* 2001;**2**:13–19.

116. Bittar RG, Rosenfeld JV, Klug GL, Hopkins IJ, Simon Harvey A. Resective surgery in infants and young children with intractable epilepsy. *J Clin Neurosci* 2002;**9**:142–6.

117. Cross JH. Epilepsy surgery in childhood. *Epilepsia* 2002;**43** (Suppl 3):65–70.

118. Markand ON, Salanova V, Whelihan E, Emsley CL. Health-related quality of life outcome in medically refractory epilepsy treated with anterior temporal lobectomy. *Epilepsia* 2002;**41**:749–59.

119. Gleissner U, Sassen R, Lendt M, Clusmann H, Elger CE, Helmstaedter C. Pre- and post-operative verbal memory in pediatric patients with temporal lobe epilepsy. *Epilepsy Res* 2002;**51**:287–96.

22

Lesional epilepsy surgery—'Spike chasing' is not necessary

MALLA BHASKARA RAO

Epilepsy surgery is the resection or modification of part of the brain with the aim of alleviating seizures.[1] With the advent of magnetic resonance imaging (MRI), there has been an increase in the use of operative procedures for lesional epileptic syndromes. In lesional epilepsy surgery, the surgical procedure is directed at the structural lesion believed to be the aetiology of the seizure disorder and complete resection of the lesion appears crucial for freedom from seizures.[2] A number of options are available to assess the completeness of resection. However, there is considerable argument as to the need for and extent of resection of regions beyond the boundaries of the lesion, as well as the role of electrocorticography (ECoG) and 'spike chasing'.[3,4] This chapter will address some of the pertinent issues with an emphasis on the structural rather than ECoG-guided resections.

A historical note

In the early days of epilepsy surgery, treatment was primarily directed at lesions.[5] John H. Jackson (1820–1903) pointed out that a chronic seizure disorder could be the initial and only symptom of a foreign-tissue lesion, such as a tumour, vascular malformation, or cicatrix. On the basis of this concept, Victor Horsley (1857–1916) performed resective surgery for epileptogenic lesions. Subsequently, with the introduction of electroencephalography (EEG) by Hans Berger (1873–1941) in 1929, Wilder Penfield (1891–1976) and Herbert Jasper (1906–1999) attempted to identify and resect the epileptogenic zones along with the lesional pathology. The status of ECoG, however, has always been uncertain. Murray Falconer (1910–1977), who pioneered the standard *en bloc* anterior temporal lobectomy at the Maudsley Hospital, always performed pre- and post-resection ECoG, but never used spike data to change the operative plan.

Pathology

Lesional epilepsy surgery is based on the assumption that the seizure disorder and the presence of a lesion are interrelated. The lesions associated with intractable epilepsy can be classified into neoplastic lesions, vascular lesions, gliotic (post-traumatic and post-inflammatory) and developmental substrates.[6] Most of these lesions are not believed to be epileptogenic per se; rather, the epileptogenicity is due to excitability of the surrounding cortex. The extent of the cortical distribution of pre-excision epileptiform activity (EA) has been found to vary substantially from patient to patient, irrespective of the type of underlying lesion, i.e. neoplasm, associated vascular malformation (AVM) or hamartoma. The potential relationships between circumscribed structural lesions and cortical epileptogenicity are numerous. Tumours have been suggested to induce epileptogenicity through infiltrative, oedematous or compressive disruption of the normal cortical architecture and metabolism, or through disconnection and subsequent denervation supersensitivity of the peri-tumoural cortex. An AVM may induce epileptogenicity in the peri-lesional cortex secondary to either local ischaemic 'steal' phenomena or haemosiderin-induced cortical damage related to a previous haemorrhage. Cortical dysplastic lesions have been convincingly shown to have an intrinsic epileptogenicity related to their abnormal cytoarchitecture. The potential of an epileptogenic lesion to induce distant EA through secondary epileptogenesis has been demonstrated in patients with neoplastic lesions.

Cavernomas lack neuronal elements and histopathological changes in the adjacent cortex would seem essential to the development of seizures. Indeed, interictal spike activity has been localized to the vicinity of cavernomas by magnetoencephalography (MEG) and excellent seizure control has been achieved through lesionectomy of the cavernoma together with the adjacent cortex stained by haemosiderin.[7] In patients with cavernoma, epileptogenesis may result from progressive, intermittent or chronic bleeding and iron deposition around the lesion. One could argue that significant micro-bleeding at a crucial stage of brain development can result in functional changes similar to those in malformations of cortical development.[8]

Pre-surgical evaluation

The presence of a lesion in a patient with refractory partial epilepsy does not invariably indicate that the lesion is responsible for the seizures.[9] Patients with long-standing temporal neocortical lesions may develop hippocampal atrophy (dual pathology).[10] The primary lesion, the secondary hippocampal sclerosis, or both may be responsible for the seizures. There is a consensus that a comprehensive epilepsy pre-surgical evaluation should be performed in patients with a lesional epileptic syndrome associated with pharmaco-resistant seizures, in order to establish a relationship between the MRI-identified lesion and the site of the epileptic brain tissue.[11] When there is discordance between the anatomical lesion and the presumed epileptogenic focus, or in patients with multiple lesions, in which case a single epileptogenic lesion is not always easy to isolate, the causal relationship between lesion and seizures needs to be established. Without question, the lesion may, on occasion, be remote or not contiguous with the ictal onset zone. This is especially a concern when the nature of the lesional pathology is more widespread, such as in focal encephalomalacia or neuronal migration disorders.[12]

For patients with epileptogenic lesions located at or near the regions of the cortex dealing with primary motor, sensory or language functions, several non-invasive tools of functional mapping have been developed. These include magneto-encephalography, $H_2^{15}O$ positron emission tomography and more recently, functional MRI.[13]

When there is a good correlation among the characteristics of the seizures, the neuro-radiological findings and the location of the EEG abnormalities, it is probable that favourable results can be obtained by performing resection of the lesion alone, without invasive preoperative work up. Invasive recordings, powerful but expensive and time-consuming techniques, are required when there is a disagreement among the clinical, anatomical and electrophysiological findings that is not resolved by ictal video-EEG and functional imaging (PET and SPECT).[14] Despite their invasive nature and the inherent risk they carry of causing morbidity, the indication for invasive recordings must be carefully evaluated for each individual case and should not be dismissed too easily. For instance, these types of recordings could be proposed not only for use in cases in which the data obtained from clinical or other investigation modalities are in disagreement, but also for lesions adjacent to the functional cortex or after failure of a lesionectomy. However, from a technical standpoint, the use of these techniques (subdural recordings or stereo-electroencephalography) can be more difficult to achieve and interpret if the patient has undergone a previous lesionectomy. Recent advances in MEG and magnetic source imaging (MSI) have been accompanied by a renewed interest in non-invasive localization of interictal spikes in the planning of epilepsy surgery, especially for extratemporal epilepsy.[15]

Surgical approaches

The surgical approach often depends on the preoperative and intraoperative identification of the particular structural substrate.[2] The operative strategy may include: (i) lesionectomy, i.e. complete lesion excision, as determined by MRI, without attempting to resect the epileptogenic zone; (ii) extended lesionectomy, i.e. resection of the lesion with margins; (iii) resection of the lesion and the epileptogenic zone; and (iv) resection of the epileptogenic zone without resecting the lesion.

The most common resection strategy involves excision of the lesion with a margin around the lesion.[6] The extent of the resection may be determined by different criteria. Radiologically, the margins can be determined by MRI signal abnormalities, by intraoperative visualization of the tissue, navigational system and intraoperative ultrasound. The histological margins of the lesion can be identified by the intraoperative frozen section evaluation of the tissue, and epileptogenic focus can be identified by the intraoperative ECoG. A combination of radiological, histological and electrocorticographic techniques may be used to determine the extent of the resection.

Incomplete resection may result if the lesion is poorly differentiated from the normal brain. The use of systems that provide 'image-guided surgical capabilities' or intraoperative imaging is likely to help solve this problem. The second cause of incomplete resection is the extension of the structural abnormalities to a functional area. Multiple subpial transections have reportedly been successful in alleviating this problem.[16,17]

Electrocorticography and 'spike chasing'

Electrocorticography refers to acute intraoperative recording. The ECoG-guided surgical approach is based on the premise that resection of the lesion, even with its immediate margins, may not be sufficient. Basically, intraoperative ECoG is an interictal recording. Therefore, it is restricted to the definition of the irritative zone and thus, has its limitations when it comes to delineating the epileptogenic zone or eloquent cortices. This technique may provide prognostic information by indicating the areas of residual electric discharges after the resection of the lesion or what was thought to be the seizure focus. It is important to remember, however, that residual spikes in adjacent areas of the brain do not reliably predict residual epileptogenicity, nor does their absence guarantee postoperative seizure control.

Intraoperative ECoG has been used for guiding the extent of the surgical resection of the epileptogenic zone, extending the resection to include all of the active interictal spikes (so-called 'spike chasing').[18] In addition, the presence of spikes in the rim of the resection or at a more distant location has been used for the prognostication of the outcome of the surgery in terms of seizures. Intraoperative ECoG is performed mostly for extratemporal epilepsies after non-invasive evaluation to determine the border of extended lesionectomy in patients with neocortical lesions distant from eloquent areas. On occasion, ECoG is a useful investigation which may provide crucial information that makes effective resection possible. It is particularly useful in the surgery of intrinsically epileptogenic lesions, like focal cortical dysplasia, as continuous ictal or ictal-like electrographic activity can be identified in 65% of patients.[19]

Intraoperative ECoG is still used in many centres, although its efficacy in determining the outcome of surgery after temporal lobe resections is debated.[3,4,20] Some authors have emphasized the importance of pre- and post-resection ECoG in guiding the extent of both medial and lateral temporal lobe resections, while others have advocated a standard operation, regardless of the ECoG findings.[4,21]

Cendes *et al.* performed ECoG before and after selective amygdalo-hippocampectomy and reported an increase in spike activity after surgical resection.[22] Spikes recorded in the unresected cortex were significantly more frequent after resection and 62% of patients had new spikes on post-resection electrocorticograms. Neither finding was predictive of postoperative seizures. That residual spikes tended to become more frequent and that new spikes appeared post-resection may represent either response to injury, disconnection from mesial structures in particular or release from the influence of any perilesional inhibitory cortex included in the resection. Schwartz *et al.* found no correlation between the presence of post-excisional spikes outside the resected area and the outcome in terms of seizures.[4] McKhann *et al.* have described the efficacy of hippocampal ECoG in predicting the extent of the hippocampal resection in temporal lobe epilepsy (TLE).[23]

The major disadvantage of ECoG is its duration, which must be limited to brief intra-operative periods. Further, it is often complicated by anaesthetic effects. General anaesthesia has a variety of effects, both of an excitatory and inhibitory nature, on the activity and these may be responsible for its limited usefulness. Inter-ictal discharges are variable in location, and intraoperative time constraints lead to sampling errors and the lack of recording of seizures.

Experience of routine ECoG is required to recognize anomalous findings. It is performed routinely at some centres, but the extent of resection has rarely been dictated by ECoG and has depended, instead, on anatomical constraints and the feasibility of complete removal of a lesion.[2,24]

Surgical outcome

Lesional epilepsy surgery has generally yielded excellent results. In a series of 195 cases, 66.6% of patients were seizure-free following lesional surgery and an additional 21.5% improved significantly.[25] The outcome is related to the preoperative duration and severity of epilepsy, as well as the type of surgical procedure. In a surgical series of 51 patients, Cohen *et al.* reported that complete remission of seizures was observed after lesionectomy in 100% of patients with only one preoperative seizure or a seizure history lasting less than 2 months; complete remission was achieved in 75%–80% of all patients with 2–5 seizures or a seizure history lasting 2–12 months; and only 50%–55% of those with more than 5 seizures or with preoperative seizure histories lasting more than a year attained complete remission.[26] A meta-analysis evaluating seizure outcome following either lesionectomy or a combination of lesionectomy and corticectomy concluded that at 2 years' follow-up, the percentage of patients with persistent seizures following lesionectomy ranged from 1.4 to 4 times the percentage of those who had persistent seizures following the combined procedure.[27] Low-grade gliomas, gangliogliomas and vascular malformations were most successfully treated with lesionectomy and corticectomy. In contrast, patients with fewer seizures before presentation, shorter preoperative seizure histories, or seizures that responded to antiepileptic medications were more likely to be seizure-free following lesionectomy alone.[25] In the case of patients with temporal lesions and intractable epilepsy, studies have shown that a simple lesionectomy without resection of mesial structures results in a low rate of control of seizures, ranging from 20%–45%. In cases of extratemporal lesional epilepsy, resection of only the lesion has yielded favourable results, with the rate of seizure control varying from 65%–95%.[28]

Several earlier studies analysed the ECoG and seizure outcomes.[3,4,19,22,29,30] With the exception of spikes in the insula, which are not predictive of postoperative seizures, there has been little agreement on the value of ECoG for temporal lobectomies. Some investigators have concluded that if there is any remaining epileptiform activity after resection, it adversely affects the outcome.[18,20,31] Others, however, have found post-resection spikes to be less useful in predicting the postoperative seizure status.[3,4] Wyllie *et al.* reported that failure to eliminate all interictal spikes defined by chronic extraoperative subdural recordings correlated with poor seizure outcomes, whereas post-resection intraoperative electrocorticographic spikes did not.[32] Extratemporal lesions may require more invasive presurgical evaluations to identify surgical candidates and various intraoperative methods including ECoG to achieve good surgical outcomes.[24,33]

Current preferences

Patients with fewer seizures before presentation, shorter preoperative seizure histories, or seizures that responded to antiepileptic medications are more likely to be seizure-free following lesionectomy alone. Excision of low-grade tumours without resection of the surrounding cortex has been reported to be associated with a good outcome.[34–36]

However, in the case of intractable seizures, the current preference in lesional surgery is extended lesionectomy, i.e. resection of the lesion with its immediate margins.[6] These margins are determined by various methods and take into account the structural substrate, and electrophysiological as well as functional considerations.

For lesions that do not involve the critical cortex, it is possible to perform a generous resection that includes the lesion and the surrounding cortex. Low-grade gliomas, gangliogliomas and vascular malformations have been treated the most successfully with lesionectomy and corticectomy. The use of histological margins has been reported in a series of patients with intractable seizures associated with glial tumours.[37]

In patients with cavernous angiomas presenting with intractable epilepsy, although the pathophysiological mechanism appears to be very focal, several series have recorded suboptimal seizure outcomes following lesionectomies.[38] This could be due to incomplete resection of the haemosiderin-impregnated area or the existence of a dual pathology, specifically when the angioma is located in the mesial temporal lobe. An accepted management strategy is to resect the surrounding damaged cortex until the normal cortex is identified. This is often accomplished by gross inspection of the surrounding tissue, although histological section analysis can also detect haemosiderin, and the preoperative MRI may be helpful as haemosiderin deposits are apparent on T2-weighted images.

In patients with AVMs presenting with occasional seizures, the seizures may be controlled by excision of the nidus, without involving the adjacent cortex. However, AVMs presenting with intractable epilepsy may have developed epileptic *foci*, which correlate with the patient's age at the onset of the seizures, duration of the seizures and location of the lesions. The surgical management of these AVMs with respect to seizure outcome is controversial. Good seizure outcomes have been reported following resection of the AVMs and additional epileptogenic cortex.[39] Intraoperative electrocorticography is sometimes performed to further delineate the extent of the cortical epileptogenic zone. This technique may provide prognostic information by indicating the areas of residual electric discharges after the resection of the vascular malformation or what was thought to be the seizure focus. It is important to remember, however, that residual spikes in the adjacent areas of the brain do not reliably predict residual epileptogenicity, nor does their absence guarantee postoperative control of seizures.

Developmental lesions, even focal cortical dysplasias, often do not have clear margins. The MRI may not reveal the entire extent of the lesion and frozen section histological analysis of cortical dysplasias may be a formidable challenge. The gross appearance of these lesions may also be difficult to distinguish from that of normal tissue. Given their developmental nature, gangliogliomas and dysembryoplastic neuroepitheliomas are frequently associated with cortical dysplasia.[40] This could explain the persistent seizures following some lesionectomies. In dealing with this pathology, wide resection of the gyrus involved is recommended rather than a pure lesionectomy. If the seizures persist, an invasive electrode study is indicated. The results suggest that in children with extratemporal dysembrioplastic neuroepithelial tumours (DNTs), complete lesionectomy alone, without invasive pre-surgical investigations, is effective for long-term control of seizures. For children with temporal DNTs not invading the amygdalohippocampal complex, extensive pre-surgical evaluations seem to be indicated.[41]

Surgery for focal cortical dysplasia (FCD) can benefit many patients, especially if complete resection of the abnormal regions is possible. The preoperative work up should include high-resolution MRI, video telemetry and EEG. It is important to recognize that the MRI findings may be normal in some cases and that the regions of histological FCD may extend beyond the abnormal areas identified on MR images. Intraoperative monitoring frequently includes ECoG and cortical stimulation for motor mapping. Sometimes, if the lesion is near the central sulcus, it includes somatosensory evoked potentials. Complete resection, however, does not necessarily predict cessation of seizures. Despite the removal of all the tissue associated with epileptiform discharges in the EEG or ECoG findings, the control of seizures has remained poor in some patients. Thus, the concept of combined resection of areas showing radiological and electrophysiological abnormalities has been emphasized.[19] The regions of dysplasia could contain normally functioning tissue, which would preclude aggressive resection and warrant avoiding significant neurological deficits.[42]

Lesions in the primary motor, sensory or language cortex may be treated with strict lesionectomy. This may be feasible only with stereotactically guided lesionectomy, corticectomy, lesionectomy guided by EEG localization and functional mapping or resection combined with multiple subpial transaction. An important surgical consideration is that developmental lesions in proximity to critical cortex should not displace or transfer function to the opposite hemisphere. Hence, in the primary cortex or speech areas, surgery can be performed under local anaesthesia to avoid or minimize neurological deficits. In the temporal lobe, strict lesion resection guided by neuroimaging may be less efficacious in controlling seizures than in other cortical regions. The minimalistic approach may be especially useful for lesions located in extra-temporal cortical regions, which are of critical importance to motor, sensory or language function.

Conclusion

Epilepsy surgery centres in the developing countries will encounter a sizable number of patients with lesional epilepsy syndromes.[43,44] Extensive pre-surgical evaluation, including invasive monitoring, and neuronavigation as well as electrophysiology-guided surgical procedures may be limited to only a few centres due to dearth of infrastructure, funding and expertise. However, centres with limited resources can also achieve excellent results by initially restricting the surgical candidacy to patients selected on the basis of results obtained from locally available, relatively inexpensive and non-invasive technologies.[45] There seems to be little justification for the higher cost of and greater time required for intraoperative ECoG when a diagnosis of mesial temporal lobe epilepsy has been made. For difficult cases, a staged approach may be an appropriate management strategy. This approach consists of excising the lesion and the surrounding epileptogenic brain tissue during an initial operation, and carrying out more extensive investigations of the remaining epileptogenicity and possibly opting for further treatment only in those uncommon cases in which seizures persist after lesionectomy.

References

1. Engel J Jr. Surgery for seizures. *N Engl J Med* 1996; **334**:647–52.
2. Awad IA, Rosenfeld J, Ahl H, *et al.* Intractable epilepsy and structural lesions of the brain: Mapping, resection strategies and seizure outcome. *Epilepsia* 1991;**32**:179–86.
3. Cascino GD, Trenerry MR, Jack CRJ. Electrocorticography and temporal lobe epilepsy: Relationship to quantitative MRI and operative outcome. *Epilepsia* 1995;**36**:692–6.
4. Schwartz TH, Bazil CW, Walczack TS, *et al.* The predictive value of intraoperative electrocorticography in resections for limbic epilepsy associated with mesial temporal sclerosis. *Neurosurgery* 1997;**40**:302–11.
5. Engel J Jr. Historical perspectives. In: Engel J Jr (ed). *Surgical treatment of the epilepsies*. New York: Raven Press; 1993:695–705.
6. Fried I, Cascino GD. Lesional surgery. In: Engel J Jr (ed). *Surgical treatment of the epilepsies*. New York: Raven Press; 1993:501–9.
7. Awad I, Jabbour P. Cerebral cavernous malformations and epilepsy. *Neurosurg Focus* 2006;**21**:E7.
8. Paolini S, Morace R, Gennaro G, *et al.* Drug-resistant temporal lobe epilepsy due to cavernous malformations. *Neurosurg Focus* 2006;**21**:E8.
9. Rougier A. The epileptic focus versus the pathological focus. *Acta Neurochir Suppl* 1990;**50**:15.
10. Cendes F, Cook MJ, Watson C, *et al.* Frequency and characteristic of dual pathology in patients with lesional epilepsy. *Neurology* 1995;**45**:20–58.
11. Cascino GD, Boon PA, Fish DR. Surgically remediable lesional syndromes. In. Engel J Jr (ed). *Surgical treatment of the epilepsies*. New York: Raven Press, 1993:77–86.
12. Olivier A, Awad IA. Extratemporal resections. In: Engel J Jr (ed). *Surgical treatment of the epilepsies*. New York: Raven Press; 1993:489–500.
13. Spencer SS. The relative contributions of MRI, SPECT and PET imaging in epilepsy. *Epilepsia* 1994; **35**:S72–S89.
14. Lüders HO, Lesser RP, Dinner DS, *et al.* Chronic intracranial recording and stimulation using subdural electrodes. In. Engel J Jr (ed). *Surgical treatment of the epilepsies*. New York: Raven Press; 1987:297–321.
15. Ebersole J. Magnetoencephalography/magnetic source imaging in the assessment of patients with epilepsy. *Epilepsia* 1997;**38** (Suppl 4):1–5.
16. Morrell F, Whisler WW, Bleck TP. Multiple subpial transection: A new approach to the surgical treatment of focal epilepsy. *J Neurosurg* 1989;**70**:231–9.
17. Dogali M, Devinsky O, Luciano D, *et al.* Invasive intracranial monitoring, cortical resection and multiple subpial transection for the control of intractable complex partial seizure of cortical onset. *Stereotact Funct Neurosurg* 1994;**62**:222–5.
18. McBride MC, Binnie CD, Janota I, *et al.* Predictive value of intraoperative electrocorticograms in resective epilepsy surgery. *Ann Neurol* 1991;**30**: 526–32.
19. Palmini A, Gambardella A, Andermann F, *et al.* Intrinsic epileptogenicity of human dysplastic cortex as suggested by corticography and surgical results. *Ann Neurol* 1995;**37**:476–87.
20. Fiol ME, Gates JR, Torres F, *et al.* The prognostic value of residual spikes in the postexcision electrocorticogram after temporal lobectomy. *Neurology* 1991;**41**:512–16.
21. Polkey CE, Binnie CD, Janota I. Acute hippocampal recording and pathology at temporal lobe resection and amygdalo-hippocampectomy for epilepsy. *J Neurol Neurosurg Psychiatry* 1989;**52**:1050–7.
22. Cendes F, Dubeau F, Olivier A, *et al.* Increased neocortical spiking and surgical outcome after selective amygdalo-hippocampectomy. *Epilepsy Res* 1993;**16**:195–206.
23. McKhann GM 2nd, Schoenfeld-McNeill J, Born DE, *et al.* Intraoperative hippocampal electrocorticography to predict the extent of hippocampal resection in temporal lobe epilepsy surgery. *J Neurosurg* 2000;**93**:44–52.
24. Richard W, Luis FQ, Andres L, *et al.* Role of electrocorticography at surgery for lesion-related frontal lobe epilepsy. *Can J Neurol Sci* 1999;**26**:33–9.
25. Engel J Jr, Van Ness PC, Rasmussen TB, *et al.*

Outcome with respect to epileptic seizures. In: Engel J Jr (ed). *Surgical treatment of the epilepsies.* New York: Raven Press; 1993:609–21.

26. Cohen DS, Zubay GP, Goodman RR. Seizure outcome after lesionectomy for cavernous malformations. *J Neurosurg* 1995;**83**:237–42.

27. Weber JP, Silbergeld DL, Winn HR. Surgical resection of epileptogenic cortex associated with structural lesions. *Neurosurg Clin N Am* 1993;**4**:327–36.

28. Cascino GD, Kelly PJ, Sharbrough FW, *et al.* Long-term follow-up of stereotactic lesionectomy in partial epilepsy: Predictive factors and electro-encephalographic results. *Epilepsia* 1992;**33**:639–44.

29. Ferrier CH, Alarcon G, Engelsman J, *et al.* Relevance of residual histologic and electrocorticographic abnormalities for surgical outcome in frontal lobe epilepsy. *Epilepsia* 2001;**42**:363–71.

30. Pilcher WH, Silbergeld DL, Berger MS, *et al.* Intraoperative electrocorticography during tumor resection: Impact on seizure outcome in patients with gangliogliomas. *J Neurosurg* 1993;**78**:891–902.

31. Jooma R, Yeh HS, Privitera MD, *et al.* Lesionectomy versus electrophysiologically guided resection for temporal lobe tumors manifesting with complex partial seizures. *J Neurosurg* 1995;**83**:231–36.

32. Wyllie E, Luders H, Morris HH. Clinical outcome after complete or partial cortical resection for intractable epilepsy. *Neurology* 1987;**37**:1634–41.

33. Schramm J, Kral T, Kurthen M, *et al.* Surgery to treat frontal lobe epilepsy in adults. *Neurosurgery* 2002;**51**:644–55.

34. Chang EF, Potts MB, Keles GE, *et al.* Seizure characteristics and control following resection in 332 patients with low-grade gliomas. *J Neurosurg* 2008;**108**:227–35.

35. Kim S, Wang K, Cho B. Intractable seizures associated with brain tumor in childhood: lesionectomy and seizure outcome. *Childs Nerv Syst* 1995;**11**:634–8.

36. Kirkpatrick PJ, Honavar M, Janota L, *et al.* Control of temporal lobe epilepsy following *en bloc* resection of low-grade tumors. *J Neurosurg* 1993;**78**:19–25.

37. Fried I. Management of low-grade gliomas: Results of resections without electrocorticography. *Clin Neurosurg* 1995;**42**:453–63.

38. Siegel AM, Roberts DW, Harbaugh RE, *et al.* Pure lesionectomy versus tailored epilepsy surgery in treatment of cavernous malformations presenting with epilepsy. *Neurosurg Rev* 2000;**23**:80–3.

39. Yeh HS, Tew JM Jr, Gartner M. Seizure control after surgery on cerebral arteriovenous malformations. *J Neurosurg* 1993;**78**:12–18.

40. Krasimir M, Olivier K, Josette M, *et al.* Surgical strategies and seizure control in pediatric patients with dysembryoplastic neuroepithelial tumours: A single-institutional experience. *J Neurosurg Pediatrics* 2008;**1**:206–10.

41. Benifla M, Otsubo H, Ochi A, *et al.* Temporal lobe surgery for intractable epilepsy in children: An Analysis of outcome in 126 children. *Neurosurgery* 2006;**59**:1203–14.

42. Wang VY, Chang EF, Barbaro NM. Focal cortical dysplasia: A review of pathological features, genetics and surgical outcome. *Neurosurg Focus* 2006;**20**:E7.

43. Radhakrishnan V, Rao MB, Radhakrishnan K, *et al.* Pathology of temporal lobe epilepsy: An analysis of 100 consecutive surgical specimens from patients with medically refractory epilepsy. *Neurol India* 1999;**47**:196–201.

44. Sarkar C, Sharma MC, Deb P, *et al.* Neuro-pathological spectrum of lesions associated with intractable epilepsies: A 10-year experience with a series of 153 resections. *Neurol India* 2006;**54**:144–50.

45. Rao MB, Radhakrishnan K. Is epilepsy surgery possible in countries with limited resources? *Epilepsia* 2000;**41** (Suppl 4):S31–S34.

Electrocorticography for epilepsy surgery—'Spike chasing' is worthwhile

P. SARAT CHANDRA, SHAILESH JAIN, MANJARI TRIPATHI

Electrocorticography (ECoG) is a neurophysiological technique for measuring electrical activity directly from the exposed brain for the purpose of localizing the suspected focus of seizure in patients who are candidates for epilepsy surgery. The basic underlying principle is to record 'abnormal' voltages directly from the brain surface, thus potentially enhancing the accuracy to localize the 'epileptogenic zone' as opposed to the conventional electroencephalogram (EEG) where there is interposition of structures such as the skin, bone, etc. between the stimulus and the recording device.

ECoG has been in use for over four decades in the surgical treatment of patients with medically refractory epilepsy.[1,2] ECoG is used essentially to confirm and delineate the site and extent of the epileptogenic process before resection. After the resection has been completed, ECoG is used to determine whether all the potentially epileptogenic tissue has been removed. However, both these roles of ECoG have been questioned.

Despite various limitations, ECoG is an important tool to localize the epileptogenic *foci* intra-operatively. It is particularly useful in mapping out the epileptogenic *foci* in neocortical epilepsies, where the relatively large cortical surface allows an optimal recording before performing the surgery. ECoG is less accurate for temporal epilepsies because recording over the (lateral) temporal surface may not exactly map the epileptogenic area. Some authors have performed ECoG for determining the precise length for hippocampal resection by placing a strip over the hippocampal surface [*see* later].

ECoG

The technique

An ECoG records the same type of cerebral potentials as a scalp EEG, except that the recordings are much better due to the absence of dispersion of signals that occur in a scalp EEG due to the presence of scalp and skull. In theory, this should allow for better localization of the origin of the epileptogenic tissue causing habitual seizures in the patient. Because of the short recording time available for ECoG and the limitations of electrode placement posed by the surgical exposure, the possibility of recording ictal events is rare. An ECoG relies on the presence of interictal epileptiform discharges for the identification of the irritative/epileptic zone, which requires careful preoperative planning.

The clinical history, EEGs (both ictal and interictal), and imaging studies need to be carefully reviewed to define the area of resection and exposure needed for adequate ECoG recordings before surgery.[2]

The technique of recording an ECoG has changed little since its introduction. Continuous, close communication is required throughout the recording between the clinical neurophysiologist and the neurosurgeon. The clinical neurophysiologist must be able to read and interpret the recording as it is being done; modifications required in the position of electrodes and montages must be done at that time. This requires that the recording apparatus be either in the operating room or in the operating room gallery with a two-way communication system in place.

A standard 16-channel EEG equipment can give adequate ECoG recordings, though a higher number of channels would be more advantageous as it would allow the use of larger grids. For example, a 64-point grid electrode (8×8) would require a 64-channel machine, though such a large number of electrode contacts are rarely required. However, a tertiary centre which regularly performs epilepsy surgeries should have this provision. As ECoG records directly from the brain, modifications in recording sensitivities, filters, and time constants will be required. Electrodes need to be able to sit on the leptomeninges and move with the pulsations of the brain. Either flexible ball electrodes mounted on a fixed horseshoe frame or a series of electrodes implanted in a soft flexible silastic grid can be used. The advantage of ball electrodes over strip electrodes is that they can be sterilized and reused, cutting down costs. Owing to the lack of adequate techniques for sterilization, silastic implanted electrodes should be used only once. The authors use large wet cotton to enhance the contact with the brain surface.

For accurate localization of the epileptogenic area, the electrodes need to be placed an equal distance apart. Montages should consist of a minimum of 4 electrodes in a straight chain. The use of montages by angulated electrode placement should be avoided as this can lead to false localization. If simultaneous recording from multiple chains of electrodes is planned, the electrodes must be placed at equal distance in both vertical and horizontal planes. This will allow for bipolar as well as referential recordings to be done. When only single chains of electrodes are used, both referential and bipolar recordings should be done simultaneously. Various referential electrode placements can be used (such as mastoid, cervical region and bone flap).

To record from the deeper structures (such as the mesial temporal regions) either a 4-contact depth electrode can be inserted through the brain to reach the deeper structure or a flexible silastic 4-electrode grid can be inserted under the temporal/frontal region. The placement of a chain of electrodes over the cortical surface at the same time as the recording allows for a better understanding of the propagation of abnormal cerebral potentials.

The total recording time is about 30 minutes, although longer times are occasionally necessary. Methohexital and alfentanil have been reported to 'activate the epileptic zone'.[3,4] These techniques should be employed only after adequate standard recordings of the exposed brain have been done. Careful interpretation of the areas of 'activation' must be made as the potential to 'activate' regions outside the true irritative/epileptic zones has been reported.[4]

In adults, the ECoG is usually recorded when the patient is in the awake state; however, in children this is often not possible. The anaesthetic agents used for the operative procedure can have significant effects on the ECoG. Sufentanil, fentanyl, alfentanil, propofil methohexital have been reported to produce epileptiform changes on ECoG, whereas halothane, barbituates and benzodiazepines may suppress the epileptic activity.[3–7] Both nitrous oxide and isoflurane have been reported to affect the ECoG, but more recent reports have suggested that this is not the case when low concentrations are used.[8,9] For these reasons, it is recommended that in patients to be maintained on nitrous oxide, isoflurane and non-depolarizing muscle relaxants be used during ECoG recordings.

Electrical stimulation of the cortex has been used during ECoG recordings to localize the area of epileptic seizure onset, as well as to map the area of cortex responsible for motor, sensory and language functions. While the ECoG is being recorded, an electrical stimulus is delivered between two ball electrodes or between adjacent silastic enclosed electrodes. This stimulus consists of a 0.5–2 nsec diphasic pulse applied at 50–60 Hz over 1–5 sec with an intensity of 0.5–2.0 mA and a voltage of 1–15 V. The site of the patient's habitual seizure aura is noted, as well as the regions of maximal after-discharges. These discharges are in the form of high frequency stereotypic paroxysms such as spikes, rhythmical sharp waves or spike wave sequences. The discharge usually ends abruptly. It may be localized or spread to multiple electrode sites.

Grading an ECoG

It should be remembered that neither the 'abnormal' voltage recorded in ECoG nor the epileptogenic focus is homogeneous. Thus, grading the ECoG is important though this is rarely done. While a number of grading systems have been described in the literature, the authors prefer the one described by Mathern *et al.*[10–12] The grading scores are:

ECoG score 1: Normal background of mixed gamma, beta and alpha frequencies of moderate-to-low amplitude (i.e. usually 20–30 mV). A few low-amplitude spikes could be observed.

ECoG score 2: Loss of fast (120 Hz) background frequencies, but otherwise a background of mixed alpha, beta and delta frequencies of low-to-moderate amplitude. Repeated but non-continuous spikes, polyspikes or paroxysmal fast activity of medium amplitude are often observed.

ECoG score 3: Mostly 6–20 Hz background frequencies with some localized nearly continuous interictal epileptiform features of moderate amplitude or persistent repetitive spiking. Very rarely, electrographic seizures were captured.

ECoG score 4: Slow (16 Hz) background frequencies with continuous synchronous features of moderate-to-high amplitude. Multiple independent epileptiform abnormalities (polyspikes, paroxysmal fast activity and electrographic seizures) could be recorded.

ECoG score 5: Slow rhythmic usually synchronous background (14 Hz), often of high amplitude. Continuous synchronized or independent high-amplitude epileptiform abnormalities in multiple cortical sites could be observed. Ictal discharges were rarely recorded but observed in surrounding cortex.

ECoG scores of 2–5 are considered abnormal and these areas should always be included within the zone to be resected. The relevance of ECoG score 1 depends on the existing situation. For instance, if there is widespread hemispheric activity consistent with ECoG score 1 activity, then 'chasing the spikes' is avoided and the maximally abnormal area is resected. If this activity is more focal and the area is amenable to surgery, then resection is guided accordingly.[10–12]

Surgery should include a wide resection, making sure that the subcortical white matter is also included. If the ECoG shows abnormal activity over the motor or sensory cortex, a subpial transaction may also be performed. A post-resection ECoG is always advised by the authors. If significant abnormal activity was still noted from the margins, further resection should be performed.

Following surgery, the patient is continued on antiepileptic drugs (AEDs) and this should not be omitted either during surgery or the same day. If the patient was receiving phenytoin or valproate, a bolus injection should be given at the time of surgery. If he/she was receiving an AED with no injectable form available, then a double dose is given in the morning through a Ryle tube which is then removed. The same is repeated at night after surgery.

The outcome is classified using the Engel grade[14] (grades I to IV, where grade I represented being completely 'seizure-free' and was included in good outcome: *see* below).

Grade I: free of disabling seizures
Grade II: rare disabling seizures
Grade III: worthwhile improvement
Grade IV: no worthwhile improvement

Validity of ECoG

To examine the validity of ECoG, a Medline literature search from 1985 to the present was done using the key words electrocorticography, ECoG, intra-operative recording, and epilepsy. As complete coverage of the medical literature for a given topic using Medline is often incomplete, a search of the references quoted in each of the articles was made. The data were reviewed by type of resection (i.e. temporal, extratemporal or lesional) and the degree of evidence in support or against the use of ECoG for each of the previously stated reasons.

Non-lesional temporal lobe resections

According to Rasmussen,[13] the removal of the 'epileptogenic zone' (the anatomical site of onset of seizure), as well as the surrounding tissue which might be potentially recruited into the critical mass of tissue, is required for a successful surgical outcome. ECoG has been reported to provide useful information for the localization of the area at the time of surgery.[11–22]

Thirty-two papers on this topic were identified by our search technique. The review of these papers revealed little evidence to establish the true value of the procedure. The published reports are mainly retrospective case studies or case series without a proper control group. Some investigators have questioned the role of this procedure.[20] The potential advantages of ECoG are mentioned below with the corresponding literature review.

ECoG records epileptiform discharges similar to those seen on surface EEG: Epileptiform discharges were reported to have been recorded from the temporal lobe in all the papers identified by our search. These waveforms were similar to those recorded from the scalp EEG, consisting of isolated spikes, brief bursts of spikes or runs of sharp waves. They were often multifocal with a wide distribution over the exposed temporal cortex. More commonly, the epileptiform discharges were reported to have been recorded from the hippocampal structures and inferiomesial surfaces of the temporal tip. To a much lesser extent, they were recorded from the lateral temporal cortices and more so from the posterior temporal cortices.[15–21] Propagation of the epileptiform discharge was commonly seen from the hippocampus, to and from the subtemporal cortex.[22–25]

Interictal delta activity may be a useful predictor to localize the epileptogenic zone: Panet-Raymond *et al.*[26] have suggested that, in addition to these epileptiform discharges, delta wave activity might also give useful information as to the location of the epileptiform tissue in patients in whom spikes were not found on ECoG [*n*=40]. However, the authors do suggest caution when using this method in individual cases.

ECoG may provide additional information not seen on scalp EEG: In theory, ECoG recordings could be expected to provide information missed on a scalp EEG especially the activity from the mesial surface of the temporal lobe. Few studies have addressed this question. Devinsky *et al.*[27] in a retrospective review of 33 patients with medically refractory epilepsy, who underwent temporal lobectomy, found 8 patients in whom the ECoG recorded epileptiform discharges not previously found by scalp EEG even with the use of sphenoidal electrodes. On the other hand, Engel *et al.*[28] noted that no additional information was obtained from the ECoG compared with the preoperative scalp EEG.

ECoG is based on the hypothesis that the interictal epileptiform activity corresponds to the epileptogenic zone: ECoG seldom records ictal events, rather the interictal epileptiform activity. The relationship between the epileptic zone (area of origin of the epileptic seizure) and the irritative zone (area of maximum interictal epileptiform discharge) is not completely understood. In particular, the degree to which the two zones overlap, especially on the ECoG recording is unclear. It has been hypothesized that the more frequent these discharges are within an area, the more likely it is that this area lies within the epileptic zone.[25] Alarcon *et al.*[25] found that the removal of this area resulted in a significantly better chance of a good surgical outcome, even if areas of less frequent discharging were left untouched. If the area of maximal discharging was not completely resected, the surgical outcome was more likely to be poor. An earlier study by Tran *et al.*[29] had found no association between surgical outcome and frequency of epileptiform discharges. This study used the visual analysis of the ECoG recordings by the electroencephalographer, whereas Alarcon had used a computerized spike detection programme.

Electrical stimulation of the cortex at the time of ECoG may be a useful technique: Electrical stimulation of the cortex at the time of ECoG has been used in further localization of the epileptic zone.[1,17] The site of reproduction of the habitual aura of the patient by electrical cortical simulation has been reported by some investigators to have strong correlation with the epileptic zone.[30–32] This was particularly the case when the area from which the responses were elicited also coincided with the region exhibiting the greatest epileptic discharge. Gloor[17] commented that this was less likely to be the case if an after-discharge occurred, especially it if spreads to distant areas. In this situation the clinical symptoms may not be related to this area of stimuli, but reflect a distant area to which the discharge had spread.

After-discharges arising from electrical cortical stimulation are of questionable value in the localization of the epileptic zone. It is not uncommon for after-discharge to issue from regions of the brain from which no epileptiform abnormalities had been recorded on ECoG.[1,17,33] The thresholds for after-discharge has been reported to show considerable variability.[20]

New epileptiform discharges can appear after the excision; when along the margin of the resection, they may be representing a cortical disturbance caused by the manipulation of the brain at the time of surgery and may not have prognostic significance. Discharges that occur some distance away from the resection margin may be more predictive of a poor surgical outcome. These differences may explain the difference in the reported use of post-resection ECoG in predicting the surgical outcome. This could not be confirmed from the reported studies as the area of residual discharge in relation to the resection margin was often unclear.

Post-resection residual spikes have shown a relationship to the outcome: The role of the ECoG in determining the surgical outcome is unclear. McBride *et al.*[34] and Engel *et al.*[28] did not find an association between the site of dominant intra-operative ECoG epileptiform discharge and the surgical outcome. Correlation between the location of discharge and underlying pathology was also not found.[28]

Bengzon *et al.*[35] noted a significant difference in the surgical outcome between patients with residual spikes compared to those with spike-free post-resection recordings. Thirty-six percent of patients who were seizure-free post-surgery had residual spikes; whereas 75% of patients who were not seizure-free had residual spikes on post-resection ECoG. These findings were similar to those reported by Penfield *et al.*,[1] Fiol *et al.*,[36] Wyllie *et al.*,[37] Drake *et al.*,[38] Tanaka *et al.*[39] and McBride *et al.*[34]

Other investigators have not been able to confirm the relationship between the degree of epileptiform discharges seen on the post-resection ECoG and the outcome.[20,40–43] This was especially the case in patients in whom selective amygdalo-hippocampectomy was done. In this situation, new epileptiform discharges were often recorded from the temporal cortex after completion of the procedure. These discharges were found to have no predictive value.[44,45]

A possible explanation for the lack of consensus on the role of ECoG in the prediction of surgical outcome may lie in the surgical procedure itself. Most centres that have reported the use of ECoG have performed standardized temporal lobe resections. Only a few centres tailored the resection according to ECoG findings.[46]

Non-lesional extratemporal resections

Evidence in support of the use of ECoG in extratemporal resections is scant (six papers). Most of the literature pertaining to this topic is related to lesional cases and will be covered in that section. Quesney *et al.*[47–49] noted that in patients whose seizures originated in the frontal lobes there was no clear relationship between the amount of epileptogenic tissue removed and a successful surgical outcome. The reason for this may lie in the anatomical and functional peculiarities of this region, which permits the epileptiform discharge to vary in location from a specific region, to multilobular or even bifrontal. Similar findings have been noted in ECoG recordings of patients with seizures arising from the centroparietal region and occipital areas.[47–49] For patients with non-lesional, medically refractory extratemporal epilepsy, the use of subdural grid electrodes may provide the answer to this question. As this procedure allows ictal events to be recorded, there is a greater possibility that the epileptic zone will be identified. Another approach may involve the use of other imaging techniques, for example positron emission tomography (PET) along with more recent techniques with magnetic resonance imaging (MRI).[50,51]

Lesional, temporal and extra-temporal resections

ECoG may be useful in deciding the excision of the epileptogenic area surrounding the lesion: The use of ECoG in patients in whom structural lesions have been identified on imaging studies remains controversial. Traditional wisdom based on the experience of the Montreal Neurological Institute holds that optimum seizure control is achieved when the lesion is removed with the surrounding epileptogenic cortex as determined by an ECoG.[49–53] This viewpoint has been supported by Pilcher *et al.*[54] who found that 11 out of 12 patients who underwent surgery for ganglioglioma were seizure-free at 3.1 years post-surgery compared with a literature control of 21 out of 39 patients (54%) with ganglioglioma in whom only the lesion was resected. They noted that the epileptogenic zone was topographically distinct from the region of the tumour-involved brain. It usually encompassed a large surface area. Non-epileptiform high-amplitude slow waves were recorded on ECoG predominantly in tumour-involved cortex, while epileptiform spike discharges were recorded over the normal-appearing cortex. They felt that these discharges represented the epileptogenic zone. The removal of this area increased the chance of a better outcome.

Berger *et al.*[55] reported a series of children and adults with intractable epilepsy, associated with low-grade tumour. Forty-one out of 45 of these patients (91%) became seizure-free. The authors did not advocate the use of ECoG in patients with lesion and occasional or new onset of seizures, but felt it should be used in individuals with medically refractory epilepsy associated with low-grade tumour. This was particularly so in children, where there was a significantly better chance of seizure control. Cohen *et al.*[56] reported similar findings in 98 patients with cavernous haemangioma. Gonzalez *et al.*[57] also reported greater control of seizures when the tumour was resected with ECoG-guided removal of the seizure focus. Drake *et al.*[38] reported the results of a series of children with structural lesions of the temporal lobe using ECoG guidance. They emphasized the concept that seizure activity often originated from the brain tissue adjacent to the tumour.

Others have not felt that ECoG guidance is necessary in this group of patients. Resections have been restricted to the tumour margins as delineated on imaging studies and at the time of surgery.[53–55] The literature states that if the lesion has not been completely removed, seizures will continue despite the removal of the 'epileptogenic zone'.[56,57]

These studies have been based on retrospective reviews of case series. Comparison between ECoG-guided resections and non-ECoG-guided resection for similar groups of lesions have not been prospectively done. Tran *et al.*[63] attempted a controlled retrospective series review in which patients with structural lesions present underwent resection of the lesion to normal tissue margins. ECoG was recorded pre- and post-resection, but not used to determine the amount of surgical resection. Patient outcome was based upon seizure-free state. ECoGs were analysed for spike distribution and spike discharge rate. Spikes were found to be over the tumour bed as well as in the surrounding tissues. Spike distribution in the pre-resection ECoG did not correlate with outcome. On post-resection ECoG, spikes were noted along the edge of the resection as well as extra-marginally in equal amounts between patients who became seizure-free post-resection and those who did not. These findings support the use of lesionectomy as the first step in seizure control in lesional cases. Like temporal cortical resections, the presence of post-resection spikes does not appear to correlate with outcome. A case may be made for the use of ECoG in patients with dual pathology to assess the degree of epileptogenesis in the distant site.[64] Clarke *et al.*[65] have suggested that even in this case, the lesion must be removed if good seizure control is to be obtained.

ECoG is useful in lesional epilepsies with subtle structural changes seen on MR imaging, e.g. cortical dysplasia: Cortical dysplastic lesions are often associated with severe, partial epilepsies of childhood and can prove refractory to medical management leading to the need for surgical resection. Palmini *et al.*[66] have reported long runs of epileptiform discharges on ECoG consisting of repetitive electrographic seizures, repetitive bursting discharges or continuous rhythmic spiking. They felt that these discharges were often co-localized with the MRI-defined lesion. The completeness of resection of the epileptiform activity on ECoC correlated with the surgical outcome. We also found that ECoG-guided resections helped in achieving a better outcome.[67] Wennberg *et al.*[68] noted similar findings in lesion-related frontal lobe resection. This would suggest a role for ECoG in these cases to determine the location and extent of resection at the time of surgery. Holmes *et al.*[69] caution that neocortical lesions on MRI do not necessarily indicate the site of ictal onset of partial epilepsy.

Conclusion

For several decades, ECoG recordings have been routinely used in the surgical management of patients with medically refractory epilepsy. Using this technique, confirmation of epileptiform activity on pre-operative scalp EEG has usually been demonstrated at the time of surgery. It also allows for direct exploration and recording of the mesial surfaces of the cerebral cortex. There have been a number of studies where post-resection ECoG have clearly documented the usefulness in determining the 'residual' epileptogenic zone and subsequently better outcome on its resection. For medial temporal lesion, tailored resections of epileptogenic tissue have been found by some authors to be useful. Whether tailored resections have better outcome than standard resections of the temporal lobe, remains unclear. In order to answer this question, a carefully designed, controlled, prospective study will need to be done, controlling for variables such as the type of resection, location and degree of epileptiform disturbance on ECoG, and outcome measures such as seizure control and psychosocial status. It is possible that the results of ECoG-guided and standard temporal resection will be very similar, when the size and extent of the surgical resection will turn out to be the same in both groups.

The role of ECoG in extratemporal and lesional resection is different from that in the case of temporal resection. The ECoG appears to be beneficial in lesional resections in patients with refractory epilepsy. Its use in new-onset cases is less clear. Also its use in patients with dual pathology remains unclear. Controlled prospective studies again would be helpful.

Extratemporal resections need to be well planned before surgery. Imaging studies such as MRI and PET have proven helpful in localizing the site of epileptogenicity. The degree of electrographic spread of epileptiform discharges suggests that chronic intracranial recordings may be needed to provide more accurate and complete information about the seizure origin than intraoperative ECoG.

References

1. Penfield W, Jasper H. Electrocorticography. In: Penfield W, Jasper H (eds). *Functional anatomy of the human brain.* Boston: Little Brown; 1954:692–738.
2. Marson CA. Depth electrography and electrocorticography. In: Aminoff M (ed). *Electrodiagnosis in clinical neurology.* New York: Churchill Livingstone; 1980:167–96.
3. Wilder B, Musella L, Van Horn G, *et al.* Activation of spike and wave discharge in patients with generalized seizure. *Neurology* 1971;**21**:517–27.
4. Keene D, Roberts D, Splinter W, *et al.* Alfentanil mediated activation of epileptiform activity in the electrocorticogram during resection of epileptogenic foci. *Can J Neurol Sci* 1997;**24**:37–9.
5. Brain J, Seifen A, Tonic–clonic activity after sufentanil. *Anesth Analg* 1987;**66**:481–3.
6. Smith M, Smith SJ, Scott CA, *et al.* Activation of the electrocorticogram by propotol during surgery for epilepsy. *Br J Anaesth* 1996;**76**:499–502.
7. Kraemer D, Spencer D. Anesthesia in epilepsy surgery. In: Engel J (ed). *Surgical treatment of the epilepsy.* 2nd edn. New York: Raven Press; 1993:527–38.
8. Hosain S, Nagarajan L, Fraser R, *et al.* Effects of nitrous oxide on electrocorticography during epilepsy surgery. *Electroencephalogr Clin Neurophysiol* 1996;**102**:340–2.
9. Fiol M, Boening J, Cruz-Rodriquez R, et al. Effect of isoflurane (Forane) on intra-operative electrocorticogram. *Epilepsia* 1993;**34**:897–900.
10. Cepeda C, Andre VM, Levine MS, *et al.* Epileptogenesis in pediatric cortical dysplasia: The dysmature cerebral developmental hypothesis. *Epilepsy Behav* 2006;**9**:219–35.
11. Cepeda C, Andre VM, Vinters HV, *et al.* Are cytomegalic neurons and balloon cells generators of epileptic activity in pediatric cortical dysplasia? *Epilepsia* 2005;**46**:S82–S88.
12. Cepeda C, Andre VM, Flores-Hernandez J, *et al.* Pediatric cortical dysplasia: Correlations between neuroimaging, electrophysiology and location of cytomegalic neurons and balloon cells and glutamate-GABA synaptic circuits. *Dev Neurosci* 2005;**27**:59–76.
13. Rasmussen T. Characterization of a pure culture of frontal lobe epilepsy. *Epilepsia* 1983;**24**:482–93.
14. Engel J. Outcome with respect to epileptic seizures. In: Engel J (ed). *Surgical treatment of the epilepsies.* New York: Raven Press; 1987:553–71.
15. Green JR, Duisberg REH, McGrath WB. Electrocorticography in psychomotor epilepsy. *Electroencephalogr Clin Neurophysiol* 1949;(Suppl 2):30–7.
16. Walker A. Electrocorticography in epilepsy. *Electroencephalogr Clin Neurophysiol* 1949;(Suppl 2):30–7.
17. Gloor P. Contributions of electroencephalography and electrocorticography to the neurosurgical treatment of the epilepsy. In: Purpun DP, Peney JK, Walker RD (eds). *Advances in neurology.* New York: Raven Press; 1975:59–105.
18. Chatrian G, Quesney L. Intraoperative electrocorticography. In: Engel J, Pedley TA (eds). *Epilepsy: A comprehensive textbook.* Philadelphia: Lippincott-Raven; 1997:1749–65.
19. Stefon H, Quesney LP, Abou-Khahl B, *et al.* Electrocorticography in temporal lobe epilepsy surgery. *Acta Neurol Scand* 1991;**83**:65–72.
20. Walker E, Lichtenstien R, Marshall C. A critical analysis of electrocorticography in temporal lobe epilepsy. *Arch Neurol* 1960;**2**:172–82.
21. Tsai M, Chatrian G, Pauri F, *et al.* Electrocorticography in patients with medically intractable temporal lobe seizures. I. Quantification of epileptiform discharge prior to resective surgery. *Electroencephalogr Clin Neurophysiol* 1993;**87**:10–24.
22. Tsai M, Chatrian G, Holubkov A, *et al.* Electrocorticography in patients with medically intractable temporal lobe seizures. II. Quantification of epileptiform discharges following successive stages of resective surgery. *Electroencephalogr Clin Neurophysiol* 1993;**87**:25–37.
23. Kanazawa O, Blume W, Girvin J. Significance of spikes of temporal lobe electrocorticography. *Epilepsia* 1996;**37**:50–5.
24. Graf M, Niedermeyer J, Schiemann S, *et al.* Electrocorticography: Information derived from

intraoperative recordings during seizure surgery. *Clinical Electroencephalogram* 1984;**15**:83–91.

25. Alarcon G, Scoane J, Binne D, *et al.* Origin and prepagation of interictal discharges in the acute electrocorticogram. Implications for pathophysiology and surgical treatment of temporal lobe epilepsy. *Brain* 1997;**20**:2259–82.

26. Panet-Raymond D, Gotman J. Can slow waves in the electrocorticogram (ECOG) help localize epileptic foci? *Electroencephalogr Clin Neurophysiol* 1990;**75**:464–73.

27. Devinsky O, Canenini M, Seto S, *et al.* Quantative electrocorticortography in patients undergoing temporal lobectomy. *J Epilepsy* 1992;**5**:178–85.

28. Engel J, Falconer M, Driver MV. Electrophysiological correlation of pathology and surgical results in temporal lobe epilepsy. *Brain* 1976;**98**:129–56.

29. Tran T, Spencer S, Marks D, *et al.* Significance of spikes recorded on electrocorticography in non-lesional medical temporal lobe epilepsy. *Ann Neurol* 1995;**38**:763–70.

30. Bernier L, Richer F, Giard N, *et al.* Electric stimulation of the human brain in epilepsy. *Epilepsia* 1990;**31**:513–70.

31. Wieser HG, Bancand J, Talairach J, *et al.* Comparative value of spontaneous and electrically induced seizures in establishing the lateralization of temporal seizure. *Epilepsia* 1979;**70**:47–9.

32. Halgren E, Walter RD, Cherlow DG, *et al.* Mental phenomena evoked by electrical stimulation of the hippocampal formation and amygdala. *Brain* 1978;**101**:83–117.

33. Ajmone MC. Electrocortigraphy. In: Remon A (ed). *Handbook of electroencephalogram and clinical neurophysiology.* Vol. 10C. Amsterdam: Elsevier; 1973:3–49.

34. McBride MD, Binnie CD, Janta I, *et al.* Predictive value of intraoperative electrocorticograms in resective epilepsy surgery. *Ann Neurol* 1991;**30**: 526–32.

35. Bengzon ARA, Rasmussen T, Gloor P, *et al.* Prognostic factors in the surgical treatment of temporal lobe epilepsies. *Neurology* 1968;**18**: 717–31.

36. Fiol M, Galis J, Torres Fernand, *et al.* The prognostic value of residual spikes in the postexcision electrocorticogram after temporal lobectomy. *Neurology* 1991;**41**:512–16.

37. Wyllie E, Luders H, Morris A, *et al.* Clinical outcome after complete or partial cortical resection for intractable epilepsy. *Neurology* 1987;**37**:1634–41.

38. Drake G, Hoffman H, Kobayashi J. Surgical management of children with temporal lobe epilepsy and mass lesions. *Neurosurgery* 1987;**21**:792–7.

39. Tanaka T, Hashizume K, Kunimoto M, *et al.* Intraoperative electrocorticography in children with medically intractable epilepsy. *Neurol Med Chir* 1996;**26**:440–6.

40. Falconer MA. Discussion. In: Baldwin M, Bailey P (eds). *Temporal lobe epilepsy.* Springfield IL: Charles C. Thomas; 1958:483–4.

41. Ajmone-Marsan C. ECOG in temporal lobe epilepsy. In: Baldwin M, Bailey P (eds). *Temporal lobe epilepsy.* Springfield IL: Charles C. Thomas; 1958:368–95.

42. Fenyes I, Zoltan I, Fenyes G. Temporal lobe epilepsies with deep-seated epileptogenic foci. *Arch Neurol* 1961;**4**:103–15.

43. Gibbs FA, Amader L, Rich C. Electroencephalographic findings and therapeutic results in surgical treatment of psychomotor epilepsy. In: Baldwin M, Baily P (eds). *Temporal lobe epilepsy.* Springfield II: Charles C. Thomas; 1958:358–67.

44. Cendes F, Dubeau F, Olivier A, *et al.* Increased neocortical spiking and surgical outcome after section amygdala-hippocampectomy. *Epilepsy Res* 1993;**16**:195–206.

45. Blume W, Parent A, Kaibara M. Stereotactic amygdala hippocampotomy and mesial temporal spikes. *Epilepsia* 1997;**38**:930–6.

46. Ojemann G. Differential approaches to resective epilepsy surgery standard and tailored. In: Theodore WH (ed). *Surgical treatment of epilepsy.* Elsevier Science Publishers; 1992:169–74.

47. Quesney LF, Munstain M, Rasmussen T, *et al.* How large are frontal lobe epileptogenic zones? EEG, ECoG and SEEG evidence. In: Channel P, Delgado-Escueta AV, Halgran E, *et al.* (eds). *Advances in neurology UN57 frontal lobe seizures and epilepsies.* New York: Raven Press; 1992:311–23.

48. Quesney LF. Extra-temporal epilepsy: Clinical presentation, pre-operative EEG and surgical outcome. In: Overwes J, Aldenkamp AL, de Boer HM (eds). *Future research in epileptology. Acta Neurol Scand* 1992:81–94.

49. Sadanova V, Andermann F, Olivier A, *et al.* Occipital lobe epilepsy: Electroclinical manifestations, electrocorticography, cortical stimulation and outcome of 42 patients treated between 1931 and 1991. Surgery of occipital lobe epilepsy. *Brain* 1992;**115**:1655–80.

50. Olson D, Chugani H, Shewman A, *et al.* Electrocorticographic confirmation of focal positron emission tomographic abnormalities in children with

intractable epilepsy. *Epilepsia* 1990;**31**:731–9.

51. Chandra PS, Salamon N, Huang J, *et al.* FDG-PET/MRI coregistration and diffusion-tensor imaging distinguish epileptogenic tubers and cortex in patients with tuberous sclerosis complex: A preliminary report. *Epilepsia* 2006;**47**:1543–9.

52. Rasmussen T. Cortical resection in the treatment of focal epilepsy. *Adv Neurol* 1975;**8**:139–54.

53. Rasmussen T. Surgery of epilepsy associated with brain tumors. *Adv Neurol* 1975;**8**:227–39.

54. Pilcher W, Silbergeld D, Berger M, *et al.* Intraoperative electrocorticography during tumor resection impact on seizure outcome in patients with ganglio-gliomas. *J Neurosurg* 1993;**78**:891–902.

55. Berger M, Ghatan BS, Haglund M, *et al.* Low grade gliomas associated with intractable epilepsy: Seizure outcome utilizing electrocorticography during tumor resection. *J Neurosurg* 1993;**79**:62–9.

56. Cohen D, Zubay G, Goodman R. Seizure outcome after lesionectomy for cavernous malformation. *J Neurosurg* 1995;**83**:237–42.

57. Gonzalez D, Elridge R. On the occurrence of epilepsy caused by astrocytoma of the cerebral hemispheres. *J Neurosurg* 1962;**19**:470–82.

58. Cascino G, Kelly P, Sharbrough R, *et al.* Long-term follow-up of stereotactic lesionectomy in partial epilepsy. *Epilepsia* 1992;**33**:639–44.

59. Eliashiv S, Dewar S, Engel J Jr, *et al.* Chronic seizures associated with temporal lobe lesions: Seizure outcome following uniform anterior temporal lobectomy. *Epilepsia* 1994;(Suppl. 8):100.

60. Kirkpatrick P, Honavar M, Janota I, *et al.* Control of temporal lobe epilepsy following enbloc resection of low grade tumors. *J Neurosurg* 1993;**78**:19–25.

61. Blume W, Girvin J, Kaufman J. Childhood brain tumors presenting as chronic uncontrolled focal seizure disorder. *Ann Neurol* 1982;**12**:538–41.

62. Fried I, Kim J, Spencer D. Limbic and neocortical gliomas associated with intractable seizures: A distinct clinico-pathological group. *J Neurosurg* 1994;**34**:815–23.

63. Tran T, Spencer S, Javidan M, *et al.* Significance of spikes recorded on intraoperative electrocorticography in patients with brain tumor and epilepsy. *Epilepsia* 1997;**38**:1132–9.

64. Jooma R, Yen H, Privetera M, *et al.* Lesionectomy versus electrophysiologically-guided resection for temporal lobe tumor manifesting with complex partial seizures. *J Neurosurg* 1995;**83**:231–6.

65. Clarke D, Olivier A, Andermann F, *et al.* Surgical treatment of epilepsy: The problem of lesion/focus incongruence. *Surg Neurol* 1996;**46**:579–86.

66. Palmini A, Gambardella A, Andermann F, *et al.* Intrinsic epileptogenicity of human dysplastic cortex as suggested by cortiography and surgical results. *Ann Neurol* 1995;**37**:476–87.

67. Tripathi M, Singh MS, Padma MV, *et al.* Surgical outcome of cortical dysplasias presenting with chronic intractable epilepsy: A 10-year experience. *Neurol India* 2008;**56**:138–43.

68. Wennberg R, Quesney L, Lozano A, *et al.* Role of electrocorticography at surgery for lesion-related frontal lobe epilepsy. *Can J Neurol Sci* 1999;**26**:33–9.

69. Holmes M, Wilensky A, Ojemann G, *et al.* Hippocampal or neocortical lesion on magnetic resonance imaging do not necessarily indicate site of ictal onset in partial epilepsy. *Ann Neurol* 1999;**45**:461–5.